STEPHEN GASCOIGNE
M.B., Ch.B., C.Ac., Dip.C.H.M.

The MANUAL OF
CONVENTIONAL MEDICINE
for
ALTERNATIVE PRACTITIONERS

Volume II

DORKING

Jigme Press

First published in Great Britain by

JIGME PRESS
20-26 South Street, Dorking, Surrey RH4 2HQ

© Stephen Gascoigne, 1994

ISBN 0 9522189 1 7

First published 1994

Printed by Antony Rowe, Chippenham, Wilts.
Cover design by Neal's Yard Desktop Publishing Studio.
Cat logo by Rob Hopkins

- CONTENTS -

Chapter

- ACKNOWLEDGEMENTS -

I owe my thanks to many people during the process of writing this book but especially to:

Eric Beckmann, Stefan Chmelik, Sarah Cleverley, Dr Tim Duerden, Andrew Flower, Hilary Gascoigne, Andra Goldman, Stuart Gracie, Stephen Guy-Clarke, Rob Hopkins, Colin, Linda and Simon of Neal's Yard Desktop Publishing Studio, Carolyn Persson, Maria Raworth, Nguyen Tinh Thong, Mark Tittle, Dr Julie Williams and all those students who have patiently allowed me to develop my ideas.

12 SPECIAL SENSES

OBJECTIVES:

At the end of this Chapter you will be able to:
List the symptoms attributable to disturbances of the eye and ear.
State when a symptom(s) would indicate a serious underlying condition.
Describe the main symptoms of diseases covered in this Chapter.
Explain the relevant management by an alternative practitioner of each disorder.

- INTRODUCTION -

Diseases of the eye are not commonly seen in the clinic. Ear disease is more frequently encountered. Many children with acute and chronic ear conditions present to alternative practitioners. Tinnitus and vertigo are also quite common. Because the eye and ear are important sensory organs, it is useful to know how problems here may manifest. In the case of eye disease, particularly, it may be necessary to seek specialist help. The situations where this is most helpful are discussed in the text but it frequently involves those symptoms which suggest a threat to sight. In an acute situation of this nature, conventional medical help may be necessary in the acute phase.

More commonly, people may present for treatment of a systemic problem and also have symptoms of eye or ear disease. The two may be considered to be unconnected by conventional practitioners. In these situations you may find it helpful to know common eye and ear diseases.

Homoeopaths often run clinics for 'acutes' and they are more likely to see conditions such as acute otitis media. It is more usual to see the chronic disorders of people with tinnitus or deafness. It is rare for people to have life-threatening disease of this area.

- EYE DISEASE -

- BASIC ANATOMY AND PHYSIOLOGY -

It is important to have a basic understanding of the structure and function of the eye. I have listed the objectives which I consider that it is useful to achieve as a preliminary to the study of eye disease. These are detailed in Table 12.1.

As a preliminary to study of eye disease you are able to:
Identify the structures of the eye
Describe the functions of these structures
Explain the mechanism of vision

TABLE 12.1: OBJECTIVES FOR ANATOMY AND PHYSIOLOGY AS PREREQUISITE FOR STUDY OF EYE DISEASE

It can be seen from a knowledge of eye function that the common symptoms which arise from disturbances are pain, redness and visual disturbances. Table 12.2 lists the symptoms which may arise from disease of the eye.

Redness
Discharge
Soreness
Visual disturbance
Blurring
Pain in eye
Spots, floaters
Double vision

TABLE 12.2: SYMPTOMS OF EYE DISEASE

- CLASSIFICATION OF EYE DISEASE -

In conventional medicine, this is made according to the site of the problem. The list in Table 12.3 is ordered in this way.

Conjunctivitis
Keratitis
Episcleritis
Scleritis
Uveitis
Posterior uveitis (choroiditis)
Cataract
Glaucoma

TABLE 12.3: CONVENTIONAL CLASSIFICATION OF EYE DISEASE

For alternative practitioners it is more useful to categorise these diseases according to their severity and their ability to harm sight. Such a method of classification is shown in Table 12.4.

MILD DISEASE
Conjunctivitis
Episcleritis
Scleritis
Posterior uveitis (choroiditis)
Cataract
Keratitis
Uveitis (iritis)
Glaucoma
SEVERE DISEASE

TABLE 12.4: ALTERNATIVE CLASSIFICATION OF EYE DISEASE

- INVESTIGATION OF EYE DISEASE -

These are specialised and carried out by opthalmologists rather than general physicians. Technical equipment can be used to examine the eye and parts of the eye. Pressure of fluid within the eye can be measured. Eye charts are well known to all as a method of checking visual acuity. All such investigations are non-invasive and would be in Category 1 as defined in Chapter 4 - Investigations. The only exception to this is the use of some eye drops and stains for particular examinations. These are temporary in their effect and of low risk.

- CONJUNCTIVITIS -

In conventional medicine this is usually considered to be infective in nature - bacterial or viral. Conjunctivitis is more likely in situations of poor hygiene or a dusty environment. A milder, recurrent form is a feature of Reiter's syndrome[1] which is a classical triad of conjunctivitis, urethritis (comparable to non-gonococcal urethritis) and polyarthritis. Allergic reactions may produce similar symptoms although the discharge then is clear or white with associated itching and nasal symptoms.

Symptoms:

The main feature is of redness which may be slight over a small area of the conjunctiva or more extensive involving the whole conjunctiva including the area lining the inside of the eyelids. There is discomfort in the eyes which usually is described as a feeling of grittiness. There is a white or, more commonly, yellow discharge in the eyes. Sensitivity to light is frequently described. The symptoms may vary in severity from person to person and some have severe problems with soreness, redness and a profuse discharge.

Complications:

COMPLICATIONS	SYMPTOMS TO LOOK FOR
Chronic conjunctivitis	Persistence of redness and discharge, grittiness, feelings of heat in the eyes

TABLE 12.5: COMPLICATIONS OF CONJUNCTIVITIS

Treatment:

This is invariably by means of local antibiotics although many cases are viral in nature. Advice is also given about bathing the eye and local hygiene.

Alternative management:

In terms of Chinese medicine, conjunctivitis is due to Invasion of Wind and Heat. If these continue to affect the eye then acute cases become chronic. Overindulgence in alcohol, overuse of the eyes, exposure to wind, poor lighting and inadequate sleep may all contribute to development of chronic state. In some people, there may be underlying Liver Blood Deficiency.

This condition is rarely serious despite the appearance and the uncomfortable nature of the symptoms. There are very effective treatments available in Chinese medicine, homoeopathy and herbalism which can remove the need for antibiotics.

- KERATITIS -

This is inflammation of the cornea which is associated with either bacteria, viruses or fungi. Bacterial disease is unusual.

Symptoms:

There is pain in the eye rather than the soreness of conjunctivitis. Watering is profuse and there is associated discomfort from light. There may be spasm of the eyelid and pupil. Redness is present but usually restricted to the circumcorneal area. It may be possible to see a corneal ulcer which will have the appearance of a grey circular area on the corneal surface.

---

[1] This condition may be familiar to homoeopaths as it is a manifestation of the sycotic miasm.

Investigations:

An ulcer on the cornea or small spots may be seen using special staining methods.

Complications:

The main worry of keratitis is impairment of vision and ultimately blindness from scarring of the cornea. Occasionally, the inflammation may involve the whole of the eye and threaten sight in this way. Symptoms to look for would include persistence and worsening of symptoms. Any visual disturbances would clearly be a cause for concern. Because of the threat to sight, effective treatment must be instituted without delay.

Treatment:

This is invariably with antibiotics or antifungal agents.

Alternative management:

The main issue for alternative practitioners is to recognise the more serious nature of this condition when compared with conjunctivitis.

- EPISCLERITIS -

This is an inflammation of the episclera. It is part of a more general autoimmune reaction and so may be seen in people with rheumatoid arthritis, systemic lupus erythematosus and so on (see Chapter 10 - Musculoskeletal System). A more severe variant is scleritis which is also described here.

Symptoms:

In cases of episcleritis, there is a localised area of redness of one eye. There is pain rather than irritation and tenderness on palpation through a closed eyelid. There is no discharge from the eye. Occasionally, both eyes may be affected.

Scleritis, on the other hand, is a more serious problem with more severe symptoms. There is pain is the forehead and sinus area also. The redness is darker than that of episcleritis with white patches. These indicate that parts of the sclera are dying.

Treatment:

Episcleritis usually settles on its own within a few weeks. Non-steroidal anti-inflammatory drugs will be given if it persists.

Scleritis is treated with high dose non-steroidal anti-inflammatory drugs and occasionally by means of corticosteroids.

Alternative management:

This condition, in its milder forms, is merely uncomfortable and treatment must be directed at the underlying systemic disease. Details of these are contained in Chapter 10 - Musculoskeletal System. Care must be taken if the more severe scleritis is suspected.

- UVEITIS -

This is an inflammation of the uveal tract[2] and is a combination of an affection of the iris - iritis (anterior uveitis) and ciliary body - cyclitis. These areas are intimately connected with function of the pupil and so a common symptom is blurring of vision.

Symptoms:

There is an acute onset of severe pain, discomfort from light and a mild to moderate degree of blurred vision. It is usually present in one eye. There is redness which is generalised as seen in conjunctivitis but with intense redness in the circumcorneal region. There is watering particularly on exposure to light but never a yellowish discharge. There is marked tenderness. There is some similarity with the symptoms of glaucoma.

Complications:

Cataract may develop some years after attacks of uveitis.

Treatment:

This is by means of corticosteroids and in severe cases, immunosuppressants or cytotoxic drugs.

- POSTERIOR UVEITIS (CHOROIDITIS) -

This is an inflammation of the posterior part of the uveal tract - the choroid. It is associated with infection, rheumatoid arthritis or gout. There is swelling and consequently disordered function of the retina.

Symptoms:

There is usually blurring of vision only due to retinal oedema and damage.

Treatment:

Local applications are given to maintain pupillary dilatation as this decreases pressure in the eye. Corticosteroids with or without antibiotics are given according to the cause.

---

[2] This comprises the iris, ciliary body and choroid. Inflammation of the iris and ciliary body is termed anterior uveitis or iridocyclitis. Inflammation of the choroid is termed posterior uveitis or choroiditis.

- CATARACT -

This is a loss of transparency of the lens. It may occur after perforating injury or disease of the eye such as uveitis. Its development without these predisposing causes in later life is known as senile[3] cataract. It leads to a distortion of vision especially for distant objects.

Cataract may develop due to various factors. These include:

- drugs. This is known as toxic cataract and may be the result of several drugs including chlorpromazine, ergotamine, corticosteroids (oral and locally in the eye), smoking, alcohol
- ultraviolet B radiation
- diabetes mellitus
- low antioxidant vitamin status[4]

Symptoms:

There is the gradual development of myopia - short-sightedness. In the case of those with hypermetropia - long-sightedness, this tends to improve. Interference with vision becomes more obvious with increasing lens opacity. Eventually only hand movements may be vaguely seen.

Treatment:

Correction of vision by means of spectacles may be possible in the early stages. It is helpful to adjust reading with good light, large print books and the like. There is no conventional medical treatment to prevent cataract or its progression. Surgery is the usual conventional treatment and is best reserved for severe cases of sight-impairment where there is interference with daily activities. Anaesthesia may be general or local.

Removal of the lens with implantation of a plastic lens may be performed at the same time. Rejection of the implant may lead to episodes of redness, soreness and visual disturbances. Only one eye is dealt with at a time. There must be a delay of several months before treating the second eye.

Eye complications of surgery include retinal detachment, uveitis, glaucoma, haemorrhage into the eye (usually minor and occasionally severe) and infection. General complications include cardiac failure, respiratory problems, stroke, diabetes mellitus, uncontrolled nausea and vomiting, acute urinary retention and acute confusional state[5].

A consequence of modern cataract surgery is opacification of the posterior lens capsule. As the opacification increases, the person begins to notice a decrease in visual function. Laser surgery is usually performed for this. Complications include glaucoma, haemorrhage, retinal detachment and corneal oedema.

- SQUINT -

A squint (strabismus) is an abnormal alignment of the two eyes. This results in an object being seen from slightly different angles by each eye. The consequence is the classical symptom of squint - double vision (diplopia). It is important to differentiate this from blurring and close questioning may be necessary to determine the exact nature of the visual disturbance. True double vision means two separate objects - side by side or one above the other.

There are considered to be several causes in conventional medicine and these are listed in Table 12.6.

---

[3] The term senile is used as an adjective for any disorder which appears after the age of 60 years.

[4] There have been suggestions that the administration of Vitamin E, C and betacarotene may prevent or reverse the formation of cataract. Varma, SD. :American Journal of Clinical Nutrition, Jan 1991 v53 n1 p335S(11).

[5] O'Day, Denis M. :American Family Physician, May 1, 1993 v47 n6 p1421(10).

PROCESS	CAUSE
Paralysis or weakness of one or more eye muscles (paralytic squint)	Injury Central nervous system disease, e.g. stroke, brain tumour Neuropathy, either single or associated with systemic disease, e.g. multiple sclerosis, thyroid disease, myasthenia gravis, diabetes mellitus
Failure of eyes to co-ordinate	This is the type requiring eye exercises and spectacles. Young children will rarely complain and soon learn to suppress one image. In older people intermittent double vision might occur when they are under stress or sedation
Alteration in angle of long-standing squint	This is one of the difficulties of treating squints in adults. Squints should be treated in early life before unwanted images are suppressed

TABLE 12.6: COMMON CAUSES OF DOUBLE VISION

Symptoms:

There is double vision as each eye is seeing an object from a slightly different angle. The long-term consequence is suppression of vision in the squinting eye. Some people may develop abnormal head postures to achieve as much reduction in the double vision as possible.

Treatment:

This is dependent upon the cause. Paralytic squint is, as its name suggests, due to paralysis of the muscles of the eye. This may occur as part of a local problem with a cranial nerve or due to diseases such as stroke or brain tumour. Management will be part of the total clinical picture.

In young children, squint may develop due to inadequate maturation of binocular vision. The vision in the affected eye may rapidly be suppressed. The most effective treatment is that which is given early. Covering of the normal eye allows the 'lazy' eye an opportunity to recover. Eye exercises are an important part of such treatment. Surgery to the eye muscles may be applied in resistant cases to adjust the angle of vision.

Alternative management:

In Chinese medicine, the frequent cause is insufficiency of Qi and Blood supplying the eye. Treatment is aimed at improving these and regulating the muscles of the eyes. Eye exercises[6] are useful for this condition.

---

[6] There are well described sets of exercises for use with many types of eye problems including short-sightedness (myopia), squint and so on. For further information see "Better Eyesight Without Glasses" by Harry Benjamin (The Health For All Publishing Company, 1943).

- GLAUCOMA -

This is a rise in the pressure within the eye. If this persists or worsens, the optic nerve can be damaged resulting in visual loss. There are several types of glaucoma.

Chronic simple glaucoma (open-angle glaucoma) develops in the middle-aged or elderly and is unusual before the age of 40 years. It affects both eyes and there is frequently a family history of the condition. It is also commoner in those with short-sightedness and diabetes mellitus.

Congestive glaucoma (closed-angle glaucoma) is found more often in people with long-sightedness. The mechanism of development is not well understood by conventional medicine.

Secondary glaucoma develops as a result of a pre-existing condition. This includes injury, uveitis, and the use of local corticosteroid drops.

Symptoms:

In chronic simple glaucoma, there may be virtually no symptoms except an occasional ache. There is an insidious, progressive visual loss which is mainly peripheral until severe.

In congestive glaucoma, the onset is more acute. There is discomfort of the eye with associated mistiness of vision and rainbow-like haloes. This may be transient but if prolonged and severe leads to discomfort in the light, watering of the eye and perhaps vomiting. There is then marked loss of vision if the pressure remains high and it may result in intractable blindness. Circumcorneal redness is a constant feature. Symptoms are worse in the dark since pressure within the eye is then greater. The condition may affect both eyes.

Treatment:

Chronic simple glaucoma can be treated by several methods. Eye drops of adrenaline or acetazolamide are commonly used. The betablocker, timolol, as eye drops can also be used. In resistant cases, surgery may be employed. This is either by an operation to drain fluid from the eye or, more commonly nowadays, by laser treatment. Eye drops have to be continued after laser treatment.

Congestive glaucoma is treated in the acute phase by dilation of the pupil as this reduces intra-ocular pressure. Surgery is always carried out at a later date.

The treatment of secondary glaucoma is by means of acetazolamide drops but frequently surgery is performed.

Alternative management:

In Chinese medicine, this is due to depletion of Kidney Yin. This causes Wind and Fire in the Liver and Gall Bladder to ascend disrupting Qi in the channels. It is reasonable to treat people with glaucoma by means of alternative medicine but it is important for monitoring of the intra-ocular pressures to be done. The normal figures are between 16 and 22 mm Hg (millimetres of mercury) with variations up to 3-5 mm which may occur over the day. The highest pressures are seen in the early hours of the morning during sleep.

I have treated people with glaucoma who had pressures up to the high 20's and low 30's and this would seem to be fine. The other things to take into account are the symptoms. It would be a cause for concern if these are marked even with relatively low pressures.

– REVIEW OF SYMPTOMS OF EYE DISEASE –

VISUAL ACUITY

This is sharpness of vision. Its measurement can be a precise guide to the severity of a condition and whether it is changing. The recorded loss of one line on the standard sight testing chart is indicative of a significant impairment.

A test with a card pierced by a pinhole will show whether or not the blurring is caused by changes in refraction[7]. If these are the cause then the visual acuity will improve when the person looks out through the pinhole, placed close to their eyes. This test will determine whether or not spectacles are likely to solve the problem. The common refractive errors are short-sightedness (myopia), long-sightedness (hypermetropia) and astigmatism. They can be corrected, more or less, by the use of spectacles and/or contact lenses.

There is a possibility that some purely visual symptoms may be the presenting symptoms of systemic disease. Anaemia, for example, may present with only visual symptoms of floaters and weak vision.

BLURRED VISION

There are several important questions to ask about this symptom:

- does it affect one or both eyes?
- is it constant or episodic?
- is it for near or distant vision?
- is it getting better or worse?

Blurring is the commonest visual symptom and the questions above will help to define its significance. It is helpful to determine the visual acuity since blurring due to short-sightedness improves when looking through a pinhole[8].

Blurring in only one eye is much more likely to be due to an eye problem particularly if of sudden onset. If it has developed slowly over months or years with no other symptoms then the most likely situation is short- or long-sightedness. In the elderly, it may also be associated with cataract formation if mainly distance vision is affected or vascular disturbances if mainly near vision is affected.

If the blurring is of sudden onset over a few weeks or days in only one eye then it is almost certainly not short- or long-sightedness. It is safest to assume, however, that the situation is potentially serious and urgent unless it suddenly recovers.

Episodic blurring is never a refractive error. In cases of multiple sclerosis the blurring lasts for many days. Migraine usually affects both eyes and occurs for the first time in younger people. More rarely the episode of blurring may be caused by interference with blood supply as in a transient ischaemic attack. This is usually described as a shutter or blind effect.

---

[7] Refraction is a term from physics. It is the change of direction in light rays when they travel from one area to another, e.g. from the air into the eye. In practical clinical terms, an error of refraction is due to abnormal lens function or eye shape.

[8] This is the basis of 'pinhole glasses' which can be part of a natural treatment for eye disorders. The pinholes cut down on peripheral light and improve central vision. Such aids, together with appropriate eye exercises, can be used to treat short-sightedness (myopia), squint and so forth.

FLOATERS AND BLURRED AREAS

Spots floating about in front of the eyes may be the first sign of failing vision in cases of short-sightedness. They are frequently first noticed during times of tiredness. Floaters are more easily seen against a white background. There is no cause for concern if no further developments occur during the first week or so.

Circulatory disturbances in the retina may cause bouts of seeing stars or flashes, particularly in at the edge of vision when tired or stressed. Floaters must be distinguished from the much rarer solitary area of blurring that does not float but moves with the eye without any time lag. This may be described as a piece missing from an object or a blurred spot. It tends to be constantly present. They are more serious than the common floater because they are often progressive or indicative of some other disorder, such as retinal disorders or neurological disease.

PAIN

Visual disturbance with pain in the eyes is always serious, and advice is urgently needed. The causes of pain in the eye include:

- iritis*
- glaucoma*
- multiple sclerosis
- shingles*
- cranial arteritis*
- ingrowing eyelash

Those of most concern are marked with an asterisk*. A painful white eye with no visual symptoms is more likely to be due to a neurological disorder, e.g. trigeminal neuralgia.

WATERING OF THE EYES

This may be due to excessive production of tears. There are several associated situations which include:

- inflammation - conjunctivitis, keratitis, uveitis
- injury - foreign bodies, chemical agents, ingrowing eyelashes
- closed-angle glaucoma
- excessive exposure to bright light

Alternatively, there may be inadequate drainage of tears which may be associated with:

- eyelid abnormalities
- blocked tear duct

Watering is common in a white, painless eye in infants, the middle aged and elderly. If there is no associated yellow discharge then it is not serious although it may be long-lasting and a nuisance. If watering is the only symptom then there is no danger to sight. Watering with discharge is treated as conjunctivitis and people will be given antibiotics.

It tends to clear spontaneously by the age of 9 months in babies. Since treatment involves a general anaesthetic and probing of the duct, it is better to wait for nature to take its course.

In middle age, probing or syringing of the duct is attempted much earlier as there is a worry about complications such as infection or in extreme cases, abscess formation in the duct. Reconstructive surgery of the duct may be necessary.

If the tear duct is open, watering is commonly caused by several possibilities. These include loss of tone in the eyelids or spasm of the lower lid leading to eversion or inversion, particularly in the elderly. This is treated by out-patient surgery.

In younger people (particularly students) excessive watering might be caused by close work and reading. The person usually describes it as watering when reading or trying to read. Eye exercises are helpful in these cases.

Watering associated with pain or photophobia may indicate corneal disease and is more serious.

DRYNESS OF THE EYES

This is reduced formation of tears and may be termed, keratoconjunctivitis sicca. It is frequently associated with autoimmune diseases such as rheumatoid arthritis[9] where it is known as Sjögren's syndrome. Such symptoms are common in middle age but little is understood about how these are caused in the absence of visual disturbance. These symptoms tend to be more common in women than men and are almost always bilateral. Some people who suffer sore or irritable eyes are the victims of an allergy - sometimes to local eye medication.

Symptoms:

There is dryness of the eyes associated with dry mouth. There may be burning in the eye and the sensation of grittiness.

Treatment:

These are by means of artificial 'tears' such as methylcellulose eye drops.

Alternative management:

In terms of Chinese medicine, this condition usually corresponds to Deficiency of Liver Blood and/or Yin. There are well-recognised treatments available to nourish Yin (fluids) within the body. Progress tends to be slow as these problems are usually deep seated.

HEADACHE

These are discussed fully in Chapter 14 - Central Nervous System. The comments I make here are specifically to do with the eyes. The headache of glaucoma usually occurs only while the blurring of vision is present, and it is seldom severe: it is often also accompanied by aching of the eye. Headaches of visual origin are extremely rare in children aged under 10. They may occasionally be caused by refractive disorders in children.

DIZZINESS

This is rarely caused solely by an eye problem. It is essential to determine what the person means by this term. The possibilities are discussed on Page 250. The situations leading to such a symptom may be sudden loss of sight in one eye, sudden loss of visual field (usually in cerebrovascular disease), or by double vision not clearly described.

---

[9] Other disorders include systemic lupus erythematosus and inflammation of the thyroid.

The Manual of Conventional Medicine for Alternative Practitioners

REDNESS OF THE EYE

A red eye does not necessarily mean a more serious situation than a white one. The extent and severity of the redness are no guide to the severity of the condition. It is the vision which is important so visual acuity needs to be checked. If a red eye is accompanied by any degree of visual disturbance then, unless the symptoms gradually improve within a few days, it would be wise to obtain an assessment from an ophthalmologist.

ALWAYS	OFTEN	RARELY
Acute glaucoma Iritis	Corneal disease Herpes zoster (shingles)	Conjunctivitis Episcleritis, scleritis Subconjunctival haemorrhage Entropion

TABLE 12.7: CONDITIONS CAUSING A RED EYE WHICH PRESENT A THREAT TO SIGHT

Spontaneous subconjunctival haemorrhage that totally obliterates the white sclera is, despite its appearance, harmless and carries no complications unless due to trauma. In that case the outcome is dependent upon the degree of injury. In other situations, it will resolve on its own. In terms of Chinese medicine, red eyes may be connected with the syndromes associated with high blood pressure as detailed in Chapter 9 - Urinary System.

Redness in one eye that is hardly noticeable may signal intra-ocular disease and a potential threat to sight. Most of the serious causes of red eye do not affect both eyes at once. One-sided redness is generally more of a danger signal.

True infective conjunctivitis is usually bilateral and not usually a serious disease in Western countries. There is always some discharge which may only be manifest as making it hard to separate the lids on waking. This distinguishes it from other conditions. Failure of these symptoms to respond may indicate corneal complications such as keratitis, especially if the person has been suffering from a systemic or local virus disease, e.g. herpes simplex, herpes zoster. Permanent visual loss is a real possibility in such cases. The redness and soreness that accompany measles have no special significance. It is important to distinguish infective or viral conjunctivitis from other forms of red eye because corticosteroid treatment will make infective conditions much worse.

Any of these symptoms occurring in a person with only one useful eye would require a greater urgency about referral than if they occur in one of a pair.

- EAR DISEASE -

- BASIC ANATOMY AND PHYSIOLOGY -

It is important to have a basic understanding of the structure and function of the ear. I have listed the objectives which I consider that is it useful to achieve as a preliminary to the study of ear disease. These are detailed in Table 12.8.

As a preliminary to study of disease of ear disease you are able to:
Identify the structures of the ear
Describe the functions of these structures
Explain the mechanisms of hearing and balance

TABLE 12.8: OBJECTIVES FOR ANATOMY AND PHYSIOLOGY AS PREREQUISITE FOR STUDY OF EAR DISEASE

From a knowledge of ear function, it is clear that the common symptoms which arise from disturbances are deafness, noises in the ear and difficulties with balance. Pain in the ear may occur particularly with acute conditions. Table 12.9 lists the symptoms which arise from disease of the ear.

Pain in the ear
Deafness
Discharge from the ear
Tinnitus
Vertigo
Deformity of the ear
Lumps around or on the ear[10]
Headaches[11]
Facial weakness[12]
Double vision

TABLE 12.9: SYMPTOMS OF EAR DISEASE

---

[10] Lumps on the ear are rare. Causes include injury, frostbite and abscess formation. Lumps around the ear may be lymphatic gland enlargement. I would remind you here of the importance in knowing the main groups of lymphatic glands and the areas they drain. Mastoid enlargement is rare nowadays and is a complication of otitis media.

[11] These are described in Chapter 14 - Central Nervous System.

[12] This is described in Chapter 14 - Central Nervous System.

- CLASSIFICATION OF EAR DISEASE -

The most appropriate way do this is according to severity and chronicity as in Table 12.10.

MILD DISEASE
Otitis externa
Otitis media
Perforation of ear drum
Ménière's disease
Otosclerosis[13]
SEVERE DISEASE

TABLE 12.10: CLASSIFICATION OF EAR DISEASE

- INVESTIGATIONS -

Examination of the auditory canal and ear drum is done with an auriscope (US - otoscope). It is helpful to have this skill as it can provide valuable information. Simple problems such as ear wax may cause impaired hearing or vertigo. They can be easily diagnosed and treated.

An audiogram is a measurement of hearing. The person is subjected to various frequencies of sound and the results charted. Both ears are tested. It has an invasiveness of Category 1 as defined in Chapter 4 - Investigations.

- MÉNIÈRE'S DISEASE -

In this condition, there are recurrent attacks of vertigo which are prostrating. There is associated tinnitus and progressive deafness. These three symptoms together are virtually diagnostic of Ménière's disease. The cause is unknown in conventional medicine but there may be a history of migraine.

Symptoms:

The most disabling symptom is a sudden attack of vertigo which is severe, of sudden onset and usually associated with nausea and vomiting. Attacks are recurrent and there is progressive deafness as the auditory nerve is damaged with each attack. Tinnitus of varying degrees and types is experienced. The person has to go to bed for a day or two and can do very little as any movement makes the symptoms worse. The deafness increases progressively and frequencies of attacks tend to decrease as the years go by. The condition can last for years and virtually rule people's lives.

Treatment:

This is with antihistamines such as betahistine which may give symptomatic relief. There is little which is available to change the course of the illness.

Alternative management:

In terms of Chinese medicine, this condition often corresponds either to Phlegm and Dampness in the Stomach interfering with the rising of pure Qi to the head or to Kidney Yin Deficiency with Liver Yang Rising. Treatment must be directed at the underlying organs to achieve improvement.

---

[13] This is described in Chapter 18 - Gynaecology in relation to hormone replacement treatment.

- OTITIS EXTERNA -

This is inflammation of the auditory canal. There are several forms which vary in intensity. They include:

- associated with systemic skin diseases such as psoriasis, eczema and contact dermatitis.
- 'swimmer's ear'
- bacterial infection

It is a simple matter to differentiate this problem from other disorders of the ear as any pain and discomfort are much worse on moving the ear.

Symptoms:

These depend upon the causes listed above and vary from mild to severe. In the case of systemic skin disease, there is evidence elsewhere of skin abnormalities. There is itching to a variable extent perhaps with scaling. In severe cases there may be weeping with a watery discharge. Conventional treatment is by means of corticosteroid drops.

In 'swimmer's ear' there is mild inflammation associated with evidence of fungal or bacterial infection. There are symptoms, after swimming, of a blocked ear with mild discomfort. This may become painful within the next 24 hours. Conventional treatment is with mixed antibiotic-corticosteroid drops.

In bacterial infection of the auditory canal there is redness, pain, enlargement of pre-auricular and post-auricular lymph glands. The canal is narrowed due to swelling. There may be a low-grade fever of around 38°C (100°F). Conventional treatment is with oral antibiotics.

- OTITIS MEDIA -

This is inflammation of the middle ear. It is usually associated with infection, bacterial or viral. It may also arise due to congestion of fluid in the middle ear where infection may have a minor role to play.

Symptoms:

These occur more commonly in children. There is the acute onset of fever, pain in the ear and decreased hearing. Occasionally, there may be mild vertigo. On examination, the ear drum is red and may be bulging towards the examiner.

Complications:

COMPLICATION	SYMPTOMS TO LOOK FOR
Mastoiditis	Persistent symptoms of otitis media for over 8-10 days, pain and swelling of mastoid.
Serous otitis media - may progress to 'glue ear' in children	Continuing impairment of hearing, crackling sounds in ear, feeling of fullness. The ear drum is opaque, dull and slightly retracted. In 'glue ear' the ear drum has a bluish appearance.
Perforation of ear drum - most heal with no complications	Increasing pain in the ear followed by discharge from the ear and relief of pain. The perforation will be visible on examination of the ear drum.
Chronic otitis media with perforated drum	Few or no symptoms usually. There may be vertigo in a cold wind. Occasionally yellow discharge from the ear but no pain or fever. The perforation will be visible on examination of the ear drum.
Facial paralysis (rare)	Weakness of one side of face with symptoms of otitis media.

TABLE 12.11: COMPLICATIONS OF OTITIS MEDIA

Treatment:

This is invariably by means of antibiotics in most areas although some conventional practitioners use decongestants, e.g. pseudoephedrine (a sympathomimetic). This is in the belief that the main problem, particularly in children, is of catarrhal congestion in the middle ear and eustachian tubes. It is important to avoid flying for at least seven days or the ear drum is at risk of perforation.

'Glue ear' is an uncommon complication of otitis media and, as its name suggests, is due to thickening of fluids in the middle ear. It may lead to damage to the delicate bones in the middle ear and severe hearing loss. 'Glue ear' is treated by means of surgical perforation of the ear drum (myringotomy) and the insertion of drainage tubes (grommets). This treatment is frequently used in those children who have evidence of chronic mucus congestion with some hearing loss. It may be combined with tonsillectomy and adenoidectomy. Some conventional practitioners now treat such cases with decongestants because surgery to the ear may cause scarring of the ear drum. Scarring is less likely if perforation occurs naturally. Such treatment, of course, does nothing to remedy the underlying problem which is the production of mucus.

Alternative management:

This is easily treated in most people by the application of homoeopathic remedies or herbal formulae. It is unnecessary in most cases to give antibiotics. I would refer you to Page 79 where the symptom of fever is analysed as to whether there is a serious underlying condition. If the symptoms do not begin to subside within 12 or 24 hours after you have started treatment, review the case and your treatment. The danger of mastoiditis is very much overplayed nowadays and it is perfectly valid to treat otitis media with alternative medicine alongside appropriate monitoring.

PERFORATED EAR DRUM

There are several causes of perforated ear drum. They include:

- injury, e.g. blow to ears ('boxing' the ears), direct to ear drum as with perforating object
- complication of otitis media

Management:

This depends upon the cause. Otitis media is treated as described above. Traumatic perforation usually heals spontaneously although direct injury may result in some infection.

Swimming is prohibited with ear drum perforation. If the perforation is small and linear it may heal within a week. If the perforation has healed then swimming may be resumed but diving is prohibited for three weeks.

Flying is no problem in the day or so after perforation as there is no pressure difference between the outside and the middle ear because of the perforation. It should be avoided for two to three weeks after this as the perforation is healing.

Large perforations and those associated with chronic otitis media may be repaired surgically (myringoplasty).

- REVIEW OF SYMPTOMS OF EAR DISEASE -

TINNITUS

This is any noise such as buzzing or ringing in the ear. There are several causes in terms of conventional medicine including:

- blockage of the auditory canal by wax
- damage to the ear drum
- otosclerosis
- Ménière's disease
- drugs. e.g. aspirin, quinine
- auditory (VIII cranial) nerve disease

In terms of Chinese medicine, this symptom may be caused by Phlegm from the Gall Bladder ascending to the head or Deficiency of Kidney Yin leading to Yang Rising.

DEAFNESS

This is partial or total hearing loss in one or both ears. It is conventionally divided into conductive and perceptive deafness.

Conductive deafness is due to a problem with the conduction of sound through the outer and middle ear. Causes include:

- ear wax in the auditory canal
- otitis externa
- otitis media
- otosclerosis

Perceptive deafness is due to a disorder of the inner ear, the auditory nerve or the centres in the brain dealing with sound. Causes include:

- congenital, e.g. congenital rubella syndrome
- Ménière's disease
- prolonged exposure to loud noise
- advancing age

VERTIGO

This has a specific meaning of a sensation of constant movement of the individual or of the environment. It is usually a spinning movement but it may be a feeling that the ground is moving. Causes of vertigo include:

- wax jammed against ear drum (mild)
- acute otitis media (mild)
- serous otitis media (mild)
- labyrinthitis
- Ménière's disease
- multiple sclerosis
- transient ischaemic attacks

Differentiation is made by the other symptoms which are present. It is important to examine the ear drum.

People may report a symptom of dizziness and it is important to identify the precise meaning. There are several possibilities:

- true vertigo as defined above'
- light-headedness as before a faint. There is no spinning and there is a feeling of floating.
- unsteadiness which leads to difficulties walking or standing. This may be a minor degree of the above two.
- rarely it may indicate depersonalisation or derealisation as may occur in the psychoses or severe neuroses.

- HOW TO RECOGNISE A SERIOUS CONDITION OF THE EYE AND EAR -

It is essential to consider visual symptoms carefully as they are always potentially graver than non-visual ones. Although discomfort or redness in the eyes seems more serious, it is the disturbance of vision which is more worrying. For this reason, it is important to know how to recognise if a symptom arises from a serious situation. You can use Table 12.12 as a guide to refer to when faced with a person who has one or more of these symptoms. I do not mention disease labels in the column on the right as I would not expect you to be able to diagnose conventionally. Seriousness can be assessed merely by reference to symptom pictures. However, you will be able to recognise that there are clinical appearances which would be diagnosed as a particular disease. For example, if you look at redness and its seriousness, you will see that this is the appearance of the more serious conditions of keratitis, iritis and glaucoma.

SYMPTOMS	WHEN TO WORRY
Redness	Circumcorneal, with visual disturbance
Discharge from the eye	Not if alone. Of concern if severe, prolonged and with pain in the eye
Soreness	Not if mild. Of concern if *pain* rather than soreness especially with circumcorneal redness
Visual disturbance	Short history, progressive, with pain, with redness
Blurred vision	Progressive
Pain in eye	With visual disturbance
Spots, floaters	If localised area of blurring
Double vision	Short history
Pain in the ear	Severe, with fever
Discharge from the ear	Long duration
Vertigo	Severe
Deformity of the ear	Severe
Lumps around or on the ear	Severe, if with redness, pain and deafness
Headaches	Progressive, severe with short history, with central nervous system symptoms
Facial weakness	With history of ear pain
Deafness	Short history, progressive
Tinnitus	Progressive

TABLE 12.12: HOW TO RECOGNISE SERIOUS CONDITIONS OF THE EYE AND EAR

- SUMMARY -

Ear conditions are common in the alternative medical clinic. Eye conditions are more often seen as a secondary complaint.

If you are treating children, it is helpful to know how to manage acute ear conditions and how to recognise complications. Other common conditions seen in children are 'glue' ear and recurrent tonsillitis.

Most eye and ear conditions are self-limiting. Know those which may lead to further problems particularly those eye diseases which may threaten sight.

13 GASTROINTESTINAL SYSTEM

OBJECTIVES:

At the end of this Chapter you will be able to:

Describe the differences between the alternative and conventional views of the gastrointestinal system.

List the symptoms attributable to a disturbance of the gastrointestinal system.

State when a symptom(s) would indicate a serious underlying condition.

Describe the main symptoms of diseases covered in this Chapter.

Explain the relevant management by an alternative practitioner of each disorder.

- INTRODUCTION -

Disturbances of the gastrointestinal system are very common in the West. Many people are seen in the clinic who have disturbances in digestive function. These may manifest as bowel disorders, disturbed appetite, nausea or vomiting, pain in the abdomen or perhaps excessive wind. Most of the underlying conditions are of relatively minor significance and reflect the close relationship between the digestive tract and the emotions. However, some conditions are more serious and it is important for the practitioner to be able to recognise the symptoms of severe disease.

- BASIC ANATOMY AND PHYSIOLOGY -

The conventional view of the gastrointestinal system is that it is merely a conduit for the passage of food and its digestion. Each part of the system has several and similar functions. These are ingestion, secretion, digestion, absorption, storage and elimination. There is merely a different emphasis in each area. For example, the mouth is mainly concerned with ingestion with some secretion and absorption. The large intestine is mainly concerned with storage and elimination with some absorption. The small intestine is mainly concerned with digestion and absorption. These processes are seen as a physical process, much the same as putting things into a food processor and churning them around.

As a preliminary to study of disease of the gastrointestinal system you are able to:

List the organs of digestion (including the 'accessory organs')

Describe the main structure of these organs

Describe the functions of the digestive system as a whole with particular reference to each of these organs

Explain how the processes of digestion are regulated

TABLE 13.1: OBJECTIVES FOR ANATOMY AND PHYSIOLOGY AS PREREQUISITE FOR STUDY OF DISEASE OF THE GASTROINTESTINAL SYSTEM

ALTERNATIVE VIEW OF THE GASTROINTESTINAL SYSTEM

Vitalistic principles presume the existence of energy as the root of any structure. In terms of the gastrointestinal system, this leads to the view that its function is not only dependent on the food eaten. It also concerns the energetic quality of food and the energy of the system itself.

Tables 13.2 and 13.3 are descriptions of the gastrointestinal system according to holistic energetic principles. These ideas are obtained from Chinese medicine but it may be that other practitioners such as homoeopaths may see similarities with their system of medicine. Clearly, when studying this list, the associations and interconnections of the gastrointestinal system are complex. It is our common experience that emotions and thoughts affect the digestive system. Homoeopathic remedies clearly show this connection in their remedy pictures. People know that certain emotional states are associated, for example, with diarrhoea or constipation. The ideas expressed in these Tables provide an explanation of these mechanisms.

ASSOCIATION	COMMENTS
Governs transformation and transportation	The Spleen[1] deals with food by transforming it into energy (Qi) and body fluid. It separates the pure from the impure, ascends the pure and descends the impure. Weak Spleen Qi leads to inadequate transformation and transportation and so to mucus formation (excess body fluids) and tiredness (lack of energy).
Controls Blood	The Spleen holds Blood in the circulation and prevents it leaking out of the vessels. Bruising may be a sign of weak Spleen Qi. Vitamin C deficiency producing bruising corresponds here.
Dominates muscles and flesh	The health of muscles and flesh are dependent upon the efficiency of Spleen function.
Raises the pure Qi	Spleen Qi ascends and so is responsible, amongst other things, for holding organs in place. Prolapse of uterus, rectum and other organs may be due to weakness of this aspect.
Residence of Thought	Overthinking and rumination may weaken the Spleen. Similarly, an imbalance of Spleen energy may affect thought. Such a connection may be observed in relation to glandular fever where Spleen Qi deficiency often predates the manifest symptoms.
Paired organ is Stomach	This connection is self-evident as food enters the Stomach to be processed.
Opens into the Mouth	Diseases of the mouth may be due to Stomach or Spleen problems such as mouth ulcers and bleeding gums. Only treating the gums and teeth is not appropriate and these organs must be addressed for the mouth to be healthy. This is why dental treatment is ineffective at treating many cases of mouth ulcers, pain in the teeth and mouth and so forth.
Manifests in the lips	The condition of the lips is a reflection of Spleen function.
Colour - yellow	The colour of Earth is yellow and foods which particularly nourish this element are such as parsnip, squash, carrot. These are generally sweet also (see below)
Taste - sweet	Each major organ has an associated taste. In this case excess sweet food can damage the Earth element. Conversely, small amounts of sweet taste nourish the Earth element
Season - sometimes described as late summer but more accurately is a centreing between each of the 4 seasons	The energy of the centre is transformative. It moves in a circular direction. In cases of imbalance, it may result in the inability to move forward as in cases of overthinking and analysis.
Element - Earth	The Element correspondence reveals the connection of Chinese medical theory to nature. Each Element is connected to the others to provide, in health, a harmonious balance.
Time - 9 - 11 a.m.	The 'time' of an organ is when its energy it at its maximum. This explains why it is best to eat a large breakfast when the energy of the digestion is strongest and not to eat late at night when it needs to rest. The time of the Stomach is 7-9 a.m.

---

[1] At first sight, there may be some confusion about the use of this word. It a consequence of translation where words are used which already have a meaning to us in the West. The Chinese word is *Pi* and its designated counterpart in the West was considered to be the spleen. This was done before our current level of knowledge of conventional anatomy and physiology. The Spleen, as this is understood in Chinese medicine, is functionally more related to the pancreas and duodenum. For these reasons, any organs which are capitalised, e.g. Spleen, refer to the Chinese medical view.

Emotions - sympathy	An imbalance of the Earth element may manifest as oversympathy or lack of sympathy. Being oversympathetic may deplete Spleen energy. This is the difference between *mother* and *smother*. Mother also applies to the Earth element - Mother Nature..
Mental aspect	Deals with the aspects of belief and faith, confidence and trust. Its paired organ, the Stomach, is to do with endurance, stamina and the ability to keep going. If there is Heat in the Stomach or its energy is scattered, there is no patience. If the energy of the Stomach is depleted, there is no endurance.

TABLE 13.2: HOLISTIC ENERGETIC VIEW OF THE DIGESTION

ORGAN	COMMENTS
Large Intestine	This organ is paired with the Lung. Its function depends largely upon the efficiency of the Lung. Mentally, it is to do with forgiveness and letting go. Its healthy functioning allows us to ease up and have a forgiving attitude. The role of the Kidney is important also as the Large Intestine is situated in the area controlled by Kidney function[2].
Small Intestine	This organ is paired with the Heart. Its function is to separate the pure from the impure. On a mental level, it is to do with awareness and sensitivity. It helps us with discernment. The ability to differentiate 'pure from impure'.

TABLE 13.3: ADDITIONAL COMMENTS ABOUT ENERGETIC VIEW OF DIGESTION

The main function of the gastrointestinal system is linked in Chinese medicine to the function of the Spleen. Spleen Qi or energy, together with that of the Stomach, is responsible for the transformation and transportation of food into energy. This is used by other organs as well as helping the formation of Blood and Body Fluids. If Spleen energy is depleted for any reason, then not only is less energy produced but also mucus is produced. This can collect in various areas of the body and cause problems. For example, in the intestines it may lead to bowel disturbances which correspond to Crohn's disease or ulcerative colitis. Mucus may pass up into the lungs and be associated with conditions such as chronic bronchitis. It may be lodged into the skin and be associated with conditions we know as eczema and so forth.

The Liver, as that organ is understood by Chinese medicine, is also important in the regulation of the digestion. The energetic associations of this are listed in Chapter 14 - Central Nervous System. The Liver is considered to deal with the free flowing of energy. Any obstruction to this in the digestive system may lead to symptoms such as belching, flatulence, bloating and abdominal pain. These connections will become more obvious when individual diseases are discussed.

The gastrointestinal system and the lungs are the main organs after birth which provide the body with energy. It is clear, therefore, why there is so much debility and ill health in the West. Food and air are two items which are very much polluted. People who live in cities and breathe in stale air with large amounts of car fumes are prone to lung disease.

Tremendous strains are put on the gastrointestinal system by eating food which is poor in quality. This may be a classical case of malnutrition when deprived of food. In the West, it is more likely to mean poor quality food due to farming techniques such as the use of pesticides and herbicides. It may be due to food processing techniques, e.g. canning, pre-cooking and freezing where old food is eaten. It may be due to cooking techniques such as microwaves[3]. Such

---

[2] A note here about colonic irrigation. This may be useful in some people with severe heat syndromes affecting the Large Intestine. In others, particularly if the energy is depleted, it will lead to further weakness. This is because the large volume of fluid passed into the Large Intestine will damage the Qi of the Lung and the Kidney. I have seen several people who have had inappropriate colonic irrigation. They were left weaker than before with evidence of more serious disease.

[3] There are two issues about the use of microwaves. One is concerning the effect of the microwave radiation on humans and particularly adverse effects on behaviour and the immune system. There was

treatment strips food of essential nutrients as well as its energy. This is dead food and cannot lead to health. When this is combined with rapid eating, irregular eating and eating when stressed, it is clear that disturbances of the digestive system, together with general debility are easily explained.

The consequence of believing that Spleen Qi drives the main system is that if we are to be healthy it is important to protect this Qi at all times. Qi is warm in nature. Therefore, Chinese medicine places great emphasis on eating warming foods[4], particularly in cold climates. The advice regarding diet in cold northern climates is to eat mainly cooked foods such as porridge in the morning and to take soups, stews and casseroles. Ginger and cinnamon in the cooking add the warming qualities of these herbs. It is essential to avoid cold fruits, particularly of tropical origin, since these are more appropriate for hot climates. In the summer, when the weather is warmer, then it is more appropriate to eat occasional salads or fruit. The ingestion of large quantities of raw, cold food can only deplete Spleen energy and in the long run lead to general weakness. This is in contrast to common advice which is heard in the West that eating raw food will mean a greater intake of vitamins and minerals into the body.

There are occasions when an intake of cold, raw food may be beneficial. This is when detoxification is appropriate. However, the use of such a technique without individualisation of the case may lead to serious consequences since there is a loss of body fluid and energy. The indiscriminate use of detoxification, particularly when linked with colonic irrigation or enemas, can deplete the body.

---

the well-documented case of microwave radiation directed at the US Embassy in Moscow in the 1960's and 1970's. This led to changes in white blood cell counts and ultimately increased rates of cancer. This and other aspects of electromagnetic radiation may be obtained from "Subtle Energy" by John Davidson (CW Daniel, 1987).

The second issue of domestic microwaves is the effect on the food itself. Microwaves cook by agitating molecules. This has the effect of depleting the Qi or energy of the food. It also tends to dry out the food as a result of this rapid stimulation. People who mainly eat microwave cooked tend to develop Spleen Qi deficiency. They may also develop Yin deficiency due to this drying action.

[4] The energetic qualities of food and how to apply these to individual cases is a complex subject. Two excellent books are "Prince Wen Hui's Cook" by Flaws and Wolfe (Paradigm, 1983) and "Chinese System of Food Cures" by Henry Lu (Sterling, 1986).

- CLASSIFICATION OF GASTROINTESTINAL DISEASE -

As can be seen from Table 13.4, the conventional classification is according to the site of the problem. The gastrointestinal system is studied in sequence from the mouth to the anus. Within each area, lists are made of the various problems which may occur. I have followed this pattern somewhat since there seems to be a fairly straightforward division into the upper and lower gastrointestinal tract. These produce symptoms in their respective areas.

Disorders of the mouth
stomatitis
Diseases of the tongue
glossitis
leukoplakia
cancer
Diseases of the oesophagus
reflux oesophagitis
cancer
Diseases of the stomach and duodenum
gastritis
duodenitis
peptic ulcer
cancer of stomach
Diseases of the small intestine
malabsorption
Crohn's disease
Diseases of the large intestine
ulcerative colitis
irritable bowel syndrome
diverticulitis
cancer
Diseases of the anus
haemorrhoids
fissure
Diseases of the pancreas
pancreatitis
cancer
Diseases of the liver
hepatitis
cirrhosis
cancer
Diseases of the gall bladder
gallstones (cholelithiasis)
inflammation (cholecystitis)

TABLE 13.4: CONVENTIONAL CLASSIFICATION OF GASTROINTESTINAL DISEASE

Those in italics are the most important.

Most disorders of the gastrointestinal system may be regarded as a disturbance of function. There may be some structural changes as with peptic ulceration or ulcerative colitis but these seem to me to be secondary to a functional disturbance. More serious disease such as diverticulitis and cancer are associated with marked physical changes and hence are more difficult to treat. Table 13.5 lists diseases according to the site of symptoms rather than organ of origin. Mild disease is placed at the top of each section.

Upper abdominal symptoms (mild disease at the top)

> Reflux oesophagitis
> Hepatitis
> Peptic ulcer
> Gall stones (cholelithiasis)
> Inflammation of gall bladder (cholecystitis)
> Pancreatitis
> Cirrhosis
> Cancer of the stomach
> Cancer of the pancreas
> Cancer of the liver

Lower abdominal symptoms (mild disease at the top)

> Anal fissure
> Haemorrhoids
> Irritable bowel syndrome
> Diverticulitis
> Inflammatory bowel disease
> > Ulcerative colitis
> > Crohn's disease
> Cancer of the large intestine

TABLE 13.5: ALTERNATIVE CLASSIFICATION OF GASTROINTESTINAL DISEASE

In terms of alternative medicine, most disorders in this system are relatively easy to treat. This is because the gastrointestinal system is, hierarchically, a relatively superficial area of the body. I would refer you to the comments I made about Levels of Health on Pages 18 and 19 of Volume 1 and especially Tables 2.2 and 2.3.

- ABDOMINAL PAIN -

As described in Chapter 7 - Cardiovascular System, there are nine main questions to ask about pain wherever its site. These are reviewed here in relation to the gastrointestinal system.

Main site:

Where is the pain? Do not just accept a vague wave of the hand but ask concisely. Make sure that there is common understanding of whatever terms are used. Ask for confirmation by pointing. Do not assume that the term 'stomach' or 'tummy' means the same thing to everyone. It can be useful to see the extent of the painful area and clues can be obtained by whether the person points with one finger or uses the whole hand to describe the site. At some stage see the area unclothed

Figure 13.1 is a diagrammatic representation of the abdomen. It is divided into several areas, each with its own name. It is important to know these since they are a common method of describing sites of symptoms. References to them are made in homoeopathic repertories, for example.

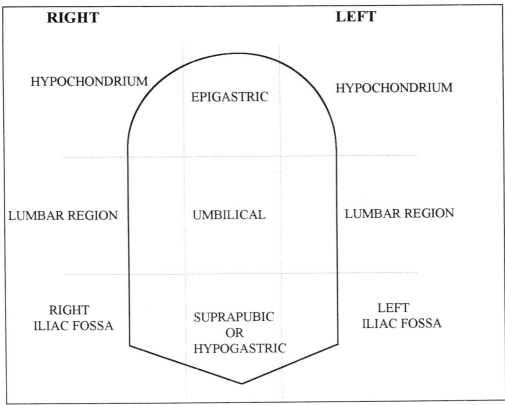

FIGURE 13.1: DIVISION OF THE ABDOMEN INTO NAMED AREAS

In conventional medicine, the site of pain in the abdomen is seen as being related to the underlying anatomical structure. Problems with organs in the epigastrium lead to epigastric pain, problems with organs in the right iliac fossa lead to right iliac fossa pain, etc. A complete list is given in Table 13.6.

AREA OF ABDOMEN	ORGANS IN THIS AREA	OTHER ORGANS WHICH MAY PRODUCE PAIN IN THIS AREA
Epigastrium	Oesophagus (lower end), stomach, duodenum, pancreas	Heart
Right hypochondrium	Liver, gall bladder	
Left hypochondrium	Spleen	
Umbilical	Small intestine	
Right lumbar region	Kidney, ureter	
Left lumbar region	Kidney, ureter	
Suprapubic (hypogastric)	Bladder (full), uterus (pregnant, fibroids)	Bladder[5], uterus
Right iliac fossa	Appendix, ureter, caecum	Fallopian tube, ovary
Left iliac fossa	Sigmoid colon, ureter	Fallopian tube, ovary

TABLE 13.6: ORGANS CONTAINED WITHIN EACH AREA OF THE ABDOMEN

---

[5] Anatomically, the bladder, uterus, fallopian tubes and ovary are situated in the pelvis. However, they may give rise to pain in the lower part of the abdomen. They cannot be palpated via the abdomen except in the case of a bladder full of urine or a uterus enlarged by pregnancy or fibroids.

Radiation:

The pain may be felt in sites in addition to the primary area. This is typical of certain conditions and certain processes. Pancreatitis pain is felt in the epigastrium and radiates *through* to the back. Cholecystitis gives rise to pain in the right hypochondrium which radiates *round* to the back and the shoulder. The pain of renal colic is felt in the lumbar region and loin and can radiate to the groin or even the knee.

It is interesting that the occurrence of back pain may not be due solely to problems with the back. This is a common mistake of conventional medicine. Back pain from organs is related to their position. They are more likely to cause this symptom if they lie outside the peritoneal cavity. Examples would be pancreas, kidney and uterus.

Character:

It can be difficult to describe the particular quality of pain but certain conditions are associated with characteristic qualities. Colic is a cramping pain which comes in waves of worsening and relief but the exact nature depends on the source organ. It is produced by hollow organs whose muscular walls are in a state of spasm such as small intestine, gall bladder, ureter, uterus and large intestine.

Colic of the gall bladder (biliary colic) or kidney (renal colic) is typically severe and does not go away completely during remissions. However, the colic of small or large intestine origin does disappear before returning some time later. This is the type of colic seen in an acute enteritis, e.g. food poisoning.

Severity:

Pain can be of any severity according to the cause or it can vary from person to person. As mentioned above biliary or renal colic is typically severe. Thresholds of pain are variable and different people will react to pain in greatly different ways. Usually, the more the severe the disease and the weaker the person then the pain is more likely to be severe and intractable.

Duration:

Ask how long the pain has been present, not only this attack but also the whole process. Is this a recent event or have there been repeated attacks in the past? Appendicitis, for example, will have a short history of not more than 24 to 48 hours although some people do have recurrent subacute attacks - the so-called "grumbling appendix". Peptic ulcers on the other hand have a chronic course of many years with flare-ups which last weeks or months.

Frequency:

How often does the pain recur? With renal colic it will be every few minutes or so, with ulcer pain it will be every day or longer, perhaps every night as in the case of a duodenal ulcer.

Time of occurrence:

This is of less importance in conventional than alternative medicine since it is an excellent way of individual differentiation. Conventional medicine sees a duodenal ulcer as being worse at night, bowel pain as being worse later in the day but otherwise changes like these are seen to be of little significance. Changes of symptoms with the weather, seasons, temperature and times of day (known as modalities) and so on are of supreme importance in alternative medicine. They serve to help differentiate many syndromes.

Modalities:

Does anything help the pain or make it worse? Ask the open question first and later suggest alternatives, if necessary, for selection. Leading questions result in information which is virtually useless in making a diagnosis. Peritonitis pain is worse for movement, peptic ulcer pain is better for vomiting, gastric ulcer is worse for eating, duodenal ulcer is better for eating, gall bladder disease is worse for eating fatty food. In alternative medicine, this is much more refined and, as mentioned above, such information as the effect of heat or cold is pretty much disregarded by a conventional practitioner.

Associated phenomena:

You should take note of any symptoms which also appear with the pain. For example, nausea with upper abdominal pain, diarrhoea with lower abdominal pain, vaginal discharge with gynaecological causes of lower abdominal pain.

From the questioning above, done in a careful and orderly way, most cases of abdominal pain can be diagnosed and examination of the abdomen would be a confirmation. Confusion can occur from the history, as with differentiating some cases of peptic ulcer from cholecystitis, but precise history-taking will minimise this.

- UPPER GASTROINTESTINAL DISTURBANCES -

In any discussion, it is important to relate symptoms to a particular dysfunction. It must be remembered that the gastrointestinal tract is essentially a hollow tube passing from the mouth to the anus. Any functional disturbance will be reflected in a particular group of symptoms. For example, disturbance of the passage of food through the gastrointestinal tract leads to constipation or diarrhoea. Reversal of the normal flow through the system leads to nausea and/or vomiting. Disturbance in flow at any particular site will lead to bloating, pain and discomfort.

The stomach is responsible for appetite and so disorders of the stomach may be associated with increased or decreased appetite. Any long lasting disturbance such as poor appetite or loss of fluid will lead to weight loss. Increased intake of food will usually lead to weight gain.

In summary, disturbances of the upper part of the gastrointestinal tract will lead to symptoms of pain, distension, appetite changes, nausea and vomiting. Disturbances of the lower part of the gastrointestinal tract will lead to pain, distension, constipation or diarrhoea. In this section I shall describe conditions which can be found in conventional textbooks. They are commonly seen and I shall summarise their symptom pictures to contrast and compare features.

- UPPER ABDOMINAL PAIN -

GENERAL OVERVIEW

This is a common symptom and may be due to many underlying disorders. Most of these are not serious in the sense of being life-threatening but frequently interfere with people's life-style, habits and activity. Essentially, I am discussing here pain in the epigastrium and right hypochondrium. Pain in the left hypochondrium does occur but it is unusual. If you look again at Figure 13.1 and its accompanying Table 13.6, you will see the organs which may give rise to pain in this area.

- OESOPHAGEAL DISEASE -

The oesophagus is a hollow muscular tube which transports food from the mouth the stomach. It has no digestive or absorptive function. Disturbances here lead to symptoms of dysphagia (difficulty swallowing), a sensation of something being stuck and pain.

REFLUX OESOPHAGITIS

This is an inflammation of the oesophagus. This condition is more common in middle age or elderly women and in those who are overweight or in pregnancy. It is associated with the passage of acid from the stomach back up into the oesophagus.

A common term which is often applied to this condition is hiatus hernia[6]. This is a technical label which refers to the passage of the upper part of the stomach through the hiatus of the diaphragm.

There are two types of hiatus hernia. There is the common 'sliding' hernia and the unusual 'paraoesophageal' hernia. The unusual type of hernia, the paraoesophageal, may be associated with dysphagia as there may be obstruction to the passage of food. However, it is rare in clinical practice.

Hiatus hernia does not produce symptoms and this is contrary to popular belief. It is the *function* of the junction between the oesophagus and stomach which is the determining factor as to whether symptoms develop. If the oesophago-gastric junction is weakened, acid can pass back up into the oesophagus. The lining of the oesophagus is vulnerable to attack as its mucus membrane is not designed to resist the effects of acid. Inflammation occurs and this leads to the classical symptoms of this condition. Such a hernia may or may not be associated with acid reflux. It can only be diagnosed by a barium meal X-ray. It is present in about one third of people over the age of 50 years and so is of no significance.

The discussion about the distinction between hiatus hernia and reflux oesophagitis is not an empty one as it may first appear. The appearances on X-ray are not especially important as many people without symptoms may have them. Many people with symptoms have no evidence of a hernia. When a barium meal is performed a person is tipped upside down specifically to see if any herniation takes place and this may be a factor in the appearance on X-ray.

The older treatment for hiatus hernia was by a surgical approach through the chest wall to fix the stomach firmly below the diaphragm. This was singularly unsuccessful and many people had exactly the same symptoms after the operation as they did before. The key is how something works, not what it looks like[7]. Its function is much more important than its structure. The preferable term to use, therefore, is reflux oesophagitis.

---

[6] A hernia describes the passage of part of the intestine outside the peritoneal cavity. This usually occurs in the groin where it is called an inguinal hernia. It may be seen in the upper thigh (femoral hernia), around the umbilicus (umbilical hernia), at the site of an abdominal operation (incisional hernia) or protrude through the hiatus of the diaphragm (diaphragmatic or hiatus hernia).

[7] Similar observations can be made about the discovery of gallstones in people with upper abdominal pain and those with back pain who may have radiological evidence of intervertebral disc prolapse. Surgical correction of the physical abnormalities frequently does *not* lead to relief of symptoms. See details of these disorders for a further discussion of these two situations.

Symptoms

The classical clinical feature of reflux oesophagitis is 'heartburn'. This is a burning sensation felt behind the sternum. It is precipitated and worsened by bending, stooping, lifting and straining. It is particularly troublesome at night when lying. There may be regurgitation of food on lying. The pain is better when the position is changed to sitting and is better after food or alkalis. Change of pain with change of posture is typical of this condition and is not really seen with any other cause of chest pain. The differential diagnosis of chest pain is described in detail in Page 117. Blood loss is frequent from the inflamed area and iron deficiency, if not obvious anaemia, is common.

Complications

COMPLICATIONS	SYMPTOMS TO LOOK FOR
Stricture (narrowing) due to scar formation	Difficulty swallowing developing over months and years, sensation of food sticking in chest
Anaemia	Pallor, tiredness, light-headedness, palpitations, anxiety
Haemorrhage	Vomiting blood

TABLE 13.7: COMPLICATIONS OF REFLUX OESOPHAGITIS

Investigations

Gastroscopy will reveal the inflamed area and barium meal may show evidence of hiatus hernia but I would refer you to the comments above. The complications of ulceration and stricture may be seen. Simple inflammation cannot be seen by X-ray procedures.

Treatment:

The conventional dietary advice given is described in the section dealing with peptic ulceration. Weight loss in the overweight is important and people are told to avoid the situations which precipitate pain. Stopping smoking is beneficial as nicotine leads to a rise in the secretion of gastric acid and so is the most important single factor in avoiding further damage. All medication taken should be reviewed as many drugs lead to upper gastrointestinal problems especially aspirin, non-steroidal anti-inflammatory drugs and corticosteroids.

There are many drug treatments available and most people will be given some form of medication. Metoclopramide causes the stomach to empty quickly and increases contraction of the cardiac sphincter. It is also used in the symptomatic treatment of nausea. It acts via the central nervous system and so its side-effects mainly appear there with symptoms similar to those of Parkinson's disease.

Antacids can neutralise gastric acid to some extent and will give immediate relief to inflammatory problems of the upper gastrointestinal tract. However, with continual usage they will lead to the production of more acid because the body tries to maintain a certain level of acidity in the stomach. Problems are experienced when people try to come off them since the stomach is exposed to the full force of an increased acid secretion.

There are various types of antacid based either on aluminium which can give rise to constipation and magnesium which can lead to diarrhoea. Ingestion of large amounts of metallic salts in this way can lead to disturbances in electrolyte concentrations in the blood giving rise to perhaps deficiency of some substances or overload with others. In view of the current thoughts about aluminium and dementia, it would seem to be unwise to continually ingest these substances.

It may be interesting here, to discuss the current thoughts about aluminium and dementia. It illustrates that despite information of a connection, the widespread use continues of prescribing compounds containing aluminium.

The main sources of aluminium are drinking water, medicines, inhaled air (small amount unless in an industrial environment) and food. It has been known for about 100 years that aluminium is toxic to the central nervous system[8].

There have been discussions for some years that aluminium may also be implicated in the genesis of dementia and related syndromes. It may lead to nerve cell deformites similar to those found in Alzheimer's disease[9]. It has been reported that aluminium is present in increased concentrations in the brains of people with Alzheimer's disease[10]. These findings have been confirmed by others[11].

Aluminium has also been shown to cause an acute dementia in people undergoing dialysis for kidney failure when present in dialysis fluid in relatively high concentrations[12].

The main source of exposure is usually the diet especially items such as tea or those which have had aluminium added, e.g. raising agents, emulsifying agents, or those foods stored in aluminium cans. The amount in drinking water provides only a small proportion of the total dietary content but such aluminium tends to be more easily absorbed and therefore a greater source of pollution. Various studies have been performed which relate aluminium in drinking water to increased rates of dementia. Of the ten studies available, seven have shown a connection[13].

A major source of exposure is the use of medicines which contain aluminium, of which the most important are the aluminium antacids[14]. These are potentially a much greater risk as the dose is much higher than that of food and drinking water. Certainly, blood levels of aluminium are raised in those who take such drugs regularly[15].

Other medicines which contain aluminium include enteric-coated aspirin and some antiperspirants[16] and deodorants that are sprayed on the skin (from which some may be absorbed).

Other sources of medically contamination include the inhalation of aluminium powder in the belief that it would protect miners from pneumoconiosis. This was used in Ontario, Canada in the 1950's. Examination shows that such exposure is related to central nervous system damage[17].

Another example of symptomatic treatment is Gaviscon which is a mixture of alginic acid and antacids. It is taken as a liquid which lies on top of the stomach contents. When acid passes into the oesophagus only the drug is in contact with the mucosa. Therefore, it protects the oesophagus from further contact with the gastric contents. It is of variable effectiveness.

The definitive conventional treatment for all conditions involving gastric acid secretion over the past 10 years or so is with histamine (H_2) blockers. Cimetidine and ranitidine decrease the amount of gastric acid secreted. They have to be given over a prolonged course to produce

---

[8] Dollken A Arch Exp Pathol Pharmacol 1897;40:98-120.

[9] Klatzo I et al, J Neuropathol Exp Neurol 1965;24:187-99.

[10] Crapper DR et al, Science 1973;185:511-13.

[11] Candy JM et al, "Regulation of transmitter function: basic and clinical aspects".Edited by Vizi ES, Magyar K (Amsterdam: Elsevier. 1984;301-6) and by Perry EK et al, Trends Neurosci 1985;8:301-3.

[12] Alfrey AC et al, N Engl J Med 1976;294:184-8 and Rozas et al, J Dialysis 1978;2:459-70.

[13] These include Martyn CN et al, Lancet 1989;I:59-62.

Michel P et al, "Alzheimer's disease basic mechanisms, diagnosis and therapeutic strategies" Edited by Iqbal K, McLachlan DRC, Winblad B, Wisniewski HM, (Chichester: J. Wiley & Sons, 1991;387-9).

Frecker MF J Epidemiol Community, Health 1991;45:307-11.

Forbes WF et al, Lancet 1991;338:1592-3.

Flaten TP. Environ Geochem Health 1990;12:152-67.

[14] There is some evidence that they are related to demented states. Leventhal GH. Dissertation presented for the Doctor of Philosophy Degree, University of Tennessee, Knoxville, 1987.

[15] House RA. J Occup Med 1992;34:1013-17.

[16] A positive association with the use of antiperspirants and dementia has been made by Graves et al. J Clin Epidemiol 1990;43:35-44.

[17] Rifat SL et al, Lancet 1990;ii:1162-5.

resolution of the inflammation. Relapses are common after stopping the drug no matter how long it has been taken. They are discussed more fully under peptic ulceration.

Surgery should be rarely considered nowadays because it is recognised that control of symptoms is poor.

Alternative management:

Treatment for this condition is very helpful when given along with appropriate dietary advice. Clearly smoking should stop. Most antacids can be taken when symptoms occur so the symptom picture can be more clearly seen..

Histamine (H_2) blockers should be approached more circumspectly as stopping them can lead to a powerful rebound of the original symptoms, whether pain or bleeding, and this can occur several years after starting them. Therefore, take care to reduce them slowly with any improvement in the person's condition.

GASTRITIS

This is inflammation of the stomach and is common. There are acute and chronic types depending upon the presentation.

With acute gastritis, there may be simple inflammation, superficial ulcers (erosions) or ulcers. Common causes include aspirin, non-steroidal anti-inflammatory agents and alcohol. They are also seen in association with stressful situations, burns, injury, kidney and liver disease.

Chronic gastritis is mainly of two types. There may be long-standing injury due to aspirin or non-steroidal anti-inflammatory agents or an autoimmune type which is associated with pernicious anaemia. The latter condition may be associated with other autoimmune diseases such as hypothyroidism and Addison's disease and in severe cases may lead onto cancer of the stomach.

Symptoms:

Acute gastritis is characterised by strong symptoms of epigastric pain and vomiting. There may be the vomiting of blood in cases of erosion or ulceration.

Chronic gastritis is considered in the conventional texts to be asymptomatic but in my experience leads to anorexia and nausea particularly in the morning. There may be vomiting of mucus. Intermittent epigastric discomfort will be experienced and there may be belching, upper abdominal distension and unpleasant taste in the mouth.

Some people with stomach disorders develop symptoms in the mouth and gums. There may be ulceration or bleeding gums and there will be signs of inflammation (gingivitis).

Investigations:

Gastroscopy will reveal inflammation. There may be ulceration in cases of acute gastritis. In chronic gastritis there is a reduced level of gastric acid and there may be evidence of anaemia with low levels of Vitamin B_{12}. A barium meal shows smoothness of the stomach lining in chronic gastritis.

Treatment:

It is important to remove the cause of the gastritis if there is one. Pernicious anaemia will be treated with Vitamin B_{12} injections for life and regular monitoring of haemoglobin levels.

Alternative management:

The comments I make in relation to peptic ulcer are relevant here.

PEPTIC ULCER

This is a generic term which is used to describe any ulcer occurring in the presence of acid. There are several possible sites. These are the lower oesophagus, stomach, duodenum, jejunum after gastric surgery and in the ileum adjacent to a Meckel's diverticulum. The latter is present in 2% of people situated 2 feet from the terminal ileum and secretes acid.

Ulceration of the lower end of the oesophagus occurs in connection with reflux oesophagitis. I shall concentrate here on ulcers of the stomach and duodenum as they are the common ones seen in clinical practice.

Around one in seven of the population in the UK develop a duodenal ulcer at some time in their life. They are two or three times commoner than gastric ulcers. Duodenal ulcers are four times more common in men whilst gastric ulcers are twice more common. There is a definite relationship between cigarette smoking and delayed healing due to an increase in gastric acid secretion.

There is often a family history of ulceration and so hereditary factors may be important. Members of the same family tend to have similar dietary and emotional features so it is not as simple as it seems.

The mechanism of ulceration in terms of conventional thought is not well understood. There are concepts of acid production versus mucosal resistance to acid. However, the main thrust of diagnosis and treatment is to look at the production of acid and this is in keeping with the philosophical viewpoint of an external force causing disease. There is some recognition that certain factors can damage the mucosa apart from acid. These include drugs particularly aspirin, emotional upsets (this is open to debate in conventional circles) and irregular eating habits. Gastric ulcers are usually associated with low acid secretion unless they are around the pylorus in which case they have more in common with duodenal ulcers. Duodenal ulcers are associated with increased acid levels. It would seem, therefore, that gastric ulcers are associated in some way with an abnormality of the stomach wall leading to decreased acid secretion and an increased risk of cancer. Duodenal ulcers are more to do with an abnormality in function where increased levels of acid lead to erosion of the mucosa.

The conventional view of peptic ulcers is that there is a strong association between aspirin, genetic factors, smoking and a family history of ulceration. It is not generally considered that factors such as non-steroidal anti-inflammatory agents, diet, corticosteroids or psychological states have much of a role to play in causing ulceration[18]. These ideas reveal much more about the state of conventional medical thought than they do about the condition of peptic ulceration.

Symptoms:

The distinction to be made between duodenal and gastric ulceration is not always an easy one. With a careful history however, it is possible to have an idea about the site of the problem.

The main symptom of any ulcer is chronic episodic pain over months or years. Some people present with the complications of the ulcer such as bleeding, perforation or obstruction of the gastric outlet because of scarring with little history of previous problems. A duodenal ulcer typically has a prolonged natural history of up to 20 years and although drugs may affect an acute situation this long natural history is unaffected. Gastric ulcers are seen as being less chronic in nature.

All ulcer pain is felt in the epigastrium directly in the middle or slightly to the right. It is localised and most people point with one finger. This is not seen with any other condition. The pain is often related to food but this can be variable. Classically, a duodenal ulcer leads to 'hunger pain', that is, pain between and before meals. It is relieved by eating and people often wake 2 to 3 hours after going to bed. Many people put on weight because they eat to relieve the pain. They keep a glass of milk and biscuits by the bed to eat in the night if there is pain. Gastric ulcer, on the other hand, leads to pain which is less regular. It comes on an hour or so after eating and rarely at night. People are afraid to eat because it leads to pain and so they usually lose weight.

---

[18] "Clinical Medicine" Second Edition, Edited by Kumar and Clark (Bailliere Tindall, 1990). See Table 4.6 on Page 189.

The pain of an ulcer is better with antacids and better with vomiting. This episodic pain continues for days and weeks and then usually disappears even with no treatment. It will recur in most cases some weeks or months later. There are commonly milder symptoms in the intervening period or some people may be very well between attacks.

Relapses of the ulcer and pain are commonly linked to alcohol intake, poor diet or emotional stress. In some cases the pain may only be felt as mild discomfort or as a distended feeling in the upper abdomen. Other symptoms include nausea, vomiting, constipation or diarrhoea, poor appetite or increased appetite, belching, abdominal distension, rumbling in the abdomen. Vomiting is not a major feature but when it does occur it relieves the pain. Severe vomiting may lead to weight loss and could indicate one of the complications of ulceration.

On examination, there is local tenderness with perhaps some upper abdominal distension.

SYMPTOM	GASTRIC ULCER	DUODENAL ULCER
Pain	Epigastrium, localised	Epigastrium
Vomiting	Yes, relieves pain	Yes, relieves pain
Effect of eating	Worsens pain	Relieves pain
Time of pain	After meals	Before meals, at night
Appetite	Often poor because afraid to eat	Good

TABLE 13.8: COMPARISON OF GASTRIC AND DUODENAL ULCERS

Investigation:

Barium meal and gastroscopy are the standard investigations and will show most but not all ulcers. Gastric function tests on secretions collected via a tube passed into the stomach may reveal changes in the levels of gastric acid. Gastric ulcers may be associated with low gastric acid output and duodenal ulcers with raised levels.

Complications:

COMPLICATIONS	SYMPTOMS TO LOOK FOR
Pyloric stenosis[19]	Copious vomiting containing food eaten 12 or more hours before, projectile vomiting, upper abdominal distension with splashing sounds
Haemorrhage	Vomiting blood, black tarry stools (melaena[20])
Perforation	Severe abdominal pain, abdominal rigidity, immobility, shock - low blood pressure, rapid pulse
Penetration into pancreas	Severe epigastric pain radiating through to back, abdominal rigidity, immobility, shock, low blood pressure, rapid pulse

TABLE 13.9: COMPLICATIONS OF PEPTIC ULCER

Treatment:

As stated above, the long term course of a peptic ulcer is not affected by conventional treatment. Any such treatment can only, therefore, be regarded as symptomatic.

There is generally no dietary advice given to people with peptic ulcers. This will clearly vary with individual practitioners but the conventional view is that diet has little, if any role, to play in the genesis and healing of ulcers.

---

[19] This is narrowing of the pylorus - the exit of the stomach. It is due to scar tissue secondary to ulceration. A rare, unrelated situation occurs in male babies causing projectile vomiting at around 3 months of age.

[20] If a peptic ulcer bleeds heavily there may be no vomiting to reveal its presence. It can be pass through the intestines where the motions take on a black tarry appearance and is known as melaena. It can be confused with the stools seen with iron medication.

Drugs such as aspirin, anti-inflammatory agents and corticosteroids are well known for causing irritation to the upper gastrointestinal tract and ulceration. Several people each year die as a result of bleeding from the stomach or duodenum caused by these drugs. No-one with a history of ulceration or indigestion should take them. It is not uncommon now to see non-steroidal anti-inflammatory drugs combined, in the same tablet, with histamine (H_2) blockers. This strange practice is similar to prescribing antibiotics with corticosteroids or antidepressants with tranquillisers. These are not uncommon events.

The only factors which have been proven to be effective by conventional medicine are the stopping of smoking, reducing alcohol intake and rest.

Despite this, drugs are the mainstay of conventional treatment especially the histamine (H_2) receptor blockers. Histamine is involved in the secretion of gastric acid and so drugs which block these receptors lead to a reduction in gastric acid secretion. The usual antihistamines, incidentally, have no effect. The two drugs used are cimetidine which has been around for about 15 years now and ranitidine, a more recent development. Four weeks of treatment leads to the disappearance of about 80% of duodenal ulcers and 70% of gastric ulcers. Most people rapidly become asymptomatic within a few days or a week of initiating treatment. There are frequently one or two exacerbations of the ulcer each year and so a repeat course of 4 weeks treatment is given. Some people relapse each time the drug is stopped and so maintenance treatment of a reduced dose each night is given either for several years or permanently. These drugs were originally only given to those people with proven evidence of an ulcer but now they are prescribed on the basis of symptoms only and relatively early. They are expensive and have some unpleasant side-effects including breast development in men. They produce a state of low gastric acid which is a consistent finding in cancer of the stomach. There is some evidence to suggest, therefore, that these drugs may lead to the development of stomach cancer.

Carbenoxolone is derived from liquorice[21] and used much less frequently since the introduction of histamine blockers. It will lead to the healing of peptic ulcers but has a high concentration of sodium. There is a risk of worsening or precipitating cardiac failure in the elderly. More likely is the development of oedema and high blood pressure.

Colloidal bismuth[22] is an older drug which actually heals as well as the histamine blockers but with a longer symptomatic response.

Before I discuss the management of these conditions, I want to mention a current fashion of diagnosing infection in the upper gastrointestinal tract. It has been discovered that an organism, Helicobacter pylori (old name - Campylobacter pylori), is present in many people. There is speculation that it may be the cause of the disorders above but there is no evidence that this is so. Nevertheless, some people may be given antibiotics. As described in Chapter 5 - Infectious Disease, any organism appears secondarily and so the use of antibiotics can only make the stomach disorder worse. Bismuth, described above, is being increasingly used as it has an action against these bacteria.

---

[21] Licorice is used in herbal medicine to treat stomach disorders. In terms of Chinese medicine, it tonifies the Qi of the Spleen and Lung.

[22] Interestingly, this is another example of conventional medicine stumbling across a commonly appropriate energetic remedy. The homoeopathic potency of bismuth has symptoms in its provings similar to those of peptic ulceration.

Failure of drug therapy leads, conventionally, to surgery. This is performed for intractable peptic ulceration, severe persistent symptoms or to prevent complications. It may be considered in several situations.

- rapid relapse after several courses of histamine blocker
- failure to heal
- interference with person's quality of life
- gastric outlet obstruction.
- gastric ulcer of uncertain nature or if persists 3 months.
- recurrent ulcer following previous gastric surgery.

Duodenal ulcers are treated by vagotomy and pyloroplasty. The vagus nerve is cut (vagotomy) to reduce gastric acid output. This also slows gastric emptying and so a drainage procedure (pyloroplasty) where the muscle is cut at the outlet of the stomach to aid gastric emptying.

Gastric ulcers are treated by partial gastrectomy, i.e. removal of the area containing the ulcer.

COMPLICATIONS	COMMENTS
Diarrhoea	Quoted in conventional textbooks as occurring in 1% after surgery. In my experience it is far higher than this and can be debilitating
Dumping	A collection of symptoms occurring after meals. They include faintness, sweating, pallor, nausea, abdominal distension and palpitations. In conventional medicine it is thought to be due to the rapid passage of food into the small intestine
Vomiting	More common after the older, more disruptive operations
Nutritional deficiencies	Iron deficiency is common after surgery. Rarer deficiencies involve Vitamin B_{12}, folate, calcium (leading to bone disease - osteomalacia - in some) and protein

TABLE 13.10: COMPLICATIONS OF GASTRIC SURGERY

Alternative management:

The causes of epigastric pain in terms of Chinese medicine are many and varied. There is a general division in to conditions of excess and those of deficiency. The energetic diagnosis in each individual case will determine the specific symptom picture, modalities and associated symptoms. This is why the descriptions given above can only ever be rough approximations. Table 13.11 is list of Chinese medical syndromes which may give rise to epigastric pain.

Spleen Qi Deficiency
Spleen Yang Deficiency
Damp-Heat injuring Spleen
Stomach Yin Deficiency
Stomach Cold
Stomach Fire Blazing
Food Stagnation in the Stomach
Blood Stagnation in the Stomach
Liver Qi attacking Stomach

TABLE 13.11: CHINESE MEDICAL SYNDROMES ASSOCIATED WITH EPIGASTRIC PAIN

Whichever system of medicine you are using, it is essential to individualise the case to obtain satisfactory results. The following case is an example of the progress which can be made, even in long-standing cases.

CASE

A man of 50 years came for treatment of his diarrhoea. He had suffered from epigastric pain for many years each Christmas. Each episode would last about a month and would settle with simple antacids. On one occasion, five years prior to his coming to see me he went to see his doctor. Because he was covered by a private health scheme, his doctor referred him to a surgeon who performed a vagotomy and pyloroplasty operation[23]. He developed diarrhoea immediately after the operation and this continued daily. Whenever he ate, he would have symptoms of light-headedness, dizziness and would have watery diarrhoea. There would occasionally be undigested food in the stools. He had lost about 21 pounds in weight in the last year and for the last 6 months had felt quite ill. His appetite was poor and he felt full quickly when eating.

His diarrhoea would be at least three times daily despite the daily prescription of a codeine derivative - loperamide. Codeine is methylmorphine. They are derived from the opium poppy and classed as narcotics. They have a primarily heating effect on the Heart and Lungs leading to the emotional and mental changes of detachment and invulnerability. The heat is passed down into the intestines and dries the stools producing the typical side-effect of constipation. This is the reason they are used for diarrhoea.

In terms of Chinese medicine, the diagnosis was Spleen Yang Deficiency. This means that the energy of the Spleen was very weak and unable to transport and transform food. The cause was the operation some five years previously. This clinical picture is commonly seen after upper abdominal surgery.

Interestingly, his tongue should have been pale, wet and swollen but at his first visit was red and thin. This is because of the heating and drying effects of the drugs.

Treatment was directed at strengthening the Spleen with acupuncture and herbs. I gave him advice to eat warming foods with the addition of ginger and cinnamon. Within one month, he had improved markedly with no watery stools and a reduced of bowel movements each day. He was able to stop his drugs quite quickly. He was left with symptoms of excessive rumbling in the abdomen but this settled over the next few months of treatment.

This case reveals several points. Firstly, even when structural damage is present it is possible for people to improve. Secondly, the conventional treatment of peptic ulcer tends to make people worse. Thirdly, be careful before having conventional treatment which is private as this may tempt overzealous practitioners to try the more expensive yet more dangerous options.

- GALL BLADDER DISEASE -

The gall bladder is a small hollow organ situated beneath the liver. Its function is to store bile secreted by the liver. Bile contains bile salts, cholesterol and the breakdown products of haemoglobin from red blood cells. It is an important method by which substances are excreted by the liver. There are two main conditions of the gall bladder. These are gallstones, (cholelithiasis) and inflammation (cholecystitis). Although I consider these separately below for the purposes of description, in reality they commonly co-exist. Gallstones in the gallbladder may produce inflammation and inflammation is a common cause for the precipitation of gallstones.

GALLSTONES

Gallstones are present in 10% of people over the age of 40 years. Most cases are seen in females. Conventionally, gallstones are considered to be commoner in people who are overweight, female and over 40 years of age. They are more commonly seen in women who have had children.

There are three varieties of stone commonly found which are classified according to their composition. Cholesterol stones make up 20%, 5% are bile pigment stones and the remaining

---

[23] Surgical procedures on the stomach and duodenum as well as the use of histamine (H2) blockers leads to depletion of Spleen Yang.

75% are mixed in nature. According to conventional medicine, the causes of gallstone formation are not well understood but seem to be related to several factors. Cholesterol is an important constituent of bile. It may be that disturbances in cholesterol metabolism or raised serum cholesterol levels may lead to the production of stones. Certainly gallstones of this type are more commonly seen in pregnancy and diabetes mellitus. Pigment stones are more common in anaemias due to red blood cell breakdown because excess bile pigment is excreted.

This does not explain the vast majority of gallstones which are present and it may be that there is some alteration in the concentration of bile constituents. Substances normally in bile are as a supersaturated solution, i.e. they are present in concentrations far exceeding normal solutions. Any small change may result in the precipitation of substances out of solution.

Symptoms:

These are variable and depend upon the site of the gallstones. In most people they cause no symptoms and merely lie in the gallbladder to be found at routine examination, in the case of an operation for another reason or at post-mortem examination. Symptoms occur when the gallstone starts to move.

If they impact at the exit of the bladder or in the cystic duct, there may be biliary colic or cholecystitis. Biliary colic is the classical symptom picture of a stone obstructing the exit to the gall bladder. Typically, pain comes on after a meal. It is severe in nature and lasts for several hours. It is the right hypochondrial or epigastric, often radiating to the right scapula. The person is restless, cannot get comfortable and there is associated vomiting and sweating. After an hour or so the pain subsides to be replaced by tenderness in the right hypochondrium. Attacks occur at irregular intervals.

If the gallstone passes into the common bile duct and obstructs, jaundice will result since bile cannot enter the duodenum. The obstructed bile backs up into the liver and spills over into the blood. This is obstructive jaundice.

Rarely the stone may ulcerate through the gall bladder wall into the duodenum or colon. Acute cholecystitis is more common with the presence of gallstones and this is described below.

CHOLECYSTITIS

This is an inflammation of the gallbladder wall. It is frequently, though not always, associated with gallstones. Inflammation is not usually associated with organisms and so is not infective in nature.

Symptoms:

Pain is more persistent in contrast to biliary colic. There are additional signs of inflammation such as fever, toxaemia, rapid pulse rate. There is also abdominal tenderness. 95% of cases are associated with gallstones. Chronic cholecystitis is typified by repeated attacks, usually precipitated by food, particularly fatty food. Abdominal distension, flatulence and/or belching are common associated symptoms.

Investigations of gall bladder disease:

Occasionally gallstones can be seen by plain X-ray examination but only about 10% are visible by this method since few contain calcium. The common investigation performed these days is ultrasound. Additional information may be gathered by oral cholecystogram, intravenous cholangiogram, barium meal and liver function tests.

Treatment:

In the acute stage, cholecystitis is treated with antibiotics, despite the common absence of bacterial infection, and pethidine for the relief of pain. After the acute phase has subsided then the gall bladder is usually removed 2-3 months later. The operation of cholecystectomy is common. It invariably leads to diarrhoea since there is an impaired ability to digest and absorb fats.

There is an increasing move to use ultrasound waves to break up the gallstones (compare with treatment of kidney stones) or to use surgery to merely open the gall bladder and remove the stones. However, since the underlying condition is not remedied using this technique, gallstones usually reappear. For this reason, surgeons may prefer to use cholecystectomy at the outset.

There is a medical treatment using bile salts to attempt to dissolve the gallstones if they are of the cholesterol type. This is long term and is of variable effectiveness. Chenodeoxycholic or ursodeoxycholic acid are the usual compounds given. They may cause liver damage and render oral contraception ineffective.

Alternative management:

The main advantage of alternative medical treatment is that it rectifies the underlying imbalance. This will prevent, or at least minimise, the development of more gallstones. There are naturopathic treatments available such as the 'liver flush' to allow the body to pass gall stones. This is a pure diet or fast over several days followed by the drinking of a pint of olive oil with lemon juice. This causes the gall bladder to contract and the gallstones to expel. In my experience it is an effective means for removing gallstones without the need for surgery.

Homoeopathy and Chinese medicine are also effective for this condition. When I was training in acupuncture in China, we saw many people treated with acupuncture, particularly ear acupuncture. In terms of Chinese medicine, this condition usually corresponds with DampHeat in the Liver and Gall Bladder.

Some people request surgery despite the alternative treatments available. The use of ultrasound to break up the stones is helpful since the gall bladder can be conserved. The subsequent use of alternative medical treatment can prevent the recurrence of more gallstones.

- PANCREATIC DISEASE -

The pancreas is a combined exocrine and endocrine organ situated behind the peritoneal cavity at the level of the duodenum and lower stomach. In this section, I am dealing with the pancreas in its exocrine function. Endocrine disturbances of the pancreas are dealt with in Chapter 15 - Endocrine System.

The pancreas secretes enzymes which have an important role in the digestion of proteins, fats and carbohydrates. It does so in response to food eaten.

PANCREATITIS

This is an inflammation of the pancreas. It is unusual but severe in its symptoms. There are considered to be various causes in conventional medicine with excess alcohol intake and associated gall bladder disease being the commonest. It may occur as part of mumps[24] in post-pubertal people when it is mild and merely uncomfortable. The symptom picture described below is of the non-mumps type.

The underlying process is not completely understood in conventional medicine. There may be several factors such as the passage of bile (an irritant) up the pancreatic duct and digestion of the pancreas itself by pancreatic enzymes. Whatever the process, the accompanying inflammation is severe and widespread.

---

[24] Homoeopaths may use the mumps nosode (a remedy made from disease products of a case of mumps) to treat pancreatic disease.

Symptoms:

The severity of the attack may vary. There is epigastric pain radiating through to the back. It can vary in strength from mild discomfort to severe pain. There is associated nausea and vomiting. On examination, the epigastrium, and perhaps the whole abdomen, is tender and rigid with rebound tenderness[25]. These signs are typical of a severe attack. There may be rapid pulse rate, low blood pressure, pallor and sweating.

Some people have milder attacks denoting a more chronic picture. Attacks of pain are milder but more frequent. The pain is epigastric radiating through to the back. Alcohol intake is often the cause of an attack. Weight loss is common together with anorexia. In long-term disease, the absorption of fat is affected leading to diarrhoea, greasy and pale stools. Some people may develop diabetes mellitus if enough of the pancreas is damaged to affect insulin production.

Investigations:

Most people with an acute attack will be admitted to hospital due to the pain and shock. Perforated peptic ulcer is the other condition which may give rise to similar symptoms. Serum amylase is the usual method of diagnosis since this is raised in pancreatitis. It needs to be 5 times normal as a rise also occurs in gall bladder disease and perforated peptic ulcer. This, together with the history and examination, is usually enough to allow a diagnosis to be made.

If there is any doubt it may be necessary to perform a laparotomy to exclude surgically correctable problems such a perforated peptic ulcer.

Treatment:

This is mainly supportive with pain relief and fluid replacement. There is no specific treatment for this condition. There is a significant mortality rate in acute episodes ranging from 1% in mild cases to 50% in severe ones.

Chronic cases are advised to stop alcohol and may be given pancreatic enzyme supplements. A low fat diet is recommended.

CANCER OF THE PANCREAS

This is an unusual type of cancer but with increasing numbers seen in the West. It is the fourth commonest cause of cancer death in the UK and US. Men are affected more than women and most people are over 60 years of age. Various reasons have been cited for the increasing incidence including smoking, alcohol and coffee.

Symptoms:

The cancer may arise either in the head or the body and tail of the pancreas. The clinical picture varies slightly depending upon its site. Cancer of the head of the pancreas leads relatively early to obstruction of the common bile duct. Jaundice without pain is the typical first symptom. Later, there is usually the development of epigastric pain or discomfort with weight loss.

Cancer of the body or tail of the pancreas leads to epigastric pain, anorexia and weight loss. The pain is typically dull, constant and boring in nature which radiates through to the back. It is often better for sitting forward or lying face down.

On examination, a lump is felt in the epigastrium in about 20% of people.

---

[25] These are the classical signs of inflammation of the peritoneum - peritonitis. Such appearances are classed as a surgical emergency. The differential diagnosis of acute abdominal pain is discussed later in this Chapter.

Investigation:

The diagnosis is usually made by ultrasound or CAT scan. Needle biopsy confirms the nature of the disease.

Treatment:

Only 1% of people with cancer of the pancreas survive 5 years. This is because the pancreas is deep within the body and comes to notice relatively late. Some surgeons perform total pancreatectomy but the operation has a mortality rate of 20%. Jaundice can be relieved by inserting a plastic tube to bypass the obstruction. This is usually performed by endoscopy.

Alternative management:

The comments I made in Chapter 6 - Cancer are relevant here.

- PERITONITIS -

This is the reaction of the peritoneum to an irritant. There may be several underlying processes such as infection as part of appendicitis or acid as part of a perforated gastric ulcer. Appendicitis is the common cause and leads to the inflammatory reaction of the peritoneum.

Symptoms:

These are usually clear cut and unmistakable. There is the sudden onset of abdominal pain. This is typically severe in nature and is worse for movement. The person lies still. The abdominal muscles over the affected area are rigid in an attempt to protect the underlying inflamed tissues. The abdomen is still and motionless. There is tenderness to the touch and this is magnified when the examining hand is suddenly removed from the abdominal wall. This is called 'rebound tenderness'. There is associated shock with rapid pulse rate and a low blood pressure. If it is secondary to a condition such as appendicitis then the initial signs are of the preceding condition.

ACUTE APPENDICITIS

This is usually seen in young people. There has been a rapid increase since 1900 and is probably related to our diet and sedentary existence. It was unheard of in Africa when the first missionaries arrived there but as Western 'civilisation' arrived so did the development of appendicitis.

Symptoms:

The symptoms are slightly different to the classical appearance of peritonitis. The underlying process is more gradual than a perforated peptic ulcer. The pain of organ inflammation tends to be non-descript and central in location. The pain becomes more severe and localised once the inflammation spreads to the parietal peritoneum lining the abdominal cavity.

There is a short history of vague central abdominal pain which migrates to the right iliac fossa over several hours. It is eventually localised to McBurney's point[26]. There is also nausea, malaise and unpleasant breath. There may or may not be vomiting. The pulse is often raised and there may be a slight fever.

On examination, there is tenderness, rigidity and rebound tenderness in the right iliac fossa. Rigidity occurs later. This typical appearance occurs in about 50% of cases. In the

---

[26] This a point on the abdomen which overlies the usual anatomical site of the appendix. It is located one-third of the way along a line connecting the anterior superior iliac spine and the umbilicus.

remainder, it varies with the location of the appendix. The differential diagnosis of pain in the right iliac fossa is discussed in Chapter 18 - Gynaecology.

Treatment:

Conventionally, this is by surgery although acupuncture is definitely effective in the early stages. Another consideration is that a significant number of appendices taken out at operation are normal so the diagnosis was clearly incorrect.

Alternative management:

In terms of Chinese medicine, this corresponds to Intestinal Abscess. It is associated with one of three syndromes - Stagnation of Blood, Accumulation of DampHeat and Toxic Heat. It is considered to be caused by several factors including irregular eating and the intake of cold and raw foods. There are treatments available and in mild cases it would be reasonable to use them. Hospitalisation is necessary in cases where toxicity is marked with fever, rapid pulse rate, severe pain with guarding and rigidity.

- LOWER GASTROINTESTINAL DISEASE -

The disorders to be mentioned now are located in the small and large intestines. They lead primarily to disturbances of bowel habit.

INFLAMMATORY BOWEL DISEASE

This term is applied to disease of the bowel where inflammation is the characteristic feature. Two diseases are included in this categorisation - Crohn's disease (also known as regional ileitis) and ulcerative colitis. They are extremely common and seem to becoming more so. You will definitely see these cases in the clinic since the effectiveness of conventional medicine is variable. Despite conventional treatment, many people continue to have distressing and disturbing symptoms.

The inflammation is caused by an autoimmune process. There is evidence of antibodies attacking the intestine. Although the two diseases are considered separately and always described differently in conventional medical textbooks, they seem to be two examples of the same process. They merely affect slightly different areas of the intestine to a differing degree.

Ulcerative colitis is commoner in 20-40 year olds whilst Crohn's disease is seen in a slightly younger age group of late teens to early 20's. Crohn's disease primarily affects the last part of the small intestine (ileum) although it can involve any part of the gastrointestinal tract from the mouth to the anus. It affects the colon in 15-20% of the cases. Ulcerative colitis, as its name suggests, primarily affects the colon but particularly the rectum.

Symptoms:

The symptoms of ulcerative colitis are commonly diarrhoea, mucus, blood, tenesmus[27], together with systemic symptoms of ill health, anorexia, tiredness. The condition frequently remits and relapses with worsenings related to dietary indiscretions or emotional stress.

The symptoms of Crohn's disease are markedly similar. Abdominal pain is more frequent in the right iliac fossa whilst the systemic symptoms such as fever, anaemia and weight loss are more severe.

Symptoms of Crohn's Disease are certainly more severe and this reflects the greater degree and depth of inflammation. In ulcerative colitis it is merely the mucus membrane which is affected whereas with Crohn's disease all three layers of the bowel wall are involved in the

---

[27] This is the desire to defaecate with no or little faeces passed. It occurs in association with inflammation of the rectum (proctitis) as here, tumour of the rectum and irritable bowel syndrome.

inflammation. Fistulae are well-recognised complications of Crohn's disease. They allow the passage of faeces from inside the intestines to other areas. These include other areas of the intestine, the abdominal wall, perineum, vagina and bladder.

Investigations:

The diagnosis of inflammatory bowel disease is primarily made by the clinical history. However, there are typical appearances which may be seen on barium X-ray examinations. A barium meal and follow-through[28] will reveal typical appearances in the case of Crohn's Disease. A barium enema is performed in cases of ulcerative colitis where colonoscopy will reveal inflammation. Blood tests reveal evidence of anaemia. There may also be deficiency of iron and folic acid.

	CROHN'S DISEASE	ULCERATIVE COLITIS
Area mainly affected	Small intestine - terminal ileum	Large intestine - rectum
Tissue affected	All three layers of the bowel wall	Mucosa only
Age group	Late teens to early 20's	20-40 year olds
Diarrhoea	Yes	Yes
Mucus	Yes	Yes
Blood	Yes	Yes
Systemic symptoms	Yes - tend to be severe	Yes - tend to be mild
Fistulae	Yes	No
Diagnosis	Barium meal and follow through	Barium enema, colonoscopy

TABLE 13.12: COMPARISON OF ULCERATIVE COLITIS AND CROHN'S DISEASE

Complications:

COMPLICATIONS	SYMPTOMS TO LOOK FOR
Skin rashes	Dark discolouration over shins, nodular, tender (erythema nodosum)
Arthritis	11% of those with Crohn's disease and 14% with ulcerative colitis. Single joints affected with no long-term damage. Look for swelling, redness, heat and pain
Liver disease	Usually asymptomatic. Look for right hypochondriac pain, nausea, anorexia, jaundice
Iritis	Pain, discomfort in the light, circumcorneal redness, blurred vision
Deep venous thrombosis	Pain in calf of leg, swelling, tenderness
Stomatitis	Sore mouth, redness
Toxicity	Fever, weight loss, severe diarrhoea
Perforation	Rare. Symptoms of peritonitis. Severe pain, rigidity of abdominal muscles, rebound tenderness, fever, shock
Kidney stones	Only in Crohn's disease. Loin pain of a colicky nature, vomiting, frequent urination, blood in urine
Cancer	Obstructive symptoms of distension and colicky abdominal pain. There is change in bowel habit, bleeding

TABLE 13.13: COMPLICATIONS OF INFLAMMATORY BOWEL DISEASE

Treatment:

The conventional medical treatment of both conditions is similar. Antidiarrhoeal agents such as codeine and its derivatives may be used to control the symptoms of loose stools.

---

[28] This is a variation of the usual barium meal. Here, the passage of barium is 'followed through' to the small intestine and X-rays taken to visualise this area.

Corticosteroids are used in more severe disease. They are applied locally by enema to treat the rectum. Oral corticosteroids are given for more systemic involvement. If corticosteroids cannot control the symptoms, immunosuppressive agents are given, e.g. azathioprine. Surgery is occasionally performed in acute emergencies only. It is well known that the removal of an affected part of the bowel in Crohn's Disease leads to spread of the inflammatory process to uninvolved areas. In addition, the development of fistulae is common. Therefore surgery should be reserved for cases of Crohn's Disease with severe complications.

TREATMENT	TREATMENT LEVEL	COMMENTS
Antidiarrhoeal agents	1	Symptomatic treatment for diarrhoea. Examples used are codeine and its derivatives, loperamide, lomotil
Sulphasalazine	2	Combination of aspirin and sulphonamide antibiotics. Also used in rheumatoid arthritis
Corticosteroid - enema	3a	Local application of corticosteroid to bowel wall
Corticosteroid - oral	3b	Systemic use
Immunosuppressants	4	Powerful drugs also used in cancer chemotherapy, e.g. azathioprine
Surgery	5	In ulcerative colitis - total colectomy with ileostomy Crohn's disease - small bowel resection

TABLE 13.14: CONVENTIONAL TREATMENT OF INFLAMMATORY BOWEL DISEASE

Alternative management:

Inflammatory bowel disease, as described here, is relatively commonly seen in the clinic. This is because conventional treatment is of variable effectiveness and people continue to have symptoms for many years. There may be relapses and remissions dependent upon dietary habits and emotional states. People may seek help at the time of a relapse or when symptoms are somewhat calmer in an attempt to prevent a flare-up.

In terms of Chinese medicine, these conditions often correspond to DampHeat in the Large Intestine. Underlying Spleen and Kidney Yang Deficiency is common as is some degree of Liver Qi Stagnation. The Intestines are a common site of emotional stagnation and manifest symptoms at times of emotional stress. It is interesting that the connection of the Small Intestine with the Heart explains how anxiety may lead to bowel disturbances. The connection between the Lung and the Large Intestine explains how feelings such as grief and loss may lead to bowel disturbances. The clearest way to illustrate these observations of Chinese medicine is to describe some cases.

CASE

A woman of 30 years came for treatment with a 15 year history of ulcerative colitis. The course of her symptoms over that time was variable but had worsened over the recent months. It had flared up again with increased work-load and some stressful situations at home. She was currently taking 20 mg prednisolone (corticosteroid) daily. She had previously been on sulphasalazine but had to stop it because it damaged her blood.

When her symptoms were severe, she would have diarrhoea up to 20 times per day with urgency, blood, mucus and undigested food. At the time of her presentation it had settled to about twice daily with slight urgency. She would still have undigested food in the stools from time to time but no blood or mucus. She had increased in weight by over 20 pounds since starting the corticosteroids. They also had increased her appetite and made her feel somewhat hyperactive and manic.

The diagnosis in terms of Chinese medicine was Spleen and Kidney Yang Deficiency, Heart Blood Deficiency and Liver Qi Stagnation. Treatment was aimed at strengthening her energy so that at some point she would be able to reduce her corticosteroids. It is important in such cases to take things slowly and you would expect to treat such people for several years. The conventional rate of reduction of prednisolone is by 1 mg per month and this is without flareups of the original condition along the way. It may sometimes to be possible to reduce slightly quicker with the support of alternative medicine but to get someone off 20 mg is slow work.

After some months of treatment, she was able to reduce her prednisolone. This was done gradually but had to be increased to cope with a flare-up after a colonoscopy. However, this flare-up lasted a shorter time than normally and was controlled with a lower dose of prednisolone. She progressed very well until after 6 months she was down to 9 mg daily. Her stools were virtually normal. She had more energy and felt strong. Along the way, the hospital had suggested to her that she should stop her corticosteroids as they had terrible side-effects long-term and go on to azathioprine. An interesting suggestion in view of the fact that azathioprine is much more damaging to the immune system. It is an immunosuppressant and used in some cancer chemotherapy treatments.

Then she had a great flare-up of her symptoms which could not be controlled by my treatment. It did help to some extent but she had diarrhoea some eight times daily with blood and mucus. She decided to increase her prednisolone to 30 mg eventually to control the symptoms and after 6 weeks she was able to begin reduction once more. I discussed reduction of corticosteroid dosage in Chapter 10 - Musculoskeletal System. It is usually preferable to continue reduction or at least maintain the same dose rather than increase. However, there are some occasions when it is necessary to seek support from the drugs and we decided that this was one of those cases. This is particularly true when the symptoms are severe and involve bleeding. It should be seen as a short-term measure and part of a general process of improvement.

She had previously told me that her symptoms were always worse in the autumn but I had attached no especial importance to this. After some discussion of what was happening, it became clear that the cause of this episode was her son starting school. The sense of loss was marked. It is interesting that the Lung, in terms of Chinese medicine, is paired with the Large Intestine and affected by grief and loss. What was more important was that she came to recognise that there was a connection with her own past. Her family had broken up when she started school and this echo had led to her recent flare-up. The fact that this had now come to consciousness was clearly therapeutic and part of the general movement towards cure.

Her treatment continues and I am sure that she will continue to improve with time, support and continued strengthening of her energy.

CASE

A man of 42 years came for treatment with a 9 year history of Crohn's disease. He had several bowel operations in the past 7 years with removal of narrowed sections. His current symptoms were diarrhoea with urgency which would contain blood and mucus when severe. He had lost some 7 pounds in weight over the years. His energy levels were low and had continual feelings of tiredness. His digestive problems actually dated back 20 years to an acute episode of diarrhoea with haemorrhoids in the Far East. This is a common story in people with Crohn's disease that symptoms develop after gastroenteritis, dysentery or related problem. When his bowels were particularly troublesome he would develop pustular spots over his lower back. His current medication was:

- Azathioprine 250 mg three times daily
- Prednisolone 10 mg daily
- Codeine phosphate 30 mg three times daily

His medication revealed the underlying severity of his condition and it is important to wait for his condition to improve before any attempt is made to alter their dosage.

The Chinese medical diagnosis was Spleen and Kidney Yang Deficiency, Blood Deficiency and DampHeat Accumulation in the Intestines.

Treatment was directed at alleviating the underlying problem, namely the weakness of the Spleen and Kidney. He improved generally with herbs and acupuncture but it was not until after 6 months of treatment did we feel confident to begin reduction of the drugs. This has now begun slowly with the most powerful reduced first[29], i.e. azathioprine.

Improvement continues but it will be many months before his medication will be withdrawn completely. Along the way there may be psychological issues to address as emotional stagnation surfaces from the Intestines. Such people need support in dealing with these as well as perhaps specific counselling.

DIVERTICULAR DISEASE

This is a condition which occurs in the colon. It is considered to be due to a weakening of the wall of the colon, perhaps associated with raised intra-colonic pressure. Small pouches (diverticuli) appear in the colon. It occurs in mid to late age with women more commonly affected than men. Symptoms are only present if there is associated inflammation and then the term used is diverticulitis.

Symptoms:

As mentioned above, symptoms are only present if there is associated inflammation. There may be a history of constipation or other bowel disturbances in those with diets lacking in dietary fibre and rich in fat and refined carbohydrates.

Pain and tenderness are common particularly in the right iliac fossa. There is constipation and/or diarrhoea. Rectal bleeding can occur and although not common it may be severe.

An inflammatory mass may appear as the process continues. This may interfere with intestinal function to the extent that intestinal obstruction may develop. In such cases, it can be difficult tell the difference between diverticulitis and cancer of the colon. Even after biopsy there may still be doubt about the diagnosis.

Treatment:

This mainly consists of symptomatic and supportive measures which include bed rest and pain killers Antibiotics are invariably given for acute episodes. Surgery may be needed in cases of intestinal obstruction and this is resection of the affected area. There is a definite correlation between the incidence of this disease and the low level of dietary fibre in the western world.

IRRITABLE BOWEL SYNDROME

This is defined as 'abdominal pain with no organic cause'. It is also known as spastic colon. The cause is uncertain in conventional medicine but it is noted that anxiety is a common associated symptom. It is considered to be commoner in women in the 20-40 age group. It is a disturbance of the function of the large intestine.

Symptoms:

There is pain in the lower abdomen which may be focussed in the right or left iliac fossa. This is better for defaecation and worse for eating. Emotional upsets may also cause an exacerbation. Abdominal distension and flatulence are associated symptoms. The pain may vary from site to site and attacks tend to be episodic and may be severe.

There may be evidence of mucus in the stools. Alternating constipation and diarrhoea is common. The stools may have the appearance of rabbit droppings or be thin and ribbon-like. Cancer of the large intestine may also present with alternating constipation and diarrhoea but it is of recent onset and tends to be progressive. Here it is intermittent and frequently related to mood.

---

[29] Details of how to reduce combinations of drugs and in which order are given in, "Prescribed Drugs and the Alternative Practitioner" by S Gascoigne (Ashgrove Press, 1992).

Investigation:

The diagnosis of irritable bowel syndrome is primarily made from the clinical picture. However, occasional investigations may be performed to exclude obstructional disease. These will be colonoscopy and barium enema.

Investigations may also be done to exclude infection in the intestines. Occasionally, symptoms may appear after an acute bowel infection.

Treatment

This is of variable effectiveness in conventional medicine. There is no effective treatment which will relieve the symptoms on a long term basis so a symptomatic approach is taken. Antispasmodics such as mebeverine or anticholinergics such as dicyclomine are common prescriptions. Diarrhoea is treated symptomatically with codeine or one of its derivatives. Tranquillisers or antidepressants are common prescriptions, particularly in women.

Alternative management:

This condition reveals the close association between the emotions and the intestines. In Chinese medicine, this usually corresponds to Liver Qi Stagnation invading the Spleen.

CASE

A woman of 25 years came for treatment of her tiredness and digestive symptoms. She had a poor appetite, lower abdominal bloating and constipation alternating with diarrhoea. In conventional medicine, this would be a diagnosis of irritable bowel syndrome. In Chinese medicine, I made a diagnosis of Liver Qi Invading Spleen. She also complained of low backache which is a common symptom of lower intestinal disorders. I treated her by strengthening her Spleen energy and relaxing her Liver energy with advice about eating warming foods and relaxation. She worked night shifts and it is common in such cases to see Stagnation of Liver Qi. She responded well to treatment which is the usual case with this condition and had no symptoms after five treatments.

HAEMORRHOIDS

These are varicose veins in the wall of the rectum. They are subdivided, conventionally, according to the symptoms which they produce.

First degree haemorrhoids are located in the lower rectum and upper anal canal. They bleed but do not prolapse. Second degree haemorrhoids prolapse on defaecation then reduce spontaneously or manually by the person. The third degree type remain prolapsed outside the anus. Their cause is usually unknown according to conventional medicine but they are associated with conditions which lead to congestion of the pelvic venous circulation. So, compression by a pelvic tumour (the commonest example being pregnancy), cardiac failure or chronic constipation are considered to be responsible in many cases.

Symptoms:

Rectal bleeding is almost universal, is bright red and usually occurs at defaecation. This is the only symptom in mild cases but in more severe types there may be itching of the anal margin, a mucous discharge and occasionally pain. The pain occurs only when the veins thrombose. The symptoms are not usually, in themselves, serious but they can be unpleasant and you must bear in mind the possible causes of this condition.

Conventionally, local treatment is given unless the occurrence of bleeding or persistent prolapse necessitates surgical intervention.

I am reminded here of a woman I treated with rheumatoid arthritis. When, she first presented for treatment, most of her joints were swollen, stiff and painful. Treatment with acupuncture resulted in a marked improvement and after about six months she remarked, 'I have not felt this well for 20 years." She commented that she was having some problems with haemorrhoids and that she was due to go into hospital the next week for an operation. I discussed this with her, informed her of the concept of suppression and said that her haemorrhoids would, with time, improve also. She decided to have the surgery.

Within two weeks her joints flared-up to become hot, swollen and painful. Some four weeks later she developed a painful, swollen right leg which I thought clinically was a deep venous thrombosis. Investigations at the hospital proved negative but for some weeks I was greatly concerned about her health. This effect of suppressive treatment is common but not always so dramatic. In conventional thought it is seen as a coincidental event or perhaps as a 'complication' occurring after surgery, drugs and other treatment. It is important to inform people of the possible consequences of conventional treatment, not in an attempt to frighten them but as part of a general education about health and healing.

Treatment:

Any serious cause as delineated above is excluded first. Creams are often prescribed for the person by their general practitioner when first attending and if the problem is not very severe. They usually contain an anaesthetic and many contain a weak hydrocortisone.

Injection therapy is given for first and second degree cases. The veins are injected with a solution of phenol which is an irritant and the walls of the veins stick together. It is a similar treatment to that of varicose veins injection. The procedure is reputed to be painless and is usually done as an outpatient. It may be repeated two or three times.

The operation of haemorrhoidectomy is done for third degree cases. It is extremely painful after the operation especially when any attempt is made to defaecate.

Alternative management:

Haemorrhoids are an indication of a constitutional imbalance affecting the large intestine. They cannot be treated locally in a curative way. The case described above reveals the possible consequences of such suppressive treatment. In terms of Chinese medicine, the usual corresponding syndrome is DampHeat Accumulation in the Large Intestine. Implicit in this diagnosis is usually some degree of Spleen Qi Deficiency, Kidney Yang Deficiency and Liver Qi Stagnation. The exact pattern will vary according to the individual.

CASE

A woman of 34 years came for treatment of her infertility. She had been trying to become pregnant for over 3 years. Conventional investigations were all normal. She had few symptoms apart from general tiredness and lethargy. Before her period she would have some soreness of her breasts and the first day or so of her period was painful. She had loose stools every day but particularly in the mornings. She had glomerulonephritis as a child and two episodes of kidney stones in the past. I made a diagnosis of Kidney Yang Deficiency. This is a common energetic problem in women with infertility. I discussed the issue of treatment for her partner at the same time as it is useful to treat both.

I treated her by strengthening her Kidney Yang and after some months, she had more energy and felt better in herself. Her bowels became normal. It was after about four months of treatment that things began to change significantly. Long-suppressed emotions started to come to the surface and she began to think about the general direction of her life and particularly her career.

At the same time she started to develop pustular spots on her back and face with constipation. Haemorrhoids also developed which were uncomfortable and itchy. These symptoms of DampHeat in the Large Intestine were now obvious because her general energy had improved and the emphasis of the pathology had moved to the surface. An adjustment of treatment to relax her Liver Qi and alleviate the Dampness and Heat in the Large Intestine resulted in improvement of her physical symptoms but also more emotional freedom.

After ten months of treatment, she feels generally well, energetic and mainly symptom-free. Although she has not become pregnant, she is emotionally more balanced and calmer. There is a sense of non-attachment to pregnancy and this may allow conception to take place.

The question of 'results' can be an issue when attempting to determine if alternative medicine is 'successful'. Her presenting complaint is unchanged but many changes have taken place resulting in an improved quality of life. A planned career change is further evidence of her altered perception and is part of her movement towards health.

ANAL FISSURE

This is a split at the anal margin which is frequently related to constipation. There is pain on defaecation and perhaps local bleeding. It is of minor significance although can be very painful. The pain is due to associated muscle spasm in the anal sphincter.

Conventional treatment is to use local creams containing local anaesthetic and corticosteroid. If this is insufficient, an operation is performed to stretch the anal sphincter under general anaesthesia.

In terms of alternative medicine, this condition may be seen as related to haemorrhoids with Heat in the Large Intestine.

- CANCER OF THE GASTROINTESTINAL SYSTEM -

Cancers of the oesophagus, stomach, caecum, colon, and rectum can be described in general terms because of their symptoms. As the gastrointestinal system is a hollow tube, the symptoms appear because of obstruction. The main symptoms are constipation, abdominal distension, colicky abdominal pain and vomiting. The emphasis of symptoms depends on the site of the cancer. Bleeding may also be seen.

In the oesophagus the first symptom is usually dysphagia - a sensation of a swallowed item becoming stuck. In the lower third of the oesophagus this is a fairly reliable indicator of where cancer is situated. Eventually there will be vomiting as the obstruction develops and an inability to take anything orally other than fluids.

In the stomach, there may have been a pre-existing ulcer and so there may be confusion between the symptoms of the ulcer and those of the cancer. Again, vomiting of blood is a major indication along with a lump on examination of the upper abdomen. There will be upper abdominal distension. Constipation develops late.

Cancers of the large bowel vary in their symptomatology according to their site. So, obstruction of the caecum will show up late in change in bowel habit because the faeces is liquid there whereas in the rectum constipation is an early sign. Distension of the abdomen is greatest the further down the bowel the cancer exists and vomiting is late in lower bowel cancer and relatively early in caecal conditions.

In the case of rectal cancer there is the added symptom of the desire to defaecate but no stools produced because of the growing mass in the rectum. This is known as tenesmus. Bleeding occurs with all the cancers but will be more obvious in the case of lower bowel cancer because it is more easily seen. It will be red in colour and probably on the surface of the stool whereas when it comes from higher up, the colour will be darker and will be mixed up with the faeces. In addition, there may be a mass in the abdomen on examination. This will be hard, fixed and probably irregular in outline, typical of a malignant lump.

The key symptoms to remember for cancer of the large intestine are change in bowel habit of recent onset with rectal bleeding.

OESOPHAGEAL CANCER

This is not a common condition and usually is seen in the 60-70 year age group. It is slightly commoner in men than women. Half of cases develop in the middle third of the oesophagus and one quarter in the lower third. In the UK there are 5-10 cases per 100,000 of the population which account for 2.5% of all cancers. There is a particularly high incidence in China and some areas of Africa and Iran.

Symptoms:

The tumour ulcerates and bleeds and can extend either up or down to cause narrowing and thus difficulty in swallowing. Progressive dysphagia is the cardinal presenting symptom starting with solids and then softer foods and finally liquids. Anyone who has these symptoms over a period of several months should be suspected of this diagnosis until proved otherwise. There is often discomfort in the chest, usually well-localised where the tumour is present. The condition worsens over several months and weight loss is common. At diagnosis, half of people have evidence of spread to local lymph nodes. Weight loss and anorexia are invariable symptoms.

It is possible to develop dysphagia as a complication of simple reflux oesophagitis. In this case, it is not progressive and there is a past history of the typical heartburn.

Investigation:

Barium swallow will show the narrowing of the oesophagus but oesophagoscopy and biopsy offer the definitive diagnosis.

Treatment:

Usually, by the time of diagnosis, there is direct invasion of surrounding structures or lymph node involvement so that surgery is impossible. Cure, in conventional terms of a 5 year survival rate, is seen in only 2% of cases. Some people have treatment by means of radiotherapy and chemotherapy which are only seen as being palliative. Operation by means of oesophagogastrectomy is only possible in a small proportion. Surgery has a high mortality and morbidity. Dilation of the obstructing cancer and the insertion of an indwelling tube may give short-term symptomatic relief.

CANCER OF THE STOMACH

This is a relatively common cancer and is the third commonest cause of cancer deaths in the UK. It is relatively low in incidence in the USA yet high in Japan. Men are more frequently affected than women. Cancer of the stomach is more likely to occur in those with low gastric acid levels. Cancer of the stomach spreads to liver, bone, brain and lung.

Symptoms:

Epigastric pain is common and is identical to that of peptic ulcer. The diagnosis of cancer is suggested by constant pain and the appearance of other symptoms. The pain may be severe. Associated symptoms include vomiting, anorexia, dysphagia (when cancer is near the entry of the oesophagus) and vomiting of blood.

Some people present with evidence of malignant spread to the liver or abdominal cavity. Such symptoms will include abdominal swelling, jaundice.

About half of people will have a lump in the epigastrium with tenderness. Weight loss is common. An enlarged lymph node may be found in the supraclavicular fossa.

Investigations:

Barium meal will reveal up to 90% of cases. Gastroscopy with biopsy is used to confirm the diagnosis. In cases to be considered for surgery, ultrasound and CAT scans are performed to detect secondary spread.

Treatment:

Surgery is associated with a 5 year survival rate of 10% which has remained the same for the past 25 years or so. 65% of cases are inoperable at the time of diagnosis. Chemotherapy is merely associated with a poor quality of life.

CANCER OF THE LARGE INTESTINE

This is the second commonest cancer in the UK yet is rare in Africa and Asia. There are increased rates of this cancer when diets are high in meat and fat but low in fibre. Ulcerative colitis may predispose to the development of large intestine cancer.

Symptoms:

The precise clinical picture depends upon the site of the cancer. In the left side there may be change in bowel habit such as constipation, alternating constipation and diarrhoea or just diarrhoea. Blood may be seen mixed in with the faeces.
Cancer of the caecum or ascending colon may merely present as an anaemia of unknown origin as the stools are liquid and obstruction occurs late.
A palpable lump may be found in some. If spread has occurred to the liver this organ may be enlarged.

Investigations:

Full blood count is performed. Diagnosis is made by barium enema with confirmation by colonoscopy and biopsy. Abdominal and rectal ultrasound are performed prior to surgery.

Treatment:

This is primarily surgical with removal of the affected part of bowel and joining of the cut ends. The overall 5 year survival rate is 50% depending upon the stage at the time of diagnosis.

CANCER OF THE LIVER

Here, I shall discuss secondary cancer of the liver which has spread from other sites. This the commonest liver cancer and is frequently the result of cancer of the gastrointestinal tract, breast and lung.

Symptoms:

These are variable and there may be none in the early stages. Liver enlargement is seen later with perhaps jaundice and discomfort in the right hypochondrium.

Investigations:

Diagnosis is made by means of CAT scan, magnetic resonance scan or ultrasound.

Treatment:

This is frequently by means of chemotherapy but with poor results. The usual result is a greatly diminished quality of life.

- DISEASES OF THE LIVER -

The liver is a large organ situated under the diaphragm in the right hypochondrium, extending partly into the epigastrium. It weighs about 3 lbs. in the average adult. The liver performs many functions, most of which are metabolic in nature. The liver has an important role in the metabolism of carbohydrate, fat and protein. It also deals with the removal of drugs and hormones by means of a detoxification mechanism. Various drugs are excreted into bile and thereby removed from the body. Substances dealt with in this way include antibiotics, e.g. penicillin, amoxycillin, erythromycin and sulphonamides, steroid hormones and thyroxine.

The liver is important for the excretion of bile salts, storage of glycogen, vitamins A, B, D, E and K and minerals - particularly iron and copper. It has a function in removing red and white blood cells from the circulation and some bacteria. It can be seen from this list that the liver, physiologically, is a very important organ. It receives substances absorbed from the stomach and intestines since it receives blood draining from the gastrointestinal system. It is, therefore, the first organ which is exposed to potential toxins.

JAUNDICE

This is a yellowish discolouration seen in the skin, mucous membranes and conjunctivae. In conventional medicine, it indicates that the amount of bilirubin in the blood is more than 30-60 mmol/l. Bilirubin is one of the breakdown products of haemoglobin and is excreted in bile. The others, iron and globin, are recycled.

Levels of bilirubin in the blood may rise as a result of three mechanisms:

- increased breakdown of red blood cells leading to increased amounts of bilirubin - pre-hepatic jaundice
- liver disease leading to inadequate handling of the bilirubin already there - hepatic jaundice
- obstruction to excretion of bile leading to a backup of bile and thence bilirubin in the body - post-hepatic jaundice

The distinction between hepatic and post-hepatic causes is not always a valid one since both factors may be in operation at the same time. However, the causation and treatment are different in each case.

PRE-HEPATIC JAUNDICE

An example of increased red blood cell destruction is haemolytic anaemia. There will be jaundice together with the symptoms of anaemia. The discolouration is typically pale yellow with normal urine and stools.

An unusual type is a congenital disorder of bilirubin metabolism. This is Gilbert's syndrome which affects up to 5% of the population. It is usually without symptoms but may be discovered on routine blood testing as a raised bilirubin level. There are no signs of liver disease but there may be a family history of jaundice.

Related disorders include Crigler-Najjar, Dubin-Johnson and Rotor syndromes. These are all rare.

HEPATIC JAUNDICE

This is the appearance of jaundice due to disturbances in liver function. It may be due to acute liver disease as in hepatitis or in more chronic conditions such as cirrhosis. These are described below.

POST-HEPATIC JAUNDICE

This is the appearance of jaundice due to an obstruction to bile flow. It may be called obstructive jaundice. Gall stones and cancer of the head of the pancreas are the two conditions to consider here.

HEPATITIS

This means, literally, inflammation of the liver. It commonly means a type which is associated with an infecting organism although strictly speaking it includes cirrhosis and other inflammatory liver disease. Viral hepatitis can be of type A, B or C. They have some differences and similarities but it is probably easier to describe them separately and then summarise their relative features at the end.

TYPE A

This is also known as 'infectious hepatitis'. It develops due to the contamination of food or water by faeces. It may also be spread by blood or body fluid contact . Various factors such as overcrowding and poor sanitation lead to greater risks as in underdeveloped countries and institutions. The incubation period is one month

Symptoms:

These are chills and fever, malaise, and anorexia. There are gastrointestinal symptoms such as nausea, diarrhoea, vomiting and upper abdominal pain. Jaundice develops with dark urine, yellow sclerae, and pale stools. The appetite gradually recovers and the nausea settles. People gradually improve in 3 to 6 weeks. Virtually everyone makes a full recovery. It is common to suffer debility for some 2 to 3 months after the infection.

Investigations:

These are performed similarly in all types of hepatitis. Liver function tests show evidence of liver impairment and there is bilirubin in the urine.

Treatment:

There is no specific treatment. The improvement of social hygiene helps to prevent attacks. Passive vaccination with human gammaglobulin is said to give 3 months protection.

TYPE B

This is known as 'serum hepatitis'. It is spread by the same methods as Type A but blood and body fluid transmission are much more common. The incubation period is 3 months.

Symptoms:

These are similar to those of Type A hepatitis except they are more severe. One in twenty people go on to develop chronic hepatitis. There are asymptomatic carriers of the disease which raises questions of public health regarding donation of blood and sexual relationships similar to those we see in the AIDS and HIV debate.

Treatment:

There is no specific treatment currently available. A trial of an antiviral drug, fialuridine, was stopped in 1993 after two people died and a third required a liver transplant. Three further people may require liver transplants in the near future. There were 20 people on the trial.

It is important to take precautions of screening transfusion blood against contamination. Human gammaglobulin is given on exposure but it is in short supply and expensive. Bed rest and an adequate diet are the most important measures taken. Corticosteroids are given if the vomiting is severe. No alcohol should be taken for 6 months after the infection and oral contraceptives are considered to be safe when the liver function tests are normal.

There are two vaccines available which are given to hospital staff as well as to travellers in areas of high risk, e.g. India. They are not compulsory for travel.

TYPE C

This is a relatively recently recognised type of hepatitis. It produces symptoms which are less severe than in cases of Type A and B. There may be the development of arthritis, agranulocytosis, aplastic anaemia and neurological disorders. Half of people with this condition go on to develop chronic inflammation in the liver. Some 20% of these develop cirrhosis.

CHRONIC HEPATITIS

This is defined as the continuation of hepatitis for longer than 6 months. There seems to be an autoimmune reaction in such people. Prognosis is poor in most with progression to cirrhosis. There are some who seem to pursue a more benign course with minimal changes in liver function and mild liver enlargement.

Alternative management:

In terms of Chinese medicine, hepatitis usually corresponds to an Invasion of Dampness and Heat creating disharmony between the Spleen and Liver. The particular emphasis depends upon the precise symptoms. Treatment by alternative medicine is definitely effective for such conditions and hepatitis is one of the diseases curable by Chinese medicine as defined by the World Health Organisation.

Treatment before travel to countries where the diseases are endemic is helpful and the avoidance of vaccination measures. It is common experience that vaccination may lead to an increased likelihood of developing symptoms not to mention the fearsome long-term consequences of such measures. The development of hepatitis in Westerners when they travel to the East, for example, is a reflection of their chronic constitutional state. Treatment after the initial attack is also helpful as it will minimise the risk of chronic liver disease.

CIRRHOSIS

This is chronic liver disease where there is death of liver cells associated with regeneration and fibrosis. There is obstruction to hepatic blood flow which leads to the typical features. The commonest causes are alcohol ingestion and post-hepatitis B infection.

Symptoms:

These are many and varied. There is enlargement of the liver at first with eventual shrinkage as scarring develops. An enlarged spleen is common. Spider naevi are found on the skin of the upper body. They are small, distended blood vessels of reddish appearance with small vessels radiating out from them. The palms of the hand become reddened. Finger clubbing is seen occasionally. Thickening of the tissues of the palm of the hand are typically seen in cirrhosis of alcoholic origin. Hormonal abnormalities lead to breast enlargement and testicular atrophy in men. There may be loss of libido and amenorrhoea.

Oedema is common and seen in the ankles. Fluid collection in the abdomen (ascites) leads to abdominal distension. There may be vomiting of blood and melaena. Itching is common.

Mental symptoms include drowsiness and confusion.

Investigations:

Liver function tests on the blood reveal raised serum alkaline phosphatase and serum aminotransferase. In severe cases, many blood tests are abnormal. Liver biopsy is frequently performed to determine the exact nature of the abnormality. Other investigations include ultrasound scan, barium meal and gastroscopy.

Treatment:

This is primarily supportive to prevent further damage to the liver. In milder cases, there may be no advice given about diet or abstinence from alcohol (unless alcoholic cirrhosis).

- REVIEW OF SYMPTOMS -

Some are of great importance both in terms of their effect on the person and their values to us to help reach a diagnosis.

PAIN

This is most important and with careful questioning a lot of information can be obtained. Subsequent examination will, in most cases serve to confirm the information gathered during the history. There are questions to ask in every case of pain and a structured approach ensures that nothing is missed. This was discussed in Chapter 7 - Cardiovascular System in relation to chest pain and at the beginning of this Chapter in relation to abdominal pain.

HEARTBURN

This is a burning pain felt in the centre of the chest behind the sternum. It may start in the epigastrium and radiate up towards the throat. Any pain in the chest should be differentiated from the pain of a heart attack.

LOSS OF APPETITE

This is known as anorexia and conventionally it is seen as occurring due to:

- psychological disorders such as depression, anorexia nervosa[30]
- stomach disease such as gastritis.
- general disease such as acute fevers or severe chronic disease as cancer

INCREASED APPETITE

This may occur with disorders of the upper gastrointestinal system depending upon the precise energetic diagnosis. In conventional medicine, the conditions to consider are diabetes mellitus, hyperthyroidism and bulimia nervosa. The first two are characterised by increased appetite with weight loss, an unusual combination. Bulimia nervosa, as with its related condition anorexia nervosa, is accompanied by disturbed perception of body image.

WATERBRASH

This is sudden filling of the mouth with saliva or tasteless watery secretions. It is seen in association with upper gastrointestinal tract disease such as a duodenal ulcer.

TASTE IN THE MOUTH

In homoeopathy and Chinese medicine, this is an important indicator of an internal organ problem. Its connection with organs in terms of Chinese medicine is shown in Table 13.15.

TASTE	ELEMENT	ORGANS
Sweet	Earth	Spleen/Stomach
Spicy (pungent)	Metal	Lung/Large Intestine
Sour	Wood	Liver/Gall Bladder
Salty	Water	Kidney/Urinary Bladder
Bitter	Fire	Heart/Small Intestine

TABLE 13.15: TASTES AND THEIR CORRESPONDING ORGANS[31]

In conventional medicine, cases of 'halitosis' or bad breath are seen as due to gum disease, dental decay or infected lung lesions such as lung abscess. In the absence of these most people who complain of bad breath, unpleasant taste in the mouth or other tastes such as metallic are labelled as being imaginative or frankly neurotic.

---

[30] The term 'anorexia' is sometimes used as shorthand for the disease anorexia nervosa which is characterised by disturbed perception of body image.
[31] The organs listed indicate their energetic nature as described in their relevant Chapters and not the narrow physical sense of conventional medicine.

VOMITING

This is a common symptom and is a more extreme form of nausea. In conventional medicine, it is seen as occurring in a wide range of differing conditions not always linked to gastrointestinal tract disease. Causes include:

- upper gastrointestinal disease
- appendicitis
- meningitis
- infections, e.g. pyelonephritis
- migraine
- pregnancy
- travel sickness
- heart attack
- drugs - prescribed and social

The appearance of material which looks like 'coffee-grounds' is characteristic of bleeding in the upper gastrointestinal tract. The blood has been altered by gastric acid and so takes on a brownish or black appearance. Iron medication can give a similar appearance. In children, vomiting may be the first indication of an infection. All children with fever and vomiting must be checked for otitis media, urinary tract infection and chest infection.

Vomiting with no preceding nausea occurs in brain tumour and is due to direct stimulation of the vomiting centre in the brain. Vomit with large amounts of food or containing food eaten a day or so ago indicates pyloric obstruction. Epigastric pain relieved by vomiting is characteristic of a peptic ulcer.

REGURGITATION

This is the appearance of recently swallowed food in the mouth but not vomiting. It usually occurs after meals but some people can perform it at will. It can have a bitter taste (bile) or acid (gastric juice). It is not common in adults but babies can have frequent episodes.

DYSPHAGIA

This means difficulty in swallowing but is also used to mean the discomfort felt when food becomes lodged in the oesophagus. It should be differentiated from globus hystericus which is a sensation of a lump felt in the midline above the suprasternal notch. This is associated with emotional symptoms and in Chinese medicine corresponds to the plum-stone throat in Stagnation of Liver Qi. It is not of structural significance although people are often concerned as to whether they have a malignant condition. Lumps felt to the side of the throat are of much more serious significance and may indicate carcinoma.

Dysphagia is seen in cancer of the oesophagus where there will be a progressive history over several months. First solid food sticks then softer food and in later, advanced cases, swallowing any liquid including saliva is impossible. The site of the sensation is an accurate representation, in the lower third of the oesophagus, of the actual site of the problem. Elsewhere the approximation is less exact. Dysphagia can also occur due to scarring of the oesophagus in cases of oesophagitis. This is not progressive as with cancer and there will usually be a history of heartburn.

FLATULENCE AND BELCHING

Symptoms of 'wind' or abdominal distension are pretty much disregarded by conventional medicine. They are considered to be due to air swallowing in anxious individuals or excessive intake of gas-forming substances, e.g. sodium bicarbonate, beans. For the purposes of easy learning, abdominal distension is seen as being due to:

- fat
- fluid
- faeces
- flatus
- foetus

Other than these, little attention is paid. However, distension of the abdomen is very common particularly in women and is very much related to the function of the Liver, Spleen and Kidney. When I was in general practice I saw many women with this problem. They would wake up in the morning with a flat abdomen and by the evening looked as if they were more than 4, 5 or even 6 months pregnant. Conventionally this is puzzling and is seen as either a neurosis or an imaginative exaggeration.

CASE

A woman of 25 years came for treatment with symptoms of abdominal distension after eating. She would develop pains in the hypochondria, flatulence and belching. Her bowels were often constipated. She had difficulty sleeping until about 1.30 am. The only medication she took was the oral contraceptive.

In terms of Chinese medicine, this is a classical case of Liver Qi Stagnation invading the Stomach and Spleen. The major contributing factor is the oral contraceptive which stagnates Liver Qi. Treatment was aimed at relaxing the flow of Liver Qi and we discussed the role of the oral contraceptive as this causes Liver Qi Stagnation.

In terms of conventional medicine, this would probably be labelled as irritable bowel syndrome. There is no understanding in conventional thought that the oral contraceptive can cause such symptoms.

CONSTIPATION AND DIARRHOEA

The conventional texts state that 10% of people have less than one bowel movement per day and 1% have less than three per week. Constipation is usually defined in terms of the frequency of bowel action as above but what is also important is the consistency of the stool. Faeces which are dry, hard or difficult to pass are an indication of constipation. Another thing to consider is the length of time it takes for material to pass through the gastrointestinal tract. Normal is around 18 hours but for most people in the West it is a lot longer than this. Although we may pass faeces every day it may be from food taken in several days ago or longer. This is related, undoubtedly, to the higher incidence of gastrointestinal tract cancer in the West.

Diarrhoea is the passage of unformed stools several times each day. The term 'loose stools' may be reserved for the passage of unformed stools only once or twice per day. Always ask about the presence of blood and mucus in people with such symptoms.

WEIGHT LOSS

This may not be a symptom to be considered in diagnosis if it is the result of a deliberate attempt to reduce weight by means of a regime of diet and/or exercise. As a symptom to be considered in the diagnosis, it will be part of a wider problem.

Anorexia or nausea and/or vomiting will lead to weight loss simply because there is a reduced intake of food. Malabsorption of nutrients as in small bowel disease, e.g. Crohn's disease or coeliac disease has the same effect. Ulcerative colitis, if severe, may lead to weight loss due to protein loss from the bowel.

Many cancers lead to loss of weight but by no means all and wasting is particularly a feature of lung and intra-abdominal malignancy.

WEIGHT GAIN

This may be a presenting symptom but is more usually part of the total case to be considered. In conventional thought it is usually seen as due to excess food intake. This is not the whole story as many people, particularly women, may be overweight and yet not overeat. The reason for this is related to the discussion at the beginning of this Chapter dealing with energetic concepts of the digestive system. If the digestive energy is depleted, any food taken may lead to increases in weight. This is more likely to occur in those who have had many years of cyclical diets, weight loss and excessive exercise. All of these practices lead to a depletion in digestive energy and the inability to transform food. Weakness and tiredness are common as well as the collection of fluid. The case I describe below is an illustration.

CASE

A woman of 41 years came for treatment complaining of being overweight for many years. She had tried many different types of diet culminating in a stomach-stapling operation the year before. Her food intake was not particularly excessive. The only time she would lose weight would be with amphetamines or a drastic reduction in calorie intake to around 800 per day. This is a common situation with women where low calorie diets are necessary thereby inducing a state of malnutrition. The recurrent cycle of dieting leads to further weakening of digestive energy and therefore greater difficulty in maintaining normal weight. The only way out of this is to increase metabolic rate. The healthy method is by means of alternative medicine which seek to correct the underlying energetic problem. Artificial methods of boosting metabolism include thyroid hormone, amphetamines and appetite suppressants[32].

Her other symptoms included low back pain, water retention and a desire for sweet food worse before the menses. In terms of Chinese medicine, her diagnosis was Spleen and Kidney Yang Deficiency. The main aim of treatment is to strengthen her Spleen and Kidney energy so that, eventually, her own energy will be able to control fluids. Her weight will then come under control. This process is slow and requires long-term treatment. Additionally, body weight, size and shape are very much the result of our innermost mental images of ourselves. Some degree of emotional and mental symptoms may arise during the course of treatment. Counselling, psychotherapy or other psychological approaches are invaluable additional methods of helping such people.

---

[32] The prescription of appetite suppressants is a potentially dangerous practice. They are stimulant in nature and rapidly lead to addiction. There are well described withdrawal syndromes. Some 400,000 people are prescribed such drugs in the UK. It costs the NHS about £1m per year. Drugs used include amphetamines, fenfluramine and dexfenfluramine.

BLEEDING FROM THE GASTROINTESTINAL TRACT

This is not a common symptom but it is important to know that some causes are of serious significance. It can manifest in several ways according to the organ involved. From the upper gastrointestinal tract blood will be seen in vomit. Coffee-grounds appearance is indicative of a small amount of blood loss from the stomach where the blood has become blackened by the action of stomach acid. Fresh red blood is seen when the loss of blood is greater and can occur with peptic ulceration or occasionally cancer. One third of people with gastrointestinal bleeding have taken aspirin in the past 24-48 hours. All the non-steroidal anti-inflammatory drugs are associated with bleeding even when taken as suppositories.

CAUSE	NUMBER PER 100 CASES
Duodenal ulcer	35
Gastric ulcer	20
Acute gastric erosion, gastritis	18
Oesophageal tear	10
Gastric cancer	6
Oesophageal varices - seen in cirrhosis	5
Others	6

TABLE 13.16: BLEEDING FROM THE UPPER GASTROINTESTINAL TRACT

Bleeding from the lower part of the gastrointestinal tract can manifest as fresh red blood if from the lower parts and as brownish or blackish if from higher up the bowel. Blood on the surface of the faeces indicates a rectal or anal problem, e.g. haemorrhoids, rectal cancer or rectal polyps. Blood mixed up with the faeces indicates a problem further up the bowel.

- HOW TO RECOGNISE A SERIOUS CONDITION OF THE GASTROINTESTINAL SYSTEM -

SYMPTOMS	WHEN TO WORRY
Nausea	Severe
Vomiting	Severe, persistent, progressive, in the very young or old, with blood, with food eaten days before, projectile
Anorexia	Severe, progressive, with mental symptoms of distorted body image
Increased appetite	With weight loss, with mental symptoms of distorted body image
Bloating	Progressive
Belching	Not serious
Flatulence	Not serious
Diarrhoea	Severe, persistent, progressive, in the very young or old, with blood, with mucus, alternates with constipation
Constipation	Severe, progressive, with blood, alternates with diarrhoea
Abdominal pain	Severe, with abdominal rigidity, with guarding, with rebound tenderness
Weight loss	Progressive, unexplained
Jaundice	Always unless mild in new-born

TABLE 13.17: HOW TO RECOGNISE A SERIOUS CONDITION OF THE GASTROINTESTINAL SYSTEM

Diseases of the gastrointestinal system are common in our society and the symptoms listed above are extremely common. It is important to know how to recognise if a symptom arises from a serious situation. You can use Table 13.17 as a guide to refer to when faced with a person who has one or more of these symptoms. I do not mention disease labels in the column on the right as I would not expect you to be able to diagnose conventionally. Seriousness can be assessed merely by reference to symptom pictures. However, you will be able to recognise that there are clinical appearances which would be diagnosed as a particular disease. For example, if you look at diarrhoea and its seriousness, you will see that this is the appearance of diseases such as severe gastroenteritis, ulcerative colitis or Crohn's disease and cancer.

- SUMMARY -

Gastrointestinal disorders are common reflecting dietary habits and emotional states.

They tend to be superficial in terms of energetic hierarchies and so relatively easy to treat.

More severe disease produces symptoms which are more serious in nature (see Table 13.17) or suggestive of obstruction.

14 CENTRAL NERVOUS SYSTEM

OBJECTIVES:
At the end of this Chapter you will be able to:
Describe the differences between the alternative and conventional views of the central nervous system.
List the symptoms attributable to disturbances of the central nervous system.
State when a symptom(s) would indicate a serious underlying condition.
Describe the main symptoms of diseases covered in this Chapter.
Explain the relevant management by an alternative practitioner of each disorder.

- INTRODUCTION -

The central nervous system is a difficult system to get to grips with because of its complex anatomy. It may also be taught in minute detail or unclearly. Many students leave with the idea that it is totally incomprehensible and that they will never go near it again. I know from my own training that it took about three or so years of medical school before some of it started to sink in and mean anything at all.

I introduce this system with a short, yet hopefully, clear description of the structure and function of the central nervous system. This may not be necessary for some of you who have grasped the essential facts but it will ensure a basic level of knowledge can be assumed. I have simplified the amount of information to that which is essential to understand terms I use later.

I have divided the system into several easily manageable portions although, obviously, they actually function as a complete whole. However, this should make it more accessible. I have also resisted using many long, difficult and irrelevant names which abound in this area of the body.

- OVERVIEW OF CENTRAL NERVOUS SYSTEM -

MOTOR SYSTEM

This is the area which deals with movement. Nerves of the motor system supply various muscles which are activated to contract. Such muscle contraction may be under voluntary control as in the case of arm or leg movements or involuntary in the case of heart muscles. The pyramidal system is another term which is applied to the motor system as it passes through the lower part of the brain. As an analogy, the motor system can be likened to the engine which moves a car. It is merely responsible for movement.

The distinction between voluntary and involuntary control is not absolute. Even so-called involuntary muscular movements are under some degree of voluntary control as we can alter our breathing within certain limits. The interest in Oriental philosophies and religions has revealed the ability to control these[1]. Involuntary muscle movements are influenced by the autonomic nervous system.

The movement of muscles is a balanced contraction and relaxation of different muscle groups. A voluntary action seemingly as simple as drinking a cup of tea involves a complex series of co-ordinated actions. As some muscles contract to move a joint in a certain direction, another muscle group has to relax. Yet another set of muscles will fix the joint around which the movement takes place. This co-ordination function is carried out by other parts of the nervous system.

There are two groups of nerve cells (neurones) which comprise the motor system. They are grouped into upper motor neurones and lower motor neurones.

The upper motor neurone consists of cells in the motor area of the cortex of the brain. Nerve fibres from these pass down into the spinal cord to connect with nerve cells. They cross over to the other side as they do so. The exact level at which this occurs is not particularly important for our purposes. Therefore, upper motor neurones in a particular area of the motor cortex control muscle movements on the opposite side of the body.

The lower motor neurone is the nerve cell in the spinal cord from which nerve fibres leave to supply particular muscle groups of that region. At the same time, sensory nerves from the muscles pass back to the spinal cord to interconnect with the lower motor neurone. This interconnection is known as a reflex arc and is continually in operation to maintain tone in the muscle. It monitors the degree of tension or relaxation in a muscle and ensures a certain degree of tone is maintained by this feedback mechanism.

The reflex arc is also the mechanism which results in tendon reflexes. These are contraction of muscles when the tendon of that muscle is tapped. The knee jerk (reflex) is commonly known but other muscles have these. If a tendon, e.g. the patellar ligament is struck there is reflex contraction of the relevant muscle, in this case the quadriceps. Thus, there is extension of the knee joint. There are also tendon reflexes at the ankle, the biceps, triceps and the supinator muscles.

---

[1] "Rainbow of Liberated Energy" by Ngakpa Chögyam (Element, 1986) contains, in the Introduction, an account of the effect of meditative practices on the EEG.

Clearly, a disorder of the lower motor neurone will lead to different symptoms from the upper motor neurone. This is mainly because of the presence of the reflex arc. The exact clinical picture will depend upon whether the lower motor neurone is partially or completely non-functional. If there is no nerve supply to a muscle the result is no movement (paralysis), absent tendon reflexes at that level and little tone in the muscle (flaccidity). Partial interruption to the nerve supply leads to weakness (paresis), reduced tendon reflexes at that level and reduced muscle tone.

If the upper motor neurone is the site of the problem then the reflex arc is still operating. A feature of the reflex arc is that it is very powerful. The normal influence of the upper motor neurone is one of sedation. The reflex arc becomes stronger when this influence is removed[2] . This is evidenced by paralysis (as the upper motor neurone is not functioning), increased tone (spasticity) and increased tendon reflexes. Wasting is minimal as the tone maintained by the reflex arc prevents this. These differences are summarised in Table 14.1

UPPER MOTOR NEURONE	LOWER MOTOR NEURONE
Weakness or paralysis	Weakness paralysis
Increased tone: spasticity	Decreased tone: flaccidity
Increased tendon reflexes	Reduced or absent reflexes in area affected
Plantar reflex - upgoing	Plantar reflex - unchanged
No muscle atrophy	Wasting of muscles
Contractures	No contractures

TABLE 14.1: COMPARISON OF APPEARANCES OF UPPER AND LOWER MOTOR NEURONE DISORDERS

The clinical appearances listed in Table 14.1 will allow you to recognise some disorders of the motor system. These can be seen in Table 14.2

UPPER MOTOR NEURONE DISORDERS	LOWER MOTOR NEURONE DISORDERS
Stroke	Polio
Brain tumour	Motor neurone disease
Motor neurone disease	Multiple sclerosis
Multiple sclerosis	Cervical and lumbar disc disease
	Peripheral nerve compression

TABLE 14.2: EXAMPLES OF UPPER AND MOTOR NEURONE DISORDERS

Table 14.3 is a summary of symptoms which may be caused by disturbances in the motor system.

Paralysis
Weakness (paresis)
Wasting
Increased muscle tone (spasticity)
Decreased muscle tone (flaccidity)
Exaggerated tendon reflexes
Reduced tendon reflexes
Absent tendon reflexes
Upgoing plantar reflex

TABLE 14.3: SUMMARY OF SYMPTOMS DUE TO DISTURBANCE IN THE MOTOR SYSTEM

---

2 Evidence of this can be seen when the influence of higher centres is removed. I am thinking of several examples here. Firstly, people who are insane or emotionally charged are very strong and may require several others to control them. Secondly, experts in various forms of martial arts can be solidly planted on the ground to the extent that several people cannot knock them over. Lastly, there are cases of mothers who have seen their children run over by cars. They have been able to lift vehicles off their children. This power at the spinal level is rarely contacted but is definitely available.

EXTRAPYRAMIDAL SYSTEM

This is the part of the nervous system which modifies voluntary motor activity. There are several parts of the brain which do this including the basal ganglia. Disorders in this area lead to disturbance in voluntary movement control. There is a classical triad of symptoms which develop. There are disturbances in voluntary movement such as slowness, disturbances in tone such as increased tone or rigidity and the development of involuntary movements such as tremor. We see these in an illness such as Parkinson's disease which is a disorder of the basal ganglia. Other, more unusual, disorders of the extrapyramidal system include Huntingdon's chorea.

To continue the analogy with a car, the extrapyramidal system can be compared with the clutch. This is responsible for the smooth control of movement. When we are learning to drive, we do so jerkily, slowly and tensely.

Involuntary movements, e.g. tremor, hemiballismus
Slow movement
Increased tone

TABLE 14.4: SUMMARY OF SYMPTOMS DUE TO DISTURBANCE IN THE EXTRAPYRAMIDAL SYSTEM

CEREBELLUM

This is responsible for the co-ordination of movement. It is important in the maintenance of posture. This may be seen as being rather passive but there is information being relayed to and from the brain and peripheries. This informs central areas about the state of tension in the body, its position in space and in relation to other parts of the body. It is the cerebellum which co-ordinates all this information and acts on it to control posture.

The cerebellum may be damaged by toxic substances including lead, alcohol and anticonvulsants. A variety of symptoms are seen including problems with posture, disturbances of walking (ataxia), head tremor, nystagmus, jerky speech, reduced tone and an intention tremor[3] .

Intention tremor
Lack of balance
Ataxia
Nystagmus
Reduced tone
Jerky movements and speech
Difficulties with co-ordination

TABLE 14.5: SUMMARY OF SYMPTOMS DUE TO DISTURBANCE IN THE CEREBELLUM

SENSORY SYSTEM

This is the area which is involved with sensation. It is the way in which we detect our external environment and inform the central areas about it. There are many types of sense organ all dealing with different qualities of sensation. In the skin, there is superficial sensation such as touch, pain, warmth, and cold. At deeper levels there is sensation of deep pain, pressure and position. Vibration is recognised by a combination of deep and superficial sensors.

Some impulses in sensory nerve fibres do not reach consciousness and these deal with reflex functions and connections with the cerebellum as in co-ordination control. The impulses in the sensory nerves pass to the spinal cord and through the thalamus in the brain to the sensory cortex.

Sensory disturbances lead to different symptoms depending on which area is affected. In the case of a peripheral nerve, complete loss of function causes numbness. This is fairly obvious. However, nerves overlap in their distribution[4] so there may be a limited area with no sensation at all.

---

[3] This is a tremor which gets worse on movement. That is, the closer you are to an object then the worse the tremor becomes.

Partial loss of function may lead, at first, to symptoms such as pain, tingling and pins and needles. The term 'neuralgia' may be applied to such symptoms. Conditions which may interfere with function in such a way are those frequently those which cause pressure on nerves. These include nerve entrapments, spinal tumour and prolapsed intervertebral disc. There may also be feelings of pain in deep structures such as muscles and ligaments supplied by the particular nerve. In severe cases, the motor part of the nerve may be affected leading to the symptoms of a lower motor neurone disorder described above.

In a neuropathy[5] there are particular nerves affected. The longest are the most susceptible so the fingers and toes are the usual areas affected. Posterior root disorders lead to loss of some types of sensation but not others. This is because some nerves cross over to the other side and others do not. This is beyond the scope of this book as we are here talking about complex neurological disease.

Disorders of central areas such as the thalamus produce pain of the opposite side of the body. It is typically unpleasant, severe and of a quality which is burning. People may develop this condition after a stroke and many such people attend pain clinics at hospitals.

Tingling
Pins and needles
Shooting, stabbing or burning pains
Numbness
Loss of perception of touch, vibration, position, pressure, heat and cold

TABLE 14.6: SUMMARY OF SYMPTOMS DUE TO DISTURBANCE IN THE SENSORY SYSTEM

REFLEXES

A reflex is a nervous system connection between a sensor and an effector organ such as a muscle or gland. There are two main points when considering the reflexes involving muscles. Firstly, there is a postural function. An example would be the reflex in a cat which always makes sure that it lands on its feet even if dropped upside down from a height. The second aim is to be protective and is evoked by stimuli to pain receptors. An example would be what happens when we touch something very hot. I need not describe the result with which we are all familiar. Rapid withdrawal is not conscious, it is at a spinal level. It comes to consciousness later.

TENDON REFLEXES

These are postural reflexes which depend on the stimulation of sensory organs within the muscle when it is stretched. The commonly known one is the knee reflex (or jerk). When the quadriceps is stretched and the tendon of the muscle tapped, the muscle will go into reflex contraction. It is a way of measuring the function of the reflex arc at a particular level in the spinal cord. Each reflex has a different level as shown in Table 14.7.

REFLEX	LEVEL
Biceps	Cervical 5 and 6
Triceps	Cervical 7
Supinator	Cervical 5 and 6
Knee	Lumbar 3 and 4
Ankle	Sacral 1

TABLE 14.7: TENDON REFLEXES AND THEIR SPINAL LEVELS

If the tendon reflex is absent, it can be assumed that there is a problem with the lower motor neurone at or above that level. If the tendon reflex is increased, there is likely to be a problem with the upper motor neurone.

---

[4] The area of skin supplied by a specific nerve is called a dermatome. Maps of such areas and the nerves supplying them can be found in anatomy books.

[5] This is disease of a peripheral nerve. There are many causes and some are discussed later.

Superficial reflexes are to do with the skin and usually involve many levels. The response is a co-ordinated movement. There are many of them and a few have clinical significance. The plantar reflex is produced at the sole of the foot. It is elicited by scraping along the lateral border of the sole and then medially proximal to the toes. At the age of one year it is normally extensor. It then becomes flexor unless an upper motor neurone lesion is present. It is then extensor in type.

The corneal reflex provokes blinking of the eyelids and has two components. Therefore, it is only present if both parts are functioning correctly. The sensory portion is via the first (ophthalmic) division of the fifth cranial nerve and the motor portion is through the seventh cranial nerve.

SPECIFIC ORGANS AND PATHWAYS

Dysfunction in a nerve supply to organs such as the rectum and bladder may herald a spinal cord compression, e.g. prolapsed intervertebral disc or spinal tumour. The bladder has a complex nervous control as it has voluntary and involuntary (reflex) mechanisms. There is a sympathetic nervous supply from the 1st and 2nd lumbar areas and this serves to relax the bladder and contract the sphincters. The parasympathetic supply is through an outflow at the second to fourth sacral level which serves to contract the bladder and relax the internal sphincter. The external sphincter is under voluntary control via 2nd to 4th sacral area.

The rectum similarly has this control. The sympathetic is inhibitory, that is it tends to stop bowel emptying ('holding on') and the parasympathetic is facilitatory ('letting go').

AUTONOMIC NERVOUS SYSTEM

Unfortunately, the word 'autonomic' conjures up a similar meaning as 'automatic' although they originate from different words in the original Greek. Autonomic implies a self-governing or regulating function. It can be affected by thoughts and emotions in a positive or a negative manner. Meditation practices are the well-known example of how our minds can affect this system. They can lead to decrease in oxygen consumption, reduction in metabolic rate and blood pressure, reduction in heart rate and changes to brain waves characteristic of a relaxed state of mind.

There are two aspects to the autonomic nervous system which have opposite functions. They are balanced in health. As with the endocrine system, it is one of the few areas, conventionally where the principles of Yin and Yang as understood by Chinese medicine may be recognised.

The parasympathetic aspect deals with relaxation and mainly involves the release of the neurotransmitter substance, acetylcholine. Drugs which are anticholinergic in nature block this area. The nerve tracts which are part of this system include parts of the cranial nerves III, VII, IX and X, and parts of the outflow from the second to fourth sacral nerves.

The sympathetic aspect is stimulatory. It mainly involves the release of noradrenaline, a neurotransmitter. Betablockers inhibit its function. The adrenal medulla is an integral part of this system as it releases adrenaline and noradrenaline and is directly stimulated by sympathetic nerves. Nerve tracts in this system arise from all the thoracic and the first two lumbar nerve roots to form the sympathetic chain. The sympathetic division plays an important role in flight-or-fight responses.

SUMMARY

From the foregoing discussion, the central nervous system is clearly a complex organ. It is not easy to accurately identify the site of any problem without an understanding of the anatomical connections of each nerve tract. This is not necessary for the alternative practitioner as you are not going to be treating a localised area. However, it is useful to gain a general idea about the underlying process and site. This may help you in deciding whether to refer or not.

There are several key questions to consider when faced with a person with neurological symptoms. Firstly, do the symptoms suggest a peripheral or central location? Secondly, are the symptoms motor or sensory in type. For example, symptoms only present in the hand can be either a central problem or a local problem in the arm or neck. Symptoms present in a hand, leg and head must be due to a central problem. A knowledge of anatomy is helpful here.

Symptoms which are only motor in type may indicate a disorder such as motor neurone disease or polio which only ever affect motor nerves. Symptoms which are only sensory in type may indicate a neuropathy which is sensory in nature such as that seen with diabetes mellitus or a mild compression, e.g. cervical spondylosis, prolapsed intervertebral disc. Symptoms which are mixed in nature may indicate a disease which affects several nerves at once, e.g. brain tumour, multiple sclerosis, more severe compression of a nerve.

The way in which symptoms appear may also give useful clues about the underlying process. Some diseases, by their nature, are rapid in onset over minutes or an hour or so. This would indicate a disturbance with blood supply as in stroke or an infection as meningitis and encephalitis. A slower process over days or weeks which is progressive would indicate a tumour. A malignant tumour would clearly develop symptoms more quickly than a benign one. A more gradual onset over months would indicate a degenerative process such as Parkinson's disease.

Some diseases have a typical history of relapses and remissions over months and years. Multiple sclerosis is an example of these.

Using these ideas, it is possible to formulate an opinion about the possible process. It may be necessary to seek referral in those cases which are rapidly changing.

- ALTERNATIVE VIEW OF THE CENTRAL NERVOUS SYSTEM -

In this section, I shall discuss the ideas in Chinese medicine which generally correspond to the central nervous system. It is difficult for Westerners to consider that there may be different explanations for a group of functions and symptoms. This is particularly true in the case of the central nervous system and the endocrine system. In Chinese medicine, there is no precise system of organs and structures which can be identified as being identical with the nervous system. This is mainly because Oriental systems of philosophy are more concerned with function than structure.

Nevertheless, there are organ systems in Chinese medicine which have a similar *function* to the nervous system. This is clearly the case since disorders of the nervous system are usually amenable to treatment by Chinese medicine. This is in direct contradistinction to conventional medicine which is usually at a loss how to address such problems.

The most important organ system of Chinese medicine to consider here is the Liver. There are several associations with this organ which I describe in Table 14.8.

Imbalances of Liver functions, may manifest in many different parts of the body. This is partly related to the role of the Liver in maintaining the free flow of Qi and also to the course of the Liver channel. This starts in the big toe, passes up the inside of the leg through the genital area. It then passes up to the breast area and connections are made eventually with the eyes and the vertex of the head.

Symptoms such as abdominal bloating, constipation, breast pain, pains around the eyes and vertex may all be related to Liver imbalances. Disease labels in conventional medicine which may be the counterpart include hernias, irritable bowel syndrome, pain in the hypochondria, pre-menstrual tension, migraine.

Disturbances in the Liver's function of allowing the free flow of qi may lead to symptoms such as stiffness, tremor, tics, convulsions and so forth. Disease labels in conventional medicine which may correspond tend to be classified as central nervous system problems.

ASSOCIATION	COMMENTS
Stores Blood	When the person is at rest and particularly when lying down, the Blood returns to the Liver. This is released during exercise and menstruation. Lack of Blood in the Liver may lead to gynaecological symptoms (see Chapter 18 - Gynaecology)
Maintains free flow of Qi	This ensures the smooth and harmonious flow of energy throughout the body and its organs
Dominates tendons and movements	This ensures the smooth movement of joints. Disturbed function leads to stiff movements, cramps, tremors
Manifests in the nails	Nails are seen in Chinese medicine as a 'by-product' of the sinews[6]
Opens into the eye	Each organ is connected to a sense organ. The function of the eye is very much related to Liver function
Paired organ is Gall Bladder	This is comparable with the conventional view that the liver and gall bladder are closely related
Colour - green	This is the colour of Spring and the Wood element
Taste - sour	Each major organ has an associated taste. In this case excess sour taste can damage the Wood element.
Season - spring	The energy of spring moves upward and outward as the branches of a tree (Wood element). This can be related to the function of the Liver in maintaining the free flow of Qi
Element - Wood	The Element correspondence reveals the connection of Chinese medical theory to nature. Each Element is connected to the others to provide, in health, a harmonious balance.
Time - 1 a.m. - 3 a.m.	The 'time' of an organ is when its energy it at its maximum. Liver imbalances may make it difficult to sleep when going to bed.
Emotions - anger	In health, this is assertiveness as befits the function of the Liver in allowing the free flow of Qi. Unbalanced, this may manifest as aggression, guilt, resentment or jealousy ('green with envy')
Mental aspect	The Liver is to do with a giving attitude. It is responsible for a kindly attitude and sharing. Its paired organ, the Gall Bladder, is responsible for decision making.

TABLE **14.8**: HOLISTIC ENERGETIC VIEW OF THE LIVER

- INVESTIGATIONS -

Any person who has a suspected condition of the central nervous system of a serious nature will have investigations performed. There are several reasons why they are done including:

- identify the exact nature of the disease
- classify how to treat the condition
- come to a conclusion regarding prognosis

The common investigations applied are listed in Chapter 4 - Investigations. I shall discuss individual situations in relation to each disease.

---

6 "The Foundations of Chinese Medicine" by Giovanni Maciocia (Churchill Livingstone, 1989)

- CEREBROVASCULAR DISEASE -

This is disease of the brain due to an interference with its blood supply. The usual problem is disruption to arterial blood supply by either haemorrhage or ischaemia (either as a result of thrombosis or embolism). The counterpart in the cardiovascular system is ischaemic heart disease leading to the clinical pictures of angina pectoris and heart attack. The comments I made in Chapter 7 - Cardiovascular System in relation to the pathological processes of atheroma, thrombosis and embolism are relevant here.

The additional process which is of importance is bleeding (haemorrhage). In the brain, this is due to a rupture of a blood vessel usually associated with high blood pressure and atherosclerosis. Primary cerebral haemorrhage is the term used to describe the process which occurs with hypertensive people where there is bleeding into the substance of the brain. This is the 'burst blood vessel', the apopleptic attack. It is of abrupt onset and can occur with exercise. It may also occur after a particularly stressful incident. There is usually a severe headache with this condition and more than 50% of people lose consciousness. The haemorrhage is often large and loss of consciousness is a sign that the condition is severe. Half of such people die within a few days.

Atherosclerosis is an extensive disease and does not affect one organ only. The way in which a person presents and the emphasis of the pathology will depend on the individual. If someone has had a stroke there may be evidence of heart disease. Conversely, if you see a person with coronary atherosclerosis there may also be evidence of damage to the central nervous system.

The common clinical condition associated with cerebrovascular disease is stroke. The precise clinical picture on the site and size or any damage and whether there are any unaffected blood vessels supplying the same area of brain.

STROKE

This is common, especially with increasing age, and is found in 1% of people over 60 years old. It causes much ill-health and leads to difficulty with mobility, dependence and rehabilitation. It occurs in 2 people per 1000 of the population each year and of these one will die as a result of this event.

Symptoms:

These are rare before the age of 40 years and uncommon before the age of 50 years.

The clinical picture usually evolves over a period of one to two hours. There is a loss of consciousness in a minority although drowsiness is common. Severe headache is unusual. The exact nature of the stroke depends on the site of the damage in the brain.

The commonest symptom is paralysis of one side of the body (hemiplegia). The face, arm and leg are affected in most cases. The side affected is opposite to the side of the problem in the brain. As I mentioned above in relation to upper motor neurone lesions, there is spasticity and increased reflexes. These features are not seen immediately but take a few days to develop as the spinal cord recovers from the 'shock' of the removal of cerebral influences.

There will be dyphasia (difficult speech) if the dominant hemisphere of the brain is affected. This is the left side in right-handed people and often the left-side in most left-handed people. Therefore, a right-sided stroke (of the body) will be accompanied by dysphasia in all right- handed people and in most left-handed people.

A milder symptom picture may present with temporary symptoms. This is named a transient ischaemic attack (TIA). There is also sudden loss of function in the central nervous system. It is followed within the hour by complete recovery. Most attacks only last a few minutes. They should be regarded as a warning of a possible stroke in the future[7].

The symptoms depend on the site of the problem within the brain. They include loss of consciousness (rare), aphasia, sensory loss and weakness (rather than paralysis) on one side of the body, difficulty swallowing, double vision and vomiting. Vertigo is common and there may be ataxia.

Visual loss is common and the typical symptom is a transient blindness which is said to be like a black curtain descending down the field of vision. It is called amaurosis fugax. Recovery is the

---

[7] Five years later, 1 in 4 are dead due to heart attack or stroke and 1 in 6 have had a stroke.

reverse of this process. The frequency of attacks is variable and they may be due to small emboli of atheroma and clot breaking off the affected arterial walls.

Prognosis:

There is a high mortality rate with stroke. Between a third and a half die within the month after an attack, usually in the first few days. This is more common with 75% of those with haemorrhage dying and less than a quarter of those with embolism or haemorrhage. A poor outcome is more likely if there is coma, squint or a severe hemiplegia. Some 10% of people have recurrent attacks of stroke. Around 30-40% of *survivors* are alive after 3 years which illustrates the severity of this condition. Common long-term problems include muscle weakness and speech difficulties.

Treatment:

This tends to be supportive immediately after the event and rehabilitation in the long-term. Any underlying disease is treated such as diabetes mellitus or hypertension. The main aim is to minimise any disability and to try and improve function. Physiotherapy plays a large part in this. It is helpful in supporting, encouraging and aiding the person gain as much mobility as possible. Massage would also be useful here. Speech therapy and psychological support are important additions.

Transient ischaemic attacks are usually treated by anticoagulants. Aspirin inhibits platelet aggregation and can be used in conditions where there is a tendency to clot formation. It is frequently used in this disease. Other drugs used include dipyridamole which has a similar function.

Alternative management:

In terms of Chinese medicine, this condition is denoted WindStroke. There are three main features of such a condition and there are similarities with many other conditions which are labelled as of central nervous system origin by conventional medicine. Essentially, there is Heat which causes the stirring of Wind. This carries Phlegm up to the orifices to cause loss of consciousness and to the channels to cause paralysis and numbness. The generation of Heat may arise from Deficiency of Kidney or Liver Yin leading to rising of Liver Yang. This is the correlation of hypertension with stroke (see Page 179). Alternatively, the Heat may arise from the excessive consumption of greasy and sweet food. Occasionally, the Wind may be of external origin in those people who are weak and Deficient.

Specifically, therapies such as acupuncture can help the paralysis and the sensory problems which people have after a stroke. Techniques such as relaxation, Tai Chi or other exercises are also beneficial.

The problems posed by this condition are frequently long-term. There is a lot of money, time and energy spent on treatment. You will see people in your clinic who have problems remaining after a stroke and alternative medicine has a lot to offer such cases. If the person has had a paralysis or a sensory problem for many years then there may seem not to be much that can be done to improve the situation. However, I have seen and heard of cases where marked improvement has occurred several years after the stroke and so the recuperative powers in the central nervous system can be strong indeed.

OTHER DISEASES LEADING TO STROKE

The clinical appearance of stroke may also be the result of other pathological processes. For example, brain tumour may lead to the death of nerve cells either due to direct pressure or to obstruction of the blood supply. Brain tumour is described later in this Chapter.

SUBARACHNOID HAEMORRHAGE

This is an uncommon condition but one which you may come across. It is haemorrhage under the subarachnoid layer around the outside of the brain. The usual source is from a ruptured aneurysm. An aneurysm is a dilatation on an arterial wall and tends to be weaker than the rest of the blood vessel. The conventional belief is that they are congenital in nature and at some time spontaneously burst to produce the typical symptoms.

Symptoms:

There is a severe and sudden headache which is usually occipital in site. It can come on so suddenly that the person may turn round because they think that they have been struck. There are signs of meningeal irritation. These are photophobia, neck stiffness and occipital headache. There will not be a fever as you would expect with meningitis or encephalitis. There may be loss of consciousness for hours or days. Vomiting is common. Impaired function of the central nervous system does not always happen and if so then clearly the condition is more serious. The danger is of a further rupture of another aneurysm.

This condition is fatal in many cases. Around 50% are dead or almost so by the time of arrival at hospital. A further 10-20% die in the next few days. The prognosis is more serious if paralysis is present or if another bleed occurs within the next few days.

Treatment:

The conventional response is dependent upon the person's age. Computerised axial tomography scans are performed under the age of 60 years and angiography in that age group if the blood pressure is normal. Less than 5% of people have a detectable abnormality..

Essentially, the management is to wait until the person's condition has stabilised. Rest and supportive treatment are important in the early stages. If an aneurysm is discovered by angiography, it will be clipped surgically.

- EPILEPSY -

Epilepsy is defined as the occurrence of recurrent convulsions or 'abnormal events'. About 3% of the population have 2 or more such attacks in their lives. Some 250,000 people in the UK take anticonvulsant drugs.

It is classified by conventional medicine according to the appearances of the attack. The symptoms are of an epileptic convulsion and the particular form varies with each type. The diagnosis is necessarily confirmed and categorised with the aid of an electroencephalogram (EEG). It is considered to be a brief disorder of cerebral function associated with disturbance of consciousness accompanied by sudden, excessive discharge of cerebral neurones. The classification is as follows:

Generalised	
	Grand mal
	Petit mal
Focal	
	Temporal lobe
	Jacksonian

TABLE 14.8: CONVENTIONAL CLASSIFICATION OF EPILEPSY

The causes are usually unknown conventionally. There may be a family history and if one or both parents have epilepsy then it is more likely to develop. It can develop secondarily to cerebral disease. The commonest conditions here are brain tumours, a head injury and cerebrovascular disease. Other situations may lead to epileptic fits and these reflect the fact that it is possible for all of us to have an attack if the conditions are right. These include hyperglycaemia, hypoglycaemia, withdrawal of drugs such as heroin and opiates and alcohol. One in twenty people with epilepsy are photosensitive and a fit can be set off by flashing lights and a flickering television or video game.

Symptoms:

I shall describe each type of epilepsy separately although you often see people who have what seems to be a mixture of types. This is difficult to explain conventionally. I treated a boy of eight once who had what was clinically petit mal and grand mal attacks but the diagnosis of the neurologist was of temporal lobe epilepsy (based mainly on the EEG finding). He was given carbamazepine, the main drug for temporal lobe epilepsy. The attacks changed in appearance only because this drug will not control his type of convulsion.

GRAND MAL OR MAJOR ATTACK.

There is a prodromal stage which can last for hours or days and is usually a change of mood. Then there may occur an 'aura' which is uncommon in this type of epilepsy and is brief. If the person does go through this stage, it may merely be an awareness that a fit is about to happen. If so, they can lie down and prepare themselves to avoid injury.

If an aura is not experienced, the person goes suddenly into a *tonic* stage. There is generalised contraction of all the muscles in the body. The person may give a 'cry' as the air is forced from the lungs and falls to the ground. There is loss of consciousness and the contraction of all the musculature is sustained for about 20-30 seconds. There is no respiration and so cyanosis develops.

This is followed by the *clonic* stage which are spasmodic contractions of the muscles. There are typical jerking movements of the face, body and limbs. It lasts for about 30 seconds and there may or may not be incontinence of urine (usually) or faeces (rarely). The person may bite their tongue either in this or the previous stage.

Finally, the attack ends in a stage of relaxation. This is a flaccid, comatose state which lapses into normal sleep. This lasts for a few minutes or half an hour. When consciousness is regained there is often a period of drowsiness and some confusion with a headache. A person should not be allowed to go home unaccompanied after an attack because of the presence of confusion and sleepiness.

PETIT MAL OR MINOR ATTACK.

This has a characteristic EEG pattern. It cannot be diagnosed medically without this. There is a transient loss of consciousness which lasts for 10 to 15 seconds. The person stares blankly. In mild cases and at the onset they may pass unnoticed. They are accurately described as 'absences'. In children it may be mistaken for inattention, learning difficulties, deafness and so forth.

TEMPORAL LOBE EPILEPSY

This is the commonest type of focal epilepsy. There are strange symptoms of hallucinations of smell, taste, hearing or sight. They are frequently unpleasant such as offensive smells or sounds of obscene words. Patients may think that people are swearing at them. There are often 'déjà vu' phenomena[8]. Déjà vu is also seen in schizophrenia and is certainly linked to altered states of consciousness although they are common in people with neither of these conditions.

Emotional changes are common. Consciousness is disturbed but not lost. There may be a situation known as automatism. This is behaviour which is not attended by conscious thought or awareness and this has medico-legal implications.

---

[8] A feeling of being in a familiar place or having done the same thing previously.

JACKSONIAN EPILEPSY

Here, there is involuntary twitching of one limb or part of a limb. It may or may not spread further. There may be loss of consciousness although it is unusual. A single part of the body is usually the first place affected such as the thumb. The shaking spreads to involve the whole limb and, rarely, the whole body. Each episode lasts for several minutes. A temporary weakness or paralysis may follow the attack.

The significance of this type of epilepsy is that it usually develops in later life and may be caused by a structural abnormality such as a brain tumour.

Investigations:

The definitive diagnosis is made with an EEG and conventional treatment cannot start until the exact type is known. Drug treatment for epilepsy suppresses the changes detectable by EEG.

Some types of epilepsy are secondary to structural problems of the brain such as tumours. Investigation will be undertaken if this is suspected. This will include brain scan - either computerised axial tomography, magnetic resonance imaging or a radio-active isotope scan.

Treatment:

There is a social stigma associated with this disease and, in general, society is not very understanding. I remember that there was a boy in my class at school who had grand mal attacks fairly regularly and he was treated miserably by the rest of us. There was little attempt to understand the condition and this seemed to be general throughout the school.

The occupation of a person may be affected as certain jobs are not considered suitable. Any job where loss of consciousness may be dangerous for the person or others is precluded. This covers such work as airline pilot, professional driving, steeplejack and working with high voltage equipment.

The regulations concerning a driving licence in the UK are that the person can hold a licence and drive if there has not been a fit awake in the previous two years. When fits occur during sleep, the convulsions must have occurred only whilst asleep and the person not to have had an attack for three years.

There are certain precipitating factors. Common ones are lack of sleep (tiredness), fevers and television or flashing lights in those who are sensitive.

The first-aid treatment of an epileptic attack is to remove the person from sources of injury such as furniture and to loosen clothing. Wait until the attack has subsided and then place the person in the recovery position until consciousness is regained. The old advice about placing an object between the teeth to protect the tongue is no longer given as the tongue will have been bitten early in the attack. If you attempt such a practice you may damage teeth or risk losing fingers!

The mainstay of conventional treatment remains drugs. Different agents are used for different types of epilepsy.

TYPE OF EPILEPSY	DRUG USED	COMMENTS[9]
Grand mal	Phenytoin	Affects the liver. Commonly used.
	Phenobarbitone	Heavily suppressesespiration
	Carbamazepine	Also used to treat neuralgias
	Sodium valproate	Commonly used. Affects the liver
Petit mal	Ethosuximide	Main side-effects on in the blood
	Sodium valproate	See above
Temporal lobe	Carbamazepine	See above

TABLE 14.9: CONVENTIONAL TREATMENT OF EPILEPSY

---

[9] All anticonvulsants may damage the blood but particularly ethosuximide and phenytoin. The latter can actually lead to lymphoma - cancer of the lymphatic system.

Alternative management:

In previous times and in other cultures, epileptics and people who could enter trance states were seen as being in touch with something powerful and perhaps useful. This is no longer true. We hide away from such things or hide them away from us. It is part of the process of treatment to perhaps allow people to reconnect with a side of themselves which is suppressed. This type of problem has similarities with some mental and emotional disturbances.

The precise manifestation of an imbalance will vary from person to person. If blockages exist in the mental and emotional levels there may be the appearance of disorders such as epilepsy, psychological disturbances and so forth. Cure is to do with transformation of these and realising that we function on all these levels. Curative treatment may well release, in the case of epilepsy, emotions which are long-suppressed. Coming to terms with these and learning how to handle them in a healthy way are the challenges of treatment.

In terms of Chinese medicine, this condition is considered in a group of mania, hysteria and epilepsy. There are common connections with these as they are all associated with the substances of Wind, Heat and Phlegm. They manifest in different ways according to the person. They may also be seen in relation to the three levels of mental, emotional and physical. Mania is a disturbance of the mental level and is described in Chapter 16 - Psychological Disorders. In Chinese medicine, this term is used broadly to include the conventional labels of schizophrenia and mania. Hysteria is a disturbance of the emotional level and is described in Chapter 16 - Psychological Disorders. Epilepsy is a disturbance of the physical level.

The treatment of these three disorders by conventional medicine may also be understood from an energetic viewpoint. Mania is treated by lithium and 'major' tranquillisers such as the phenothiazines. Hysteria is treated by 'minor' tranquillisers such as the benzodiazepines. Epilepsy is treated by anticonvulsants (of which the benzodiazepines are one example). These interrelationships are shown in Table 14.7.

DISORDER	CONVENTIONAL TREATMENT	COMMENTS
Mania	Lithium, antipsychotics such as 'major' tranquillisers	Sedative to the mental level. Side-effects are damage to the central nervous system causing tardive dyskinesia similar in its manifestation to Parkinson's disease
Hysteria	'Minor' tranqullisers	Sedative to the emotional level. Withdrawal may lead to mania (mental level), anxiety (emotional level) or convulsions (physical level)
Epilepsy	Anticonvulsants	Sedative mainly to physical level. Side-effects include damage to the central nervous system

TABLE 14.10: CONVENTIONAL TREATMENT OF MANIA, HYSTERIA AND EPILEPSY

Treatment by alternative medicine is effective for epilepsy but it will almost always be complicated by the administration of anticonvulsants. Sudden withdrawal of these is dangerous and must not be attempted. Some 40% of people with epilepsy can withdraw their drugs and have no problems, presumably because the original exciting cause has gone. The difficulty we have with each person is that we do not know if they are one of the 40%.

Treatment must be accompanied by an awareness that hidden issues on a psychological level may arise. These can be dealt with as they appear but a general atmosphere of support and openness is helpful. It is beneficial to avoid as much stimulation as possible particularly drugs including coffee, regular relaxation, a healthy diet especially avoiding greasy, sweet and spicy food. In this way it is certainly possible to gradually reduce medication after people's health begins to improve. How far you can go will vary from case to case.

- MULTIPLE SCLEROSIS (DISSEMINATED SCLEROSIS) -

This is the main example of a group of diseases which is associated with loss of the myelin sheath (demyelinisation) around the nerve fibre. This sheath of fatty material is essential for normal nerve function. The loss of myelin leads to abnormal function of whichever nerve or nerves are affected.

It occurs in one in 2000 people and the cause is unknown. There are about 250,000 people with multiple sclerosis in the US.

It occurs in geographical clusters and is commoner in the North and West of Europe, UK, northern United States, Canada, Iceland, Tasmania and southern New Zealand. This may be an association with damp and cold conditions. Certain dietary changes may lead to improvement and seem to support this. I describe them later. It is more common in those areas where people have a high intake of animal fats.

Conventionally, there are considered to be genetic or autoimmune mechanisms involved. There is evidence from the study of disease incidence and antibody levels to suggest that multiple sclerosis may be linked to latent viral infections in the body. These, in susceptible people, disrupt the immune system so that it attacks the nervous system. Many viruses have been implicated but especially the measles virus[10]. This has implications for vaccination procedures which are the deliberate introduction of such material into the body. Recent evidence indicates that 30-60% of new attacks of multiple sclerosis occur soon after a common cold, influenza or other viral illness.

Symptoms:

Initially there is an episode of symptoms reflecting a neurological disorder. The exact nature depends on the nerves involved as any nerve in the body can be affected. Typically, this includes an acute weakness of one or more limbs, the appearance of pins and needles or numbness, double vision or blurred vision (common), vertigo, loss of balance. Most people recover within one to three months of the onset of symptoms. There is a recurrence after a variable period of time and this is usually within two years.

In some people, the disease enters a stage of gradual increase in disability without remission. Most people recover almost to normal but after each relapse there is a further degeneration in function and so the result is a step-wise deterioration. Half of affected people enter a chronically progressive stage.

The motor dysfunction is of an upper motor neurone type. It is typically worse after a hot bath. There is often loss of balance and an intention tremor[11]. Sensory affections are common and include tingling, electric shock-like sensations and numbness. Mental changes also take place and the common one is depression. It is said in conventional texts that euphoria can also occur. As this is a side-effect of corticosteroid therapy, I think that it is much more likely to be as a result of such treatment than of the disease itself.

It is considered to be a progressive and chronic disease and 5% die within 5 years. In the rest there is a variable course. A significant proportion (up to one third) has only the first attack. These are then lost to medical follow-up so the conventionally held view of almost certain deterioration is not valid.

Investigations:

There is no single investigation which can lead to a definite diagnosis of multiple sclerosis. The diagnosis is made from the clinical history and an exclusion of diseases causing similar symptoms such as brain tumour.

The investigations which are performed provide circumstantial evidence but must be considered in the light of the total picture. They include lumbar puncture and examination of cerebrospinal fluid, tests of visual evoked potential and scanning of the nervous system. This latter is by means of magnetic resonance imaging (MRI) or computed tomographic (CT) scanning.

---

[10] Kinnunen, Esko; et al. Archives of Neurology, July 1990 v47 n7 p743(4).

[11] This is a tremor which increases with movement as the object is approached. It is typical of a coordination difficulty due to cerebellar involvement.

The MRI scan, in particular, is seen as a more sensitive indicator of the presence of areas of demyelination. However, it is not positive in all and many things may give rise to the same appearances.

Treatment:

In conventional terms, there is nothing which is considered to be curative. Corticosteroids are frequently given as it is believed to lead to a more rapid and complete recovery of a relapse. This is a matter for debate even in conventional circles. There is no documented evidence of benefit from long-term corticosteroid use. It tends, instead, to lead to serious side-effects such as osteoporosis, fluid retention, hypertension and cataracts.

One consideration is to attempt the relief of spasticity through drugs. These are of variable effectiveness. Urinary incontinence is common and an in-dwelling catheter may be necessary. Kidney infections are common as a result of the underlying urinary problem and the presence of the catheter.

An important aspect is support for the relatives as this disease is tremendously tiring for the carers.

Alternative management:

You will definitely see people with this condition as they look for alternatives to the approach of conventional medicine. One issue to be considered is the effect upon the person of the label itself. As described above there is a wide range of variable courses of the disease. However, when a doctor in a white coat in a hospital tells you that you have multiple sclerosis, that you will end up in a wheel-chair, and that there is nothing that can be done to cure you, these are very powerful messages to you not to get better. Even if there were nothing wrong, many people would end up in that state.

There is currently an advertisement in the UK for an organisation which purports to help people with multiple sclerosis. It shows a woman's back with a tear in the photograph down the length of the spinal column and a spine-chilling! (literally) message about the effects of the disease. These are often self-fulfilling prophecies.

This is a difficult disease to treat as far as the alternative practitioner is concerned. This is particularly so since many people seek treatment when the disease is well established. It is important to have several approaches. Diet seems to be a major factor and especially the avoidance of animal fat[12]. This would fit in with the observation that multiple sclerosis occurs more commonly in damp[13] areas such as the UK and the North and West of Europe. Some people also benefit from removing gluten from the diet. I have known people who started to improve with treatment and then relapse after eating dairy products or meat. These foods tend to produce Dampness within the body, in terms of Chinese medicine. It is such observations which lead people to take oils such as linoleic oil and evening primrose oil for this condition[14].

My approach to a person with multiple sclerosis is similar to someone with cancer. There are frequently psychological factors which play an important part in the genesis and the continuation of the disease. Relaxation is very beneficial as well as looking at those emotional and mental factors which may be of importance.

In terms of Chinese medicine, this condition is usually seen as Wind in the Channels which may be due to several causes. There may be WindDamp directly invading the Channels and Organs. Otherwise, there is Deficiency of Kidney, Spleen or Liver leading to Wind because of Qi and Blood Deficiency. Phlegm and Dampness gather in the tissues giving rise to stiffness and numbness. Long-

---

[12] A survey of 134 people with multiple sclerosis over a course of 34 years showed that a low-fat diet leads to significantly less deterioration and lower death rates from the disease. It works best at an early stage of the disease. Swank, R.L., et al. Lancet, July 7, 1990 v336 n8706 p37(3). Also, Swank, R.L. Am J Med Sci 1950;220:421-30. Also, Swank R.L. Nutrition 1991;7:368-76.

[13] Here I am relating the intake of foods which generate mucus in the body with the climatic factor of dampness.

[14] This has been confirmed by studies such as Millar JHD, et al Br Med J 1973; 1:765-8 and Bates D, et al Br Med J 1978;2:1390-1.

term the tendons and ligaments are damaged. Usually, the milder the symptoms, the harder it is to treat. People with heat symptoms tend to do better because there is more energy in the system.

It is definitely possible for people to improve and I know of people who are leading a full and active life after a diagnosis of multiple sclerosis. When the disease has progressed and there is paralysis and other neurological symptoms, there is still much to offer. Treatment can help alleviate the worst of the pain or tingling. It can help the weakness. It can help the urinary and bowel problems of incontinence or impaction. You would expect the person to continue with symptoms but with an improved quality of life and comfort.

- PARKINSON'S DISEASE -

This is one of a group of diseases where there is a disturbance in the function of the extrapyramidal system. This system is like the clutch on the car and serves to act as a control of movement. Abnormalities here lead to three typical groups of symptoms. There is disturbance of voluntary movement, the appearance of involuntary movements and an alteration in the muscle tone. Another disease of the same part of the brain is Huntington's chorea.

In Parkinsonism, there is impairment of voluntary movement, rigidity and tremor. If these three symptoms co-exist in an elderly person then the diagnosis is usually made. The incidence is around 1 in 1000 of the population and this rises to 1% in the over 60 year old age group. The pathological lesion is in the basal ganglia and involves a relative lack of the transmitter substances of that part of the nervous system. There are several causes in conventional terms:

- unknown in 75%
- post-encephalitis especially encephalitis lethargica
- prescribed drugs such as the phenothiazines used in schizophrenia, Alzheimer's disease and senile dementia
- head injury

Symptoms:

There is the gradual development of a tremor in the fingers and the forearms. It is slow in nature and is described as pill-rolling. The person looks as though they are rolling a pill between the thumb and index finger. Tremor of the head is rare. It is worse at rest and improves with purposeful movements such as attempting to pick up something. This is in contrast to the tremor of cerebellar disease which gets worse the closer the hand moves to an object (intention tremor). The tremor of Parkinson's disease is typically worse with stress and with embarrassment.

The rigidity in the muscles is due to increased muscle tone. It is of a 'cog-wheel' type where passive movement of the arm, for example, reveals the intermittent nature of the rigidity. There are often fixed abnormalities of posture and the body appears to be in a permanent state of flexion. Movement is slow and there is a delay in the initiation of movements. It is difficult for a person to start to walk from standing or to stand from the sitting position. It is as if the person has slowed down and almost stopped and that people walk in slow motion. Conversely, it is not possible to control the speed of walking and people may gather speed when walking downhill. There is a typical gait which is short and shuffling because the legs cannot be picked up very well. The voice is quiet.

This is a severe, degenerative disease of the central nervous system. One in five people cannot cope independently with normal living and have to be supported in some way by family, friends or the health services.

Treatment:

This is aimed at the cause if known but this is a minority of people. The main aim of treatment is to minimise the worst symptoms of the disease. This is primarily with drugs designed to correct the chemical abnormalities in the affected area of the brain.

DRUG	TREATMENT LEVEL	COMMENTS
Anticholinergic, e.g. benzhexol, orphenadrine	1	Rarely used since the advent of L-dopa. Lead to dry mouth, blurred vision and retention of urine.
L-Dopa	2	Early use is associated with worsening of the symptoms in the long-term. There is an 'on-off' phenomenon where either the drugs do not work or they have strong side-effects. This can occur with no warning and a constant drug dosage. Originally L-Dopa seemed to revolutionise the treatment of Parkinson's disease. People who had been almost seized up for years started to walk and move. However, they cause many side-effects and limitation on the dose used is the appearance of these.
Bromocryptine	3	Used when L-dopa is ineffective. The dosage is restricted by the appearance of side-effects.
Surgery	4	This is the implantation of brain cells obtained from aborted foetuses. This has ethical implications.

TABLE 14.11: CONVENTIONAL TREATMENT OF PARKINSON'S DISEASE

Alternative management:

In terms of Chinese medicine, this condition usually corresponds to Liver Blood Deficiency with Wind. Phlegm accumulates in the channels and muscles leading to stiffness and slow movement. The conventional drugs have a heating effect and mainly affect the Liver and Heart. The heating effect of the drugs is to dry the Phlegm and to help movement but leads to side-effects of restlessness and sometimes worsening of the tremor. Long-term, of course, they cause Liver Blood Deficiency and so can only worsen the disease.

- CEREBRAL TUMOUR -

This causes 2% of deaths at all ages so it is not that uncommon. The tumour is frequently a secondary development from a cancer elsewhere in the body but it can be a primary growth.

Benign tumours may develop in the brain and these will present with similar symptoms to those of malignant tumours. However, malignant tumours grow more quickly and symptoms develop more rapidly with clear progression. The treatment of both types may be the same. The main restriction for surgery is the site of the tumour. Some are not amenable to removal as the operation would cause too much damage. Consequently, radiotherapy and chemotherapy may be given.

An exception to the above is the meningioma. This is a slow growing benign tumour on the meninges, the membrane which surrounds the brain. This can be removed surgically without damaging internal structures.

Symptoms:

These are considered to be due to two factors. Firstly, there is the local effect on neighbouring tissues. Secondly, there is increased pressure as the tumour grows inside the rigid bony skull.

Local effects are due to pressure on adjacent brain tissue. Therefore, there are symptoms dependent upon the particular nerve tract which is affected. This will obviously depend on the site of the tumour in the central nervous system. There could be problems with motor nerves, sensory nerves, cerebellum and other areas. Symptoms here include weakness or paralysis, numbness, tingling, pins and needles, difficulties with balance, fits. The clinical syndromes seen include stroke and epilepsy.

The pressure inside the skull increases because there is no outlet for the cerebrospinal fluid. As the tumour expands in size the pressure rises. This leads to a headache which is described as diffuse. It is worse for activities such as bending, coughing or straining. It is worse on waking and when lying flat. There is often clouding of consciousness which varies from a mild degree of listlessness and drowsiness to deep coma. There may be the development of generalised epileptic attacks. Also, there is often dizziness and, typically, vomiting with no preceding nausea due to direct stimulation of the vomiting centre in the midbrain.

Investigations:

The approach to this condition will depend on whether it is a primary or a secondary tumour. As I described in Chapter 6 - Cancer, the presence of a secondary cancer means that the only treatment in conventional medicine can be palliative. There will be no attempt to cure (in the conventional meaning of the word). Therefore, the number of investigations will be limited as surgery will not be an option.

If the cancer is primary, or suspected to be so, investigations will be carried out with several aims in mind. In conventional medicine, it is important to locate the exact anatomical site and to determine the histological appearances. This information defines the type of tumour and this will enable a decision to be made about whether surgery is a viable proposition.

Treatment:

It is generally considered that surgery with or without radiotherapy offers the only hope for people with cerebral tumours. There are less than 50% of people with malignant tumours alive one year later.

Dexamethasone, a corticosteroid, is frequently used to shrink the tumour and any surrounding oedema. This may lead to short-term relief of symptoms as the underlying progress is not affected. It can be helpful for people to improve their level of consciousness in order to settle their affairs and connect with family relationships.

- ENCEPHALITIS AND MENINGITIS -

This is inflammation of the substance of the brain and the lining around the brain, respectively. They are considered together as they lead to similar symptoms. In conventional medicine, there are considered to be several causes of meningitis including:

- infection by bacteria, virus or fungus - encephalitis is almost always associated with viruses
- drugs
- dyes used in radiology
- blood - see subarachnoid haemorrhage

Symptoms:

Both meningitis and encephalitis produce similar symptoms with meningitis having the more severe clinical picture. There is fever, severe occipital headache, photophobia and vomiting. Irritability and desire for quiet are common. The presence of a rash should be looked for and indicates severe disease.

Neck stiffness is found on examination which progresses to opisthotonos and eventually convulsions. These symptoms are obvious when the disease has progressed. Recognition at an early stage is essential if complications are to be avoided. The symptoms frequently follow an upper respiratory tract but may occur directly. If there is any suspicion of meningitis, appropriate measures must be taken immediately. The death rate in treated cases is 15%.

Encephalitis and viral meningitis have similar symptoms but milder. The exception is encephalitis caused by the herpes simplex virus which is severe and has a death rate of at least 20%.

Complications:

COMPLICATIONS	SYMPTOMS TO LOOK FOR
Venous sinus thrombosis or cerebral oedema	Drowsiness, squint
Septicaemia	Low blood pressure, rapid pulse, pale, ill and sweaty
Convulsions	Loss of consciousness, epileptiform attacks

TABLE 14.12: COMPLICATIONS OF MENINGITIS

Headaches are common after meningitis and encephalitis. In severe cases, there may be intellectual impairment.

Treatment:

This is invariably with antibiotics after examination of cerebrospinal fluid obtained by lumbar puncture. They must be given early in the course of bacterial meningitis to prevent or minimise the occurrence of complications. Herpes simplex encephalitis is treated with intravenous acyclovir.

Alternative management:

The main differentiation to be made is with meningism. This is the appearance of vague symptoms of neck stiffness, photophobia and headache with a fever. It is not serious and does not progress. If there is any suspicion of meningitis, antibiotic treatment and hospitalisation are necessary.

The occurrence of meningitis is due to general weakness of the immune system. Prevention depends on providing optimum situations for healthy childhood - see Chapter 19 - Children's Health.

In terms of Chinese medicine, this condition corresponds to Extreme Heat generating Wind. It is a consequence of pathogenic influences passing directly into deep levels of the body.

- SPINAL CORD DISORDERS -

CERVICAL SPONDYLOSIS

This is a condition of chronic cervical disc degeneration. The term is applied to a particular appearance of the X-ray. It becomes commoner with age. Many cervical spine X-rays in people over the age of 35 or 40 years will show some evidence of degeneration. Again we have a situation where many people have abnormal investigations but only a few will have symptoms.

It is not the disc spaces which give rise to pain but associated muscle spasm. There are many causes of muscle pains especially in the neck and so it may be inappropriate to assume that it is cervical spondylosis on the basis of an x-ray. This is why treatments by acupuncture, osteopathy, massage, aromatherapy and the like can frequently be beneficial.

Symptoms:

The overriding feature is of a pain in neck. It may, in severe cases, radiate to the area of supply of the nerve associated with the affected disc degeneration. These are usually the 5th, 6th, 7th and 8th cervical nerve roots. The pain in the neck is felt under the occiput and may radiate over the head into the forehead. There is often pain across the shoulders into the joint itself and in severe cases will radiate down the arm. There may be decreased tendon reflexes as this is a lower motor neurone problem.

On examination, the neck is stiff and there are reduced movements in the cervical spine. It may be worse in one direction than the others. There will also be tenderness under the base of the skull and in the trapezii muscles. The pain is worse for movement and especially those movements which involve use of the arms or neck. Therefore, window cleaning, carrying bags or weights, knitting, hanging curtains or washing and so on may lead to more pain.

Investigations:

An X-ray of the cervical spine may reveal degenerative changes in people with neck pain.

Treatment:

The main treatment is with drugs and physiotherapy. A collar is often used to restrict the movements in the cervical spine but only serves to help prevent the actions which cause pain. It will weaken the muscles in the neck and so, as with corsets for lumbago and sciatica, I usually tell people to only use them for specific situations.

Physiotherapy, in my experience, may make the problem worse and must be applied with care. Traction may be used in this condition and will do nothing for the spasm of the muscles of the neck but will lead to problems in the thoracic musculature. Also, treatment with heat or cold can make be unhelpful as there is no attempt to individualise the case and ensure that it is the sort of condition for which these may be appropriate.

The main drugs used are the group of non-steroidal anti-inflammatory agents which are described in detail in Chapter 10 - Musculoskeletal System. Therefore, little benefit will be obtained and there is the risk of very serious side-effects from these drugs.

On occasion, people may be prescribed 'muscle relaxants'. These are invariably benzodiazepine tranquillisers such as diazepam. They are rapidly addictive and when prescribed for pain can only lead to depression.

Alternative management:

In terms of Chinese medicine, this condition is due to Stagnation of Qi and Blood in the Channels. There may be several causes of this and underlying conditions. In an acute situation, particularly in those with strong energy, there may be an Invasion of Cold, Wind or Dampness. Injury may also play a part in some.

When the condition is more long-term, there may underlying syndromes of Blood Deficiency. There may be associated tingling and numbness in the arms and hands. There are similarities here with carpal tunnel syndrome and repetitive strain injury. Tension and worry can generate neck pain and there may be connection with Stagnation of Liver Qi. The Gall Bladder channel passes over the shoulders and up into the back of the head and Stagnation here can give rise to pain due to a problem in its paired organ, the Liver. Remember that the acupuncture point, Gall Bladder 21 in the trapezius muscle is connected with the uterus. Women may exhibit pain here due to a uterine imbalance.

LUMBAGO-SCIATICA

Lumbago is low back pain and is usually felt in the lumbar region. Sciatica is pain in the distribution of sciatic nerve and so is felt in the buttock and down the back of the leg. It may pass into the calf and foot in severe cases. The exact distribution of the pain depends on the particular nerve root affected but essentially it is either down the back or the side of the leg.

I have seen people develop pain in the back of this type with minimal trauma such as opening the boot of a car or washing the windscreen of a car. The onset may be sudden as in, "My back has gone, doctor". It may be gradual over a period of days or even weeks. The lumbago may precede the development of sciatica by months or years.

In a case of compression of the nerve root, there are considered to be for two main reasons:

- prolapsed intervertebral disc ('slipped disc')
- spinal tumour - primary or secondary (rare)

With prolapsed intervertebral disc, there is degeneration of the discs from the early 20's onwards. The disc is considered to herniate outwards and press onto the nerve. This can be due to trauma such as twisting the spine while flexed, e.g. lifting a heavy object incorrectly or in childbirth.

Symptoms:

In the case of lumbago, there is low back pain which is brought on by bending. It may be better for heat or warmth. There is often tenderness over the lumbar musculature. Sciatic pain radiates down the leg in the distribution of the affected nerve root. It usually starts in the buttock and is felt down the back or side of the leg. It is typically worse for coughing, sneezing and movement. It may be difficult to move the leg and some people have excruciating pain and cannot move at all. Some people have sensory symptoms of 'pins and needles' or numbness.

In severe cases there will be evidence of motor involvement of a lower motor neurone type. There is weakness of the muscles of the affected nerve root. There are weak calf muscles and foot drop, i.e. inability to dorsiflex the foot in the case of 5th lumbar affection. There are weak quadriceps muscles and no knee tendon reflex in the case of 4th lumbar affection.

In the case of spinal cord compression from a spinal tumour the symptoms will be more severe, there will be a combination of motor and sensory nerve loss and the symptoms will be progressive. There will be little, if any, improvement with treatment.

Investigations:

The main investigation will be that of myelography. It will reveal if there is any compression of the nerve root and where this is present. Plain X-ray may reveal degenerative changes in the lumbar spine but these are so common that they cannot be relied upon to be the 'cause' of the problem. Similar comments were made in relation to cervical spondylosis.

Treatment:

The first thing which people are told to do is rest. This is total initially in the case of severe pain or with sciatica and rest in bed is advised as the best way of attaining this. This may be continued for 2 to 4 weeks and then back strengthening exercises for the next 10 to 14 days. A spinal support or surgical corset may be given.

If there is no improvement then surgery will be considered in order to remove the compression of the disc on the nerve root. Laminectomy[15] does not remove the disc but relieves the pressure. The same will also be considered if the condition is recurrent.

Further surgery in resistant cases may be spinal fusion. All surgical procedures tend to further weaken the back and can lead to great difficulties in treatment by alternative medicine.

Alternative management:

In terms of Chinese medicine, there are two main syndromes which are seen. In people with strong energy, these symptoms are due to Stagnation of Qi and Blood in the Channels due to an Invasion of Wind or Damp or Cold. This is the type of situation where people develop acute lower back pain and find it difficult and painful to move. Treatment can lead to immediate relief. It is the situation where acupuncture and osteopathy have a well-known reputation for almost miraculous improvement.

Whilst I am on the subject of osteopathy, there are far more indications, of course, for its use than merely backache. There are many conditions which benefit from manipulation and it is outside the scope of this book to list them all. Nevertheless, osteopathy provides an effective treatment for musculoskeletal conditions of many types.

In terms of back pain, the Alexander technique is extremely helpful for remedying long-term postural problems. This may necessarily be on-going in order to correct spinal deformities. It works on very subtle levels and can be almost meditative in its methodology.

In weaker people, and this is the common situation in the West, there is usually an underlying syndrome of Kidney Deficiency. This is because the Kidney is responsible for the functioning of the lower back and knees. Treatment, in most cases therefore, needs to be directed at underlying issues of Kidney function as outlined in Chapter 9 - Urinary System. Strong treatments of this condition may lead to worsening of symptoms as the energy is not strong enough to cope. Gentle tonifying treatments are more appropriate and need to be applied long-term. In the short term, the back pain may not change much but you will be looking for improvement on inner levels first.

---

[15] In my experience, many people who undergo laminectomy gain little relief. Relapses are common in the months after surgery. A study of workers who had undergone laminectomy showed that they were six times more likely to develop back injuries. James R, et al Journal of Occupational Medicine, May 1990 v32 n5 p468(5).

- DISEASES OF THE PERIPHERAL NERVES -

MONONEUROPATHY

This is disease of a single nerve. It is usually due to injury or compression. A typical example of this is carpal tunnel syndrome which is described in Chapter 10 - Musculoskeletal System. Another common situation is injury of the ulnar nerve at the elbow, the radial nerve in the axilla[16] or the peroneal nerve at the knee. The clinical picture is one of a lower motor neurone weakness with sensory loss. They may take up to 4 to 6 weeks to recover.

A multiple form is seen in systemic diseases. These include:

- diabetes mellitus
- autoimmune disease, e.g. systemic lupus erythematosus, polyarteritis nodosa, temporal arteritis, rheumatoid arthritis
- sarcoidosis
- AIDS

- DISORDERS OF THE HEAD AND FACE -

TRIGEMINAL NEURALGIA

This condition occurs mainly in the elderly and is of unknown cause in conventional medicine. It is also known as 'tic douloureux'.

Symptoms:

There is pain in the face in the distribution of the fifth (trigeminal) cranial nerve. Maxillary and/or mandibular divisions are usually affected. It is rarely felt around the temple or eye and most people have pain over the upper and lower jaws. Particular areas which are troublesome are the gums, the edge of the nostril and in front of the ear. The pain is characteristically severe and sharp or stabbing. It occurs in episodes where there will be pain every day and probably all day for several days, weeks or months. It is sharp in nature and can be excruciating. There are often trigger areas where contact such as washing, brushing the teeth or eating will set off attacks of pain. There are remissions when the pain goes but these become shorter and shorter as time passes.

Treatment:

This is usually with carbamazepine, an anticonvulsant. It is frequently used for any neuralgic condition. It works to a variable extent and there are side-effects on other parts of the central nervous system. I treated a woman with this condition who, whenever she took this drug, would develop weakness in her legs and would have to use a wheelchair.

Some people may be given benzodiazepines or phenytoin. The aim of all the drug treatments is to sedate the central nervous system and damp down its activity.

Surgical destruction or injection with alcohol may be used in intransigent cases to destroy the nerve function. This leads to numbness in the face.

In terms of Chinese medicine, the usual syndromes which correspond are WindHeat Invasion, Fire in the Liver and Stomach or Yin Deficiency with Yang excess.

CASE

A woman of 53 years came for treatment of left-sided facial pain. This had begun some 3 years previously. She complained of pain in front of her left ear to around the left eye and affecting the

---

[16] This is known as 'drunkard's' palsy as it occurs after falling asleep with the arm over the back of a chair.

upper lips and left lower jaw. This gradually worsened and developed into a paralysis of the left side of her face. She also had double vision and floaters in the visual field. All her symptoms were worse at the end of the day.

Her other symptoms included dry mouth, palpitations, poor appetite, heartburn, intestinal bloating and cramps, diarrhoea and constipation, frequent urination and cold limbs. Her Chinese medical diagnosis was Spleen and Kidney Yang Deficiency with Blood Deficiency. The symptoms in her face had developed as a result of weakness and this needed to be remedied before any improvement would be seen. It is common to see facial pain and symptoms in people with Stomach or Spleen (digestive) weakness. This is because the Stomach channel begins under the eye and passes downwards over the face on its way to the Stomach.

I treated her with acupuncture and herbs. She gradually began to feel more energetic and her digestive symptoms improved. She received treatment over the course of six months. At the end of that time she felt generally better. Her digestive symptoms had eased and her urination was less frequent. Her facial pain was somewhat lessened. The main difficulty here is the paralysis which has been present for some years. It may be that it will not improve but she will be happy if the pain is a lot easier as it is this which is causing most problems.

FACIAL PARALYSIS (BELL'S PALSY)

This is a disorder of the seventh cranial nerve of unknown cause. It is considered to be associated with oedema of the facial nerve as it passes through the facial canal in the base of the skull and this may be associated with a viral infection. Men are just as likely as women to suffer and it can come on at any age.

Symptoms:

There is a one-sided facial paralysis where the person cannot close the affected eye. The mouth is drawn over to the opposite side and saliva and fluids may escape from the corner of the mouth. There is paralysis of the upper and lower parts of the affected side of face. The taste may be affected over the front two-thirds of the tongue. It typically lasts for several weeks and then subsides. Some people (15%) are left with a chronic weakness where wasting will be evident. There is considered to be recovery in 85% of cases after 2 to 3 weeks which is usually complete after 2 to 3 months. Recovery may take many months.

This is an example of a lower motor neurone type of paralysis. If the forehead muscles are normal on both sides then the facial paralysis is of the upper motor neurone type as will occur in a stroke and the approach to this will be completely different. It is important to make this differentiation.

Treatment:

There is little which is effective since the cause is not known. Corticosteroids are often given in a short reducing course. Around 60 mg daily are given at first, reducing to zero over a week or 10 days. In some cases, adrenocorticotrophic hormone (ACTH) may be injected to stimulate the person's own corticosteroid levels. Care is taken to reduce or prevent problems of corneal damage as the eyelid cannot close on the affected side.

Persistent cases are treated by cosmetic surgery perhaps with an attempt to reactivate the nerve by joining it to a normal nerve.

Alternative management:

In China, it occurs in large numbers in the spring and is due to the winds that appear at that time of year. Certainly people often report that it came on after they were in a draught. In terms of Chinese medicine, this is a case of WindCold Invasion affecting the channels of the face. In the West, there is almost always an underlying deficient condition which allows for this invasion.

A case of facial paralysis with facial pain is described above.

- HEADACHE AND MIGRAINE -

This is a pain in the head. It is very common and no-one probably does not suffer from this at some time in their lives. Many people have recurrent problems. An occasional one is probably a 'normal' reaction to many influences either physical or emotional. However, if they become severe or frequent, they indicate a chronic imbalance.

There are many different associations with the symptom of headache. In conventional medicine, the search is for an underlying physical cause which can then be treated and most of these are situated in parts of the head or neck. The vast majority of causes are seen in Western medicine as being non-serious. The exceptions to this are cerebral tumour, meningitis and cerebral vascular problems.

Cranial arteritis is seen in the elderly. Such headaches tend to be severe and diffuse. Temporal tenderness is only one manifestation. They are usually severe enough to be troublesome at night and interfere with sleep.

Pain can be referred from eye diseases such as glaucoma and iritis. They are frontal in site and there are the signs of the underlying disease. 'Eye strain' is conventionally considered to be uncommon. However, some people who overuse their eyes, especially in conditions of poor lighting and when tired will develop headaches.

Nasal or sinus disease can produce pains in the head and these can be severe. The most usual sinus to be involved is the maxillary. Pain is felt either in the face with tenderness over the sinuses There will also be the other symptoms of sinusitis.

Dental conditions can cause headaches. They are usually frontal and again can be in the face. Tapping on the suspected tooth will produce pain. Such causes of pain are notoriously difficult to pin down on occasion and I have known people have recurrent dental surgery in an attempt to track down the source of the pain.

Aural conditions lead to headaches as in cases of otitis media or mastoiditis.

Cervical spondylosis is commonly associated with headaches. They are usually occipital in site. The pain is felt at the back of the neck, up into the head and can on occasions radiate into the frontal area. It can be severe with limitation of movement of the neck and perhaps creaking and cracking.

A cold stimulus on the soft palate leads to a frontal headache in the so-called 'ice-cream headache'.

Neuralgias in the head and face typically cause severe pains. Trigeminal neuralgia is usually in the face although if the ophthalmic division of the nerve is affected then it will be felt further up the head. It is classically episodic and sharp. It occurs in paroxysms and is intractable. The pain of post-herpetic neuralgia however is continuous and burning in quality. It follows on from herpes zoster of the face and here it is usually severe.

Meningeal irritation is one of the conditions which indicates a serious and possibly life-threatening situation. The three diseases to bear in mind are encephalitis, meningitis and subarachnoid haemorrhage. The pain is generalised but is worse occipitally. It is continuous, of an aching or boring quality and there are signs of 'meningism'[17]. This is evidence of meningeal irritation and exhibits itself as photophobia and neck stiffness. The neck stiffness can be elicited by raising the neck and trying to put the person's chin on their chest. This will produce marked pain in the occiput and will reveal a lot of neck stiffness. A fever is often in evidence with the first two conditions.

Investigations:

This depends on the history. As can be seen above, conventional medicine considers about two or three conditions particularly serious and so the person will be investigated if these are suspected. Otherwise, treatment is instituted with no further action being taken.

---

[17] A difficulty arises in diagnosis because meningism of a lesser degree may be seen in children with upper respiratory infections and fever. The symptoms are mild and do not progress. This situation and early meningitis can be confused in the unwary.

MIGRAINE

These are periodic headaches which are typically one sided in site. The term migraine is derived from 'hemicrania'- one side of head. In conventional medicine, migraine is considered to be due to a disturbance in blood flow to the brain. There is firstly constriction of blood vessels followed by vasodilatation. It is the constriction in the blood vessels which is associated the visual symptoms and dilatation leads to the classical headache. This explanation explains the emphasis in conventional treatment of using drugs which affect blood flow. Three-quarters of people with migraine have a family history of this condition.

Symptoms:

Visual disturbances such as flashing or coloured lights are a common association. There may be vomiting during an attack. There are several precipitating factors where the headaches are more likely to occur. They are more likely around the time of menstruation, with flashing lights, emotional stress, anxiety and with certain foods. They usually occur between puberty to middle life and come in paroxysms.

An attack is different for each person but typically it starts with visual symptoms as above. In severe cases there may even be pins and needles or weakness of one part or half of the body. This can last for up to half an hour. Then the pain starts, usually in one spot around the temple and spreads to the whole of one side of the head. It is severe, throbbing and there may or may not be vomiting. There is usually a degree of photophobia. There is often pallor, sweating and an attack may be so severe that the person may be prostrated. Many people end up in bed and have to lie in a darkened room. Tiredness is a common association and some people may feel weakened for a day or so after an attack. They typically occur at periods of relaxation and so weekends and the first few days of a holiday are common times for migraine.

Treatment:

It is helpful for some people to avoid triggers especially if it is something specific such as red wine or prawns. Drugs are frequently used conventionally. They may either be those which are designed to prevent attacks or to be given during an attack.

TREATMENT	TREATMENT LEVEL	COMMENTS
Diuretic	1	Aims to reduce fluid retention. Variable effectiveness. Described in detail in Chapter 7 - Cardiovascular System
Paracetamol with buclizine	2	Simple analgesic with antihistamine
Ergotamine	3	Powerful drug which constricts arteries. When used in excess it may cause gangrene
Tranquilliser	4	Used on the assumption that there is an emotional basis. Rapidly addictive and causes depression when used for pain
Clonidine	5	Also used in high blood pressure and flushing attacks. Dangerous to stop suddenly
Betablocker	5	Described in detail in Chapter 7 - Cardiovascular System. Weakens the digestion, heart and kidneys
Sumatriptan	5	New, powerful drug. When used frequently it tends to lead to more migraine attacks presumably due to a depleting effect
Methysergide	6	Powerful drug related to lysergic acid diethylamide (LSD). Causes fibrosis in the abdomen with horrific consequences. Must not be given for more than 6 months continuously. Must be withdrawn slowly

TABLE 14.13: CONVENTIONAL TREATMENT OF MIGRAINE

Alternative management:

The conventional label of migraine is a loose collection of many different energetic entities. In terms of Chinese Medicine there are common associations with Stagnant Liver Qi, Stomach Heat or Liver Blood Deficiency. With imbalances of the Liver there may be a particular association with emotional disturbances or the menses. In the case of Stomach Heat, the headaches will be worse with dietary factors such as red wine, chocolate and shellfish - all of which are heating energetically. Liver Blood Deficient headaches tend to be worse with standing, overwork and during or after menstruation.

The typical site of the headache will tend to be temporal with Liver pathologies and frontal with a Stomach imbalance. Associated symptoms include irritability and visual disturbances with Liver imbalances. This type of headache will be precipitated or exacerbated by the oral contraceptive which Stagnates Liver Qi. This connection is discussed in detail in Chapter 18 - Gynaecology.

Vomiting is common if the Stomach is primarily involved. Clearly the Stomach and Liver functions are closely interwoven as combinations of these symptoms may occur and I discuss some such connections in Chapter 13 - Gastrointestinal System.

CASE

A woman of 32 years came for treatment of her migraine headaches. These had begun at the age of 15 years but had been worse for the past 9 years. They took the form of right-sided headaches mainly around the right eye. Occasionally, the pain would pass back to the right side of the occiput. Nausea and sometimes vomiting always occurred with the headache. She had attacks twice each month but also had what she described as ordinary headaches more often. These would affect the temples and forehead for several days each week.

Her general energy was low and particularly so in the afternoon. She had low back pain regularly and a tendency to loose motions. Her periods tended to be heavy at the beginning with some cramping pains. The diagnosis, in terms of Chinese medicine, was Spleen Qi Deficiency with Damp Accumulation and Liver Qi Stagnation.

I treated her with acupuncture and herbs together with general advice about diet to strengthen the digestive energy and relaxation. She worked long hours in the city with much travelling each day. Gradually, after a couple of months treatment she began to feel better with more energy and less headaches. Her migraines declined in number to once per month before the period and then stopped completely. After 6 months of treatment she felt well with only occasional headaches when she was overtired or particularly stressed.

CASE

A woman of 35 years came for treatment of her migraine headaches. These had been off and on from the age of 13 years. They resumed whenever she felt particularly stressed. Her energy was slightly low. The migraines took the form of pain in the occipital region which passed over the head to above the left eye. She would have associated nausea and dizziness. Her other symptoms included abdominal bloating and slight oedema before her periods.

In terms of Chinese medicine, this is Liver Qi Stagnation with Spleen Qi Deficiency. Her energy was not so low as in the case described above. This was reflected in treatment as she responded very quickly. Her headaches disappeared after three treatments and she continued for a short while to consolidate her progress. She had also had other alternative medical treatments in the past and this helps people to respond more effectively.

- HOW TO RECOGNISE A SERIOUS CONDITION OF THE NERVOUS SYSTEM -

Diseases of the central nervous system are common in our society and the symptoms listed below are extremely common. It is important to know how to recognise if a symptom arises from a serious situation. You can use Table 14.14 as a guide to refer to when faced with a person who has one or more of these symptoms. I do not mention disease labels in the column on the right as I would not expect you to be able to diagnose conventionally. Seriousness can be assessed merely by reference to symptom pictures. However, you will be able to recognise that there are clinical appearances which would be diagnosed as a particular disease. For example, if you look at headache and its seriousness, you will see that this is the appearance of a brain tumour.

SYMPTOMS	WHEN TO WORRY
Headache	Progressive, severe with short history, with other central nervous system symptoms
Tremor	Severe, progressive
Numbness	Severe, progressive
Paralysis	Always
Tingling	Severe, progressive
Dizziness	Severe, progressive
Convulsions	Always
Loss of consciousness	Not if short duration with specific trigger (see Page 105)
Stiffness	Severe
Pain	Severe

TABLE 14.14: HOW TO RECOGNISE A SERIOUS CONDITION OF THE CENTRAL NERVOUS SYSTEM

- SUMMARY -

Conventional anatomy and physiology of the central nervous system are complex.

The essence of physiology is the important aspect and this knowledge of function can provide most of what an alternative practitioner needs to know.

Symptoms of central nervous system dysfunction are similar in many varied disorders. It is their development and timing which are the important factors in determining the underlying process.

Conventional medicine is not particularly effective at treating such disorders.

Alternative medicine can offer people real benefits, sometimes to a surprising degree, in central nervous system disease.

You must know the presenting symptoms of the life-threatening conditions, i.e. meningitis, brain tumour.

15 ENDOCRINE SYSTEM

OBJECTIVES:

At the end of this Chapter you will be able to:
Describe the differences between the alternative and conventional views of the endocrine system
Describe the main symptoms of diseases covered in this Chapter
Explain the relevant management by an alternative practitioner of each disorder
Describe the issues of treating endocrine system disease complicated by hormone replacements

- INTRODUCTION -

The endocrine system is one of the few areas of the body where there is a recognition of balance by conventional medicine. There are control mechanisms which serve to maintain bodily functions within narrow limits. In addition, hormones from the same or different organs may have effects which are opposite to each other. These need to be in balance for the body to function efficiently. For example, in the case of blood sugar control, insulin and its opposite hormone, glucagon, are partially responsible for maintaining sugar levels in the blood within closely determined limits. Other hormones such as corticosteroids, adrenaline and noradrenaline also have a part to play in this. This is helpful for alternative practitioners as ideas of balance are vital features of alternative medicine.

In endocrine disturbances, there may be an overactivity or an underactivity. Each of these represents a particular extreme and there are close relationships with symptom pictures recognised in Chinese medicine. Homoeopaths may recognise remedy pictures in the descriptions given later. In terms of Chinese medicine, the duality of Yin/Yang philosophy can be recognised in the extremes of imbalances seen in endocrine disorders. For example, overactivity of the adrenal gland can be recognised as an excess of Yang energy and underactivity of the adrenal gland as a lack of Yang energy, i.e. a Yin state. These comments are amplified when discussing each disease in turn.

There has been rapid progress recently in the conventional investigation of endocrine disease. It is now possible to determine blood levels of many hormones and so gross dysfunction can be diagnosed more accurately. Disorders which are the result of too little of the respective hormone being released into the circulation are treated by replacement. Other endocrine disorders are due to overactivity and treatment, conventionally, comprises either destruction of the gland, partial removal or the use of a chemical which blocks the action of the hormone released.

The issue for alternative practitioners is when you see people who either have severe disease or who take replacement hormones. Endocrine disease of a severe degree may be life-threatening. Care must be taken with such cases. If hormone replacements are stopped or reduced without adequate checks on blood levels there may be quite serious problems. For example, it is manifestly dangerous for a person with diabetes mellitus taking daily insulin injections to reduce or stop insulin without effective treatment of the underlying condition. This is true for all endocrine abnormalities.

An additional situation to consider is the general effect of alternative medical treatment on a person's hormone balance. Alternative treatments do not treat one specific area. It is necessary to bear in mind the effect on endocrine hormones whatever the presenting complaint. There are significant numbers of people taking regular hormone replacements[1] who will come for treatment of what they consider to be an unrelated problem. Alternative medicine will have the effect of improving endocrine function. Reduction of prescribed replacement hormones will be necessary to avoid overdosage. Monitoring is of prime importance to ensure that such situations are handled safely and appropriately.

- BASIC ANATOMY AND PHYSIOLOGY -

I want to spend some time describing the essential features of the endocrine system. In addition, I shall introduce some information which may be new to you but will hopefully serve to make some connections with alternative medical views. The information which is useful to know prior to study of the endocrine system is summarised in Table 15.1.

As a preliminary to study of disease of the endocrine system you are able to:
List the organs contained in the endocrine system
State the hormones secreted by each organ
Describe the function of these hormones
Explain the homeostatic mechanisms and feedback systems of the endocrine system

TABLE 15.1: OBJECTIVES FOR ANATOMY AND PHYSIOLOGY AS PREREQUISITE FOR STUDY OF DISEASE OF THE ENDOCRINE SYSTEM

The endocrine system is composed of the hypothalamus, pituitary and various end organs[2], the most important of which, for clinical purposes, are the thyroid, ovaries, testes and adrenal glands. All these organs are interconnected and are influenced by feedback mechanisms of control.

Hypothalamus
Pituitary
Pineal
Thyroid
Parathyroid
Pancreas
Adrenal
Ovary
Testis

TABLE 15.2: ENDOCRINE ORGANS

---

[1] By hormone replacement in this Chapter, I am referring to the prescription of a hormone in a deficiency disease. Hormone replacement therapy may be used to refer to oestrogen and progesterone supplements during or after the menopause. This is something quite different and is discussed in Chapter 18 - Gynaecology. This phrase is somewhat of a misnomer since it is not a replacement. Menopause is not a disease state and low oestrogen levels at this time are not a deficiency disease.

[2] An end organ of the endocrine system is one which is stimulated by the pituitary gland to produce a hormone. The hormone has an effect on body tissues/metabolism.

The hypothalamus can be considered as the centre. It releases hormones which influence the pituitary. This, in turn, secretes hormones to stimulate a relevant end organ. For example, thyrotrophic releasing hormone (TRH) is formed in the hypothalamus and stimulates the production by the pituitary of thyroid stimulating hormone (TSH). Consequently the thyroid gland is stimulated into action in response to circulating levels of TSH. The thyroid gland releases thyroxine (T_4) and tri-iodothyronine (T_3). These circulating levels of T_3 and T_4 have an effect on the hypothalamus.

If the circulating levels of T_3 and T_4 are low, the hypothalamus increases its production of TRH. If circulating levels of T_3 and T_4 are high, the hypothalamus reduces the secretion of TRH. In this way, levels of T_3 and T_4 are kept within normal limits. There are similar *negative feedback* mechanisms for the adrenal gland, testes and ovaries. The parathyroid and pancreas have a different mechanism as they produce hormones in response to blood levels of the substances they control. Therefore, the parathyroid responds to blood calcium levels and the pancreas to blood sugar levels.

The secretion of hypothalamic hormones is dependent upon a wide variety of stimuli of nervous, metabolic, physical and hormonal origin. The hypothalamus is the interface between the endocrine system and the central nervous system. It is the means by which external events influence the endocrine system. It responds to changes in temperature, to the amount of light in the environment and to psychological factors. There is a great similarity to the Chinese view of the human being where natural life cycles and the environment have important roles to play in human health.[3] These are the beginnings of understanding in conventional thought that perhaps there is a relationship between these. Such ideas are very much at a primitive stage in conventional medicine and have not developed into available treatments. They will, hopefully, lead to increased understanding by conventional practitioners of insights which have long been recognised by alternative systems of medicine.

The endocrine glands may also be considered from the viewpoint of the chakras. The base chakra relates to the testes and ovary, the adrenals relate to the chakra around the kidney area, the pancreas is in the solar plexus, the thymus relates to the heart chakra, the thyroid is in the throat chakra, the pituitary relates to the brow and the pineal to the crown.

- CLASSIFICATION OF ENDOCRINE SYSTEM DISEASE -

The most important organs to consider, in terms of clinical significance, are the thyroid, ovary, testis and adrenal. Pathologies of the ovary are discussed in Chapter 18 - Gynaecology. In conventional medicine, the classification centres on the physical organ which is responsible for the imbalance. This is shown in Table 15.3.

It can be seen from this Table that, there is no mention of hypothalamic disorders as they are extremely difficult to diagnose. Therefore, the interconnections between the hypothalamus and the external environment and psychological state are completely missed by most conventional practitioners. The main treatments applied to the diseases listed are by affecting the end organ, for example, thyroid or adrenal. This is a classical case of suppression, in any terms, since the root is not treated. The administration of external hormones will only serve to suppress the function of the endocrine system. Hyperthyroidism (overactivity of the thyroid gland), for example, is a result of a

---

[3] 'The three months of spring .. It is desirable to sleep at night, get up early in the morning, take a walk in the yard, to loosen up hair and relax the body ... The three months of summer .... It is desirable to sleep at night and get up early in the morning, to have no dislike of sunlight, possess no will of anger so that things will bloom beautifully and so that energy will move outward through perspiration as if in love with the outside world ....The three months of autumn .... It is desirable to sleep early and get up early with the crowing of the rooster, to maintain a peaceful will in order to slow down the killing effects of autumn, to constrict the energy of the spirits in order to calm down the energy of the autumn, to refrain from moving outward in order to clean up the energy of the lungs .... The three months of winter ...... It is desirable to sleep early and get up late, to await the arrival of sunlight, so that the will remains dormant as if hiding or pretending, not unlike someone with private intentions, not unlike someone with all his desires already fulfilled.' "Neijing" Volume 1, Chapter 2. Translation by Henry Lu.

psychological disturbance. Removing part of the gland surgically or destroying the gland by radioactivity does nothing to resolve the underlying imbalance.

Pituitary gland
    Tumours of the pituitary
    Pituitary overactivity
    Pituitary underactivity
        Diabetes insipidus
Thyroid gland
    Hyperthyroidism
    Hypothyroidism
    Goitre
    Hashimoto's thyroiditis
    Subacute thyroiditis
    Tumours of the thyroid gland
        Benign tumours
        Carcinoma
Pancreas
    Diabetes mellitus
Adrenal gland
    Adrenal Cortex
        Overactivity
            Cushing's syndrome
            Hyperaldosteronism
        Underactivity
            Addison's disease
    Adrenal Medulla
        Phaeochromocytoma

TABLE 15.3: CONVENTIONAL CLASSIFICATION OF ENDOCRINE DISEASE

Those in italics are the most important clinically.

A more practical classification, from the point of view of an alternative practitioner, would be to consider the severity of the disorder and its rapidity of change. Thus, a disease such as diabetes mellitus which may produce rapid deterioration in health would be more severe than hypothyroidism which presents a much slower clinical progress. In this way it is possible to produce a classification as in Table 15.4

MILD DISEASE

Hyperthyroidism
Hypothyroidism
Cushing's syndrome
Diabetes mellitus
Diabetes insipidus
Addison's disease

SEVERE DISEASE

TABLE 15.4: ALTERNATIVE CLASSIFICATION OF DISEASE OF THE ENDOCRINE SYSTEM

- DIABETES INSIPIDUS -

This is an uncommon disease but is useful to mention since it may be confused with diabetes mellitus which is described later. Diabetes, the word, refers to the passage of large volumes of urine and before urine testing was available the distinction between these two diseases was made by tasting the urine. People with diabetes insipidus pass large quantities of urine which is bland to the taste whilst those with diabetes mellitus pass large quantities of urine which is sweet.

In conventional medicine, there are two types of diabetes insipidus. A cranial type is associated with an inadequate production of antidiuretic hormone (vasopressin) by the pituitary gland and a renal type due to the kidney unresponsive to the effects of vasopressin.

All types of diabetes insipidus are rare. The cranial type may result from pituitary tumour or after meningitis and head injury. Occasionally a genetic defect is seen. Diabetes insipidus due to kidney unresponsiveness may be genetic, heavy metal poisoning or treatment with lithium.[4]

Symptoms:

There are the characteristic symptoms of frequent urination, the persistent passage of large quantities of pale urine and constant thirst. The person may pass up to 20 or more litres of urine in 24 hours. The urine is clear in appearance. Eventually as dehydration develops there will be confusion and eventually fits and unconsciousness.

Investigations:

The usual way of diagnosing cranial diabetes insipidus is to withhold water and measure the specific gravity of urine which does not rise in this disease. It will do so if vasopressin is given. The main distinction to be made is between this condition and diabetes mellitus.

Treatment:

This is usually with the long acting type of vasopressin, desmopressin (DDAVP). It is given intranasally or intramuscularly. The dosage in each case is individually assessed depending upon how much urine is produced. Other drugs which may be used in treatment include thiazide diuretics, carbamazepine or chlorpropamide. Thiazide diuretics remain the only effective drug therapy for renal diabetes insipidus and reduce urine volume in this condition by about 50%.

- THYROID GLAND -

The thyroid gland produces two hormones, thyroxine (T_4) and tri-iodothyronine (T_3) which control the rate of the metabolism. Production of these hormones is influenced by thyroid stimulating hormone (TSH) produced by the pituitary gland. The gland itself is situated over the thyroid cartilage in the neck and upper end of the trachea. It may be palpable in women with no other indications of thyroid imbalance. Embryologically, the thyroid gland originates in the pharynx between anterior and posterior sections of the tongue. It migrates downwards to its eventual position in the throat along the thyroglossal duct. If this duct persists beyond foetal life, cysts may occasionally develop in children. This connection between the thyroid gland and the tongue, throat and larynx is explored later in the section on alternative management of thyroid disease.

The two main clinical syndromes of the thyroid gland are overactivity and underactivity. They provide excellent examples of the need for balance within the body to prevent the appearance of the extremes of excess production or underproduction of hormones. Both syndromes are primarily autoimmune in nature in that the body produces antibodies against the thyroid gland. In overactivity of the thyroid gland, hyperthyroidism, these antibodies serve to stimulate the thyroid gland. In underactivity of the thyroid gland, hypothyroidism, these antibodies are destructive in nature. The natural history of thyroid disease is firstly to respond to the autoimmune disturbance by stimulation and then by exhaustion. This is a common feature of all organs in that the first stage of disease is of

---

[4] Lithium is used in the treatment of manic depression.

overactivity to be replaced eventually by non-reaction. I would remind you here of the comments I made about immune system disease on Page 192 and in Table 10.1.

HYPERTHYROIDISM[5]

This is overproduction of the thyroid hormones, thyroxine (T_4) and/or tri-iodothyronine (T_3). There are frequently associated autoimmune disorders such as diabetes mellitus and pernicious anaemia.

Hyperthyroidism is common. It affects about 1 in 20 women at some time in their lives, usually between 15 and 20 years of age. Men are rarely affected with nine times more cases seen in women. There are increased levels of thyroid hormone in the blood so levels of thyroid stimulating hormone are reduced sometimes to extremely low levels. This is an attempt by the pituitary to reduce the amount of stimulation to the thyroid gland. There is invariably an associated goitre[6].

In most people with hyperthyroidism, the thyroid gland is either generally overactive or there are several nodules which are overproductive of thyroid hormones. The latter cases are known as toxic nodular goitres. They tend to occur in older people whilst the general overactive type with diffuse goitres is seen in young people.

Symptoms:

The symptoms of hyperthyroidism are conventionally explained as due to an overproduction of thyroid hormones. These are responsible for controlling the metabolic rate, i.e. the amount of energy consumed by the body. A by-product of energy usage is heat and so many of the symptoms are related to this.

There are feelings of heat with intolerance to heat, sweating, increased appetite yet weight loss, raised heart rate, palpitations, diarrhoea, tiredness, anxiety, tremor of the fingers. It is common for the thyroid gland to be enlarged (goitre). It is usually a soft, diffuse swelling of both lobes.

There are other features which are difficult to explain conventionally. These include exophthalmos, pretibial myxoedema[7], finger clubbing[8], reduced fertility, menstrual irregularities and muscle weakness.

Exophthalmos is a protrusion of one or both eyes. It can be detected in most cases by observing the white sclera above and below the iris. Exposure of the cornea may result from eyelids failing to close properly leading to keratitis. There is a grittiness in the eye and excessive watering. The conjunctivae can become red and swollen. Double vision can be present because of the weakness of extraocular muscles. It is first detected when the person is asked to look upwards and outwards.

In some, exophthalmos may precede the development of the symptoms of hyperthyroidism by some months or years. The conventional treatment of hyperthyroidism has no effect on exophthalmos which would again confirm that the underlying process is unaffected by such treatment.

The natural history of hyperthyroidism is variable. Some people recover within a few months or a year whilst other have more persistent problems. A few develop a 'thyrotoxic crisis' which is uncommon now with drug therapy given to all. This is a state of severe mental and physical exhaustion with delirium, delusions or mania, dehydration, palpitations, oedema and fever. The person is literally 'burning up'.

Complications:

COMPLICATIONS	SYMPTOMS TO LOOK FOR
Cardiac failure	Oedema, breathlessness
Thyroid (thyrotoxic) crisis	Extremely rapid heart rate, high fever, severe agitation

TABLE 15.4: COMPLICATIONS OF HYPERTHYROIDISM

---

[5] It can also be referred to as thyrotoxicosis. The term, Grave's disease is reserved to describe hyperthyroidism of an autoimmune nature.

[6] Goitre is a swelling of the neck due to thyroid gland enlargement.

[7] This is thickening of the skin over the tibia. Confusingly, hypothyroidism may also be known as myxoedema.

[8] This is described on Page 162.

Investigations:

There are raised levels of thyroxine (T_4) and tri-iodothyronine (T_3) with reduced or virtually absent levels of thyroid stimulating hormone. There is a wide range of normal and errors occur so several estimates are the ideal. The presence of minor symptoms with blood levels near normality may not need immediate conventional treatment. It is easy, on occasions, for conventional practitioners to assume that a diagnosis is one of hyperthyroidism and to initiate treatment. However, it is the complete picture that is more important and as with all investigations, single estimations should be viewed as only one aspect of the case. A radionuclide scan of the thyroid may be used to assess the appearance of the thyroid gland.

Treatment:

The aim of conventional treatment is to achieve normal blood levels of thyroid hormones. There are three methods of doing this.

Antithyroid drugs:

Antithyroid drugs block the function of the thyroid gland and thereby reduce the amount of thyroid hormone produced. A commonly used example is carbimazole in the UK and its relative, methimazole, in the US. Propylthiouracil is occasionally used in the event of allergy to carbimazole.

Antithyroid drugs are given initially for 3 to 4 weeks, according to the severity of the condition and the size of the goitre. Thereafter, the dose is reduced according to symptoms. The aim is to maintain a normal thyroid state with as little medication as possible. The normal dosage of carbimazole is between 5 and 30 mg daily.

Overtreatment with antithyroid drugs will result in increased thyroid stimulating hormone production by the pituitary and an increase in thyroid size. Carbimazole may be given as sole treatment or as a preparation for surgery. If used alone, these drugs are given for at least 1 year and restricted to people who do not have a large goitre.

Just under half of people treated in this way remit and do not require further treatment. The probability of relapse after 6-12 months treatment with antithyroid drugs is more likely in the presence of autoimmune disease.

Antithyroid drugs may produce toxic effects. The commonest is a rash and the most serious are blood disorders, agranulocytosis being the most frequent. Routine white cell counts are of little value in its early detection as it occurs with dramatic suddenness. People taking these drugs must be told to report a sore throat and to stop the drug immediately until it is clear whether agranulocytosis has occurred or not.

Betablockers are commonly given in addition to specific antithyroid drugs to reduce symptoms of palpitations, increased heart rate, anxiety, tremors, sweating and so forth. These are merely symptomatic in their action and have no influence on the thyroid gland itself.

Surgical treatment:

This is usually applied if the person is too young for radioactive iodine or antithyroid drugs have failed. People with large goitres may be offered surgery no matter what their age. Men are considered to relapse more often after antithyroid drug treatment and so may be considered for surgery earlier rather than later.

The amount of thyroid gland which is removed at operation is based upon an assessment made by the surgeon. Clearly the function of the thyroid gland is reduced after partial removal and about 4 out of 5 people who have a partial thyroidectomy have no problems for around 3-5 years. In 15% there will either be a recurrence of the hyperthyroidism or hypothyroidism will develop after the operation. This latter situation requires the administration of thyroxine supplements.

Local effects of surgery to the thyroid may include damage to the recurrent laryngeal nerve which occurs in a small percentage of people and will produce temporary hoarseness. The normal function of both vocal cords should be confirmed before surgery and checked after surgery. The parathyroid glands, which are usually situated in the substance of the thyroid gland, may be temporarily damaged by the surgery or occasionally removed leading to disturbances of calcium metabolism. Damage to the parathyroid glands may lead to persistent low calcium levels in the blood and so long-term follow-up should include checks for cataracts and any mental disturbance. Damage to the recurrent laryngeal nerve and the parathyroid glands are very common after second operations on the thyroid gland and so are rarely performed. The appearance of hyperthyroidism after surgery is always treated with radioactive iodine.

Radioactive iodine:

The aim of treating the thyroid gland with radioactive iodine is to destroy a proportion of the gland. Iodine is concentrated in the thyroid gland as it is an integral part of the thyroid hormone molecule. Administration of radioactive iodine means that radioactivity is concentrated in the thyroid gland and this destroys the thyroid cells. It is mainly used for people over the age of 40 years and certainly when having children is no longer a likelihood. It may also be given to young people who have been sterilised or if they have an associated condition which shortens life expectancy. The actual dose to be administered is difficult to calculate accurately for various technical reasons. Regular review is essential until such time as the person has become hypothyroid and is on a suitable life-long replacement dose of thyroxine. As with surgical treatment, there is no attempt to affect the underlying process. The overall incidence of hypothyroidism may be of the order of 50% at seven years depending on the dosage given.

Alternative management:

If overactivity and underactivity of the thyroid gland are considered together, clearly there is a gradual process of disease with these two being merely extremes. The first response is of overproduction. This is in common with many bodily functions where an imbalance firstly manifests as an overstimulation. Underactivity develops as time passes and the gland becomes exhausted. The natural history, therefore, of thyroid gland disease is for hyperthyroidism to wane as time goes by, to be replaced at some later date by hypothyroidism. Since the conventional treatment of hyperthyroidism usually involves removal or destruction of part of the gland, hypothyroidism is a more likely consequence. Whilst the majority of people who become hypothyroid after surgery do so within the first six months or a year, there is a low but steady further incidence with each year after surgery. Because of this, all people who have received conventional treatment for hypothyroidism must have annual checks of circulating thyroid hormones.

In terms of Chinese medicine, this condition results from emotional distress or frustration. These feelings prevent the energy of the Liver and Spleen from flowing through the channels and Fire is generated which depletes the Yin of the Heart. This causes Phlegm to accumulate which gradually obstructs the channels of the neck, thereby leading to goitre. It is interesting at this point to note that enlargement of the thyroid gland (goitre), as well as disturbances in the thyroid function are common some 6 to 12 months after an emotional shock.

The throat area is clearly associated with communication and I would remind you of the comments I made above with regard to the position of the thyroid and its embryological origin. I would also suggest that this is why thyroid diseases are much more common in women than men Women may well know what feelings they have but have difficulty expressing them. Society generally teaches women not to express their thoughts and feelings. This energy then becomes blocked and causes pathology in the neck and throat area.

It is certainly valid to treat people who have hyperthyroidism by means of alternative medicine but you should be aware of the complications of hyperthyroidism and their symptoms. Severe cases need to be treated with more care and monitored more closely.

CASE

A woman of 51 years came for treatment after diagnosis of hyperthyroidism about 18 months previously. Her current medication was carbimazole 7.5 mg daily. Her main complaints were low energy, irregular periods with intermenstrual bleeding and headaches around the right eye. The headaches would be more likely to appear before a period and worse if she was under stress. They could last three days and involve pain around the right ear and arm.

In terms of Chinese medicine, I made a diagnosis of Blood Deficiency particularly of the Heart and Kidney Yang Deficiency. I treated her with herbs and acupuncture. She improved quickly with normalisation of her periods within a month. Her energy gradually improved and she began to take more exercise. A check on her thyroxine level showed this was normal. She reduced the carbimazole to 5 mg daily and then 2.5 mg daily over the course of the next few months as she was beginning to feel cold and tired. This drug clearly damages the Yang in order for it to change the symptoms of hyperthyroidism.

She found that she was beginning to be a little anxious and overactive with the dosage of 2.5 mg daily and so she settled on 5 mg for a while. She continues to receive treatment and feels well. In the forthcoming months I am expecting improvement to continue and for her to further reduce the dose of carbimazole.

HYPOTHYROIDISM

This is underactivity of thyroid gland function. It is occasionally due to pituitary disease but the common situation in clinical practice is autoimmune disease where there may be a history of hyperthyroidism. This relationship is discussed above. There may, in some cases, be damage to the gland by the conventional treatment of hyperthyroidism, i.e. drugs, surgery or radioactive iodine. Some cases develop spontaneously with no previous history of overactive thyroid function.

Hypothyroidism is primarily seen in women and there is almost always an associated goitre. Inflammation may be an important feature where the label of thyroiditis may be applied (see below).

An uncommon cause of hypothyroidism nowadays is due to iodine deficiency. This is more common in areas situated a long way from the sea. Iodine, essential for the normal functioning of the thyroid gland, is found in abundance in seafood, seaweed[9] and the like. The connection between such a clinical appearance and mountainous areas was noted by the Chinese during the Sui dynasty in the 6th Century AD. 'Derbyshire neck' is the term used in the UK and reflects the distance of this English county from the sea. Such a development is unusual now due to the addition of iodine to table salt. The first response of the body to reduced iodine intake is goitre and eventually symptoms will appear due to underactivity of the thyroid function.

Symptoms:

The commonest situation is in adult life where there is a decreased metabolic rate. The consequence of this is a general slowing of physical and mental functions. There is a feeling of coldness and sensitivity to cold. Associated features include dry skin, coarse, dry hair, constipation, gain in weight, tiredness and vague generalised pains. The outer third of the eyebrows becomes thin and sparse.

Menstrual disturbances are common and mental symptoms, such as forgetfulness, lack of concentration and eventually confusion are common. There may be tingling of the fingers and there is a general appearance of pallor. In severe cases, the face and eyelids become swollen, sweating is absent and the voice is husky. The pulse is slow and tendon reflexes delayed. In some, there is the appearance of psychotic symptoms such as hallucinations and delusions. The end stage of the mental symptoms is coma. Body temperature is low. In the early stages of hypothyroidism, the symptoms may be attributed to the ageing process by conventional practitioners. It is true there may be some confusion when symptoms first develop. Later, the diagnosis is more clear.

In children and especially infants it may be difficult to recognise. There may be poor performance at school and a lack of interest in games. In infants there may be constipation and poor feeding, a general 'failure to thrive' and a failure to attain the usual developmental milestones at the appropriate age. The development of the brain is dependent on thyroid hormones and so a delay in diagnosis at this stage may lead to permanent mental impairment.

---

[9] In Chinese medicine, there are various types of seaweed available as herbal remedies. They have the effect of transforming Phlegm which is considered to collect to form goitre.

Investigations:

There are reduced levels of thyroid hormones in the blood and a raised level of thyroid stimulating hormone. There may be thyroid antibodies in the blood.

Treatment:

This is with thyroxine supplementation which initially is given at a low dose and increased gradually over several weeks. The normal maintenance dose is 0.15 to 0.2 mg per day[10]. Annual checks of thyroxine levels are necessary to ensure that supplementation is adequate as the underlying disease process may be progressive.

There are a significant number of people who present to medical practitioners with non-specific symptoms of tiredness, gaining weight, coldness, depression and the like and they may be subjected to evaluation of thyroid hormone levels. Thyroxine may be given to such patients, even if the thyroxine level in the blood is at the low end of normal. In addition, you may still see some people who are given thyroid hormone on the basis of being overweight. That is clearly an inappropriate way in which to treat such problems and the administration of thyroid hormones leads to a reduction in the person's own thyroid gland function. Over the course of the next year to 18 months, the dosage of thyroxine will be increased as the person's own production declines. They may not have had a thyroid deficiency to begin with but they certainly end up with one.

CASE

A woman of 37 years came for treatment after a diagnosis of hypothyroidism. She had a baby of 6 months and had been well during the pregnancy except excessive weight gain. After the birth, which was uneventful, she developed tiredness and lethargy. She had not particularly lost weight since the delivery. Her appetite was generally poor and she tended to suffer from constipation. Her Chinese medical diagnosis was Spleen Qi Deficiency, Kidney Yang Deficiency and Blood Deficiency.

Pregnancy is a tremendous drain on Blood and Qi which, in some women, can lead to symptoms. It is important, if possible, to treat women before conception, certainly during pregnancy and after delivery. This case is typical, however, in that most people seek help when they develop overt signs of ill-health.

Her thyroxine level was 35 nmol/l four months before treatment and 21 nmol/l two months before. She was advised to take thyroxine but sought alternative medical help in an attempt to deal with the problem. I gave her herbs and acupuncture and she felt generally better with more energy. We decided not to repeat the blood test as this would not have changed the management of the case and because she was symptomatically improved. The thyroxine level was checked ten months after treatment began and was normal.

GOITRE

This is any enlargement of the thyroid gland. It is commoner in women. When seeing a person with such a condition, it is important to consider certain factors:

- size
- shape
- consistency
- symmetry
- irregularity of surface
- mobility of the thyroid - the thyroid normally moves on swallowing
- presence or absence of enlarged lymph glands in the neck
- are there symptoms of underactivity or overactivity of thyroid function? Blood tests may help in this regard but use them as a guide not as an absolute statement.

---

[10] This may be expressed as micrograms (mcg or μg). The equivalent is 150 to 200 mcg (μg) per day.

Thyroid enlargement is usually noticed due to its appearance since symptoms are absent or minor in most cases. In some, where the enlargement is marked, there can be difficulty in swallowing or breathing because of pressure on the oesophagus or trachea.

In general, thyroid enlargement can be classified according to several criteria. These are:

- generalised or local
- presence or absence of pain
- presence or absence of symptoms due to thyroid function disturbance
- soft or hard

There are various causes of goitre in conventional medicine and these are listed in Table 15.5 with comments about such classification.

CAUSE OF GOITRE	COMMENTS
Puberty	Diffuse enlargement. No associated symptoms
Pregnancy	Diffuse enlargement. No associated symptoms
Hyperthyroidism	Diffuse enlargement, firm. Symptoms of hyperthyroidism
Hypothyroidism	Diffuse enlargement, firm, rubbery. May be soft or hard. Symptoms of hypothyroidism
Thyroiditis	Diffuse enlargement which is painful. Fever and malaise.
Drugs	Female sex hormones[11], sulphonylureas
Iodine deficiency	Smooth, soft enlargement
Cancer	A single lump, painful, short history, enlarged lymph glands in the neck
Cysts and benign tumours	Lumps in the thyroid - one or several. If several then unlikely to be cancer

TABLE 15.5: CAUSES OF GOITRE

Investigations:

These will include thyroid function tests, mainly estimations of thyroxine (T_4), tri-iodothyronine (T_3) and thyroid stimulating hormone. Radioactive scans of the thyroid are done in many cases since the thyroid will concentrate the radioactive substance in an active area. Ultrasound scans can also give information about whether an enlarged area within the thyroid is solid of cystic. Cystic areas are rarely malignant. Biopsy of the thyroid gland using a needle is an increasingly used technique.

Treatment:

This depends upon the cause.

HASHIMOTO'S THYROIDITIS

This is a firm, diffuse enlargement of the thyroid gland which may or may not be associated with underactivity of the thyroid gland. If this is the case, then I would refer you to the section dealing with hypothyroidism.

Symptoms:

There may be aching in the gland and mild dysphagia depending upon the extent of the enlargement. It is most common in middle aged women and is autoimmune in nature. Virtually all people with this condition have antibodies to thyroid tissue in their blood.

---

[11] There is an energetic connection between the neck and the pelvis which explains why suppression of ovarian function may lead to thyroid enlargement. It is important to review all medication in cases of goitre.

Treatment:

This is by means of thyroxine (0.2-0.3 mg daily) to reduce the functioning of the gland and so lead to a reduction in size. Corticosteroids are given in addition to treat the autoimmune aspect.

SUBACUTE (DE QUERVAIN'S) THYROIDITIS

This is a painful condition of the thyroid usually associated with enlargement. It is considered to be associated with a viral infection. Thyroid function is reduced and may recover spontaneously or persist.

Treatment:

This is treated in the same way as Hashimoto's thyroiditis.

Alternative management of goitre:

The main point to make here is that the symptom of goitre must be only part of the complete case. The exact management will depend upon the case. In terms of Chinese medicine, goitre is associated with living in the mountains and a long distance from the sea. This observation was noted in the 6th Century AD and corresponds with the modern view of low iodine levels.

In Chinese medicine, there is also a belief that goitre is related to emotional causes where emotional distress interferes with the flow of Qi, allowing Dampness and Phlegm to coagulate and obstruct the channels. In this situation it would be important to transform the Phlegm rather than to disperse it (break it up) since the Phlegm accumulation represents a gathering of the emotions. The use of local needles in the neck may disperse the swelling and stronger treatments can break up the stagnation. This can, however, lead to the sudden release of strong emotional states which overwhelm the person.

It is valid to treat goitre by means of alternative medicine but expect progress to be slow, particularly in terms of the actual size of the gland. In my and other practitioner's experience, results tend to be very good. You will have be more circumspect in underactivity or overactivity of thyroid function and if cancer is a possibility.

TUMOURS OF THE THYROID GLAND

Benign tumours may produce thyroxine and so produce a syndrome identical to hyperthyroidism described previously. They are removed surgically.

Cancer of the thyroid gland is uncommon. It accounts for 1% of all cases of cancer in the UK and about 400 deaths per year. In advanced cases, it can be recognised by its hardness, irregularity and adhesion to surrounding tissues. There may be associated glandular enlargement. In early cases it may present as a single nodule which is seen as being non-functional (a "cold" area) on radioisotope scan.

Treatment:

This is by means of total thyroidectomy together with thyroxine replacement. Local radiotherapy is also used if there is secondary spread. The majority of thyroid tumours spread locally and then to the lung or bone. Prognosis is variable depending on the exact type.

Alternative management:

I would refer you to Chapter 6 - Cancer for those comments are relevant here. The thyroxine supplementation in this situation cannot be reduced or discontinued as there is no thyroid gland remaining to be stimulated.

- DIABETES MELLITUS -

In conventional textbooks, diabetes mellitus is usually placed with disorders of metabolism. I have chosen to put it here since it is a disturbance of endocrine function. The term 'diabetes' means excessive urination and 'mellitus' is derived from the Latin for honey. Colloquially, it may be known as 'sugar diabetes' to serve as a distinction from the rarer diabetes insipidus.

The primary feature of diabetes mellitus is raised blood sugar levels. This is the result of an inadequate production of insulin by the pancreas. The key to understanding this disease is to appreciate the ways in which the body balances blood sugar levels.

Simply stated, carbohydrates taken into the body can only be absorbed as simple sugars[12]. More complex carbohydrate sources such as starches and complex sugars have to be broken down into simple sugars before absorption can occur. These are absorbed into the blood and used as a source of energy either immediately or stored as glycogen in the body for use at some later date. The body attempts to maintain blood sugar levels within fairly narrow limits (3.5 to 6.0 mmol/l).

Insulin is secreted by the pancreas in response to circulating levels of blood sugar. The effect of insulin is to allow glucose to enter the cells more readily and to facilitate the storage of glucose as glycogen, i.e. reduce blood sugar levels. Conversely, low levels of insulin lead to the breakdown of glycogen stores to glucose and a reduced ability of the cell to absorb sugar. The net result is an increase in blood sugar levels.

Other hormones play a role in regulating blood sugar levels. Glucagon from the pancreas with adrenaline and corticosteroids from the adrenal glands have the effect of raising blood sugar levels. Adrenaline and corticosteroids are released in response to stressful situations and so blood sugar will rise as a result. Similarly, if the blood sugar is low, these hormones are released and so people feel anxious, sweaty, irritable with a rapid pulse.

In the West, diets are not particularly healthy in most cases due to a high intake of carbohydrates especially of the refined type. In addition, there are irregular eating habits and the use of stimulants such as alcohol, nicotine and caffeine.

The long-term intake of refined carbohydrates, together with the use of stimulants, causes large swings in blood sugar. The blood sugar rises quickly because a diet rich in refined carbohydrate leads to rapid absorption of sugars. Large amounts of insulin are produced in response. A rapid fall in blood sugar follows as there are no complex carbohydrates to be broken down more slowly and to allow gradual absorption of sugar.

The low points of blood sugar are known as hypoglycaemic episodes. They are associated with feelings of hunger, sweating, anxiety, irritability and agitation as stress hormones are released in an attempt to normalise blood sugar levels. Commonly, a mid-meal snack or sugar food will be taken at this time to relieve such symptoms. This causes another peak in blood sugar level with the consequent release of insulin. Clearly, on a daily basis, there are large amounts of insulin produced by the pancreas and adrenaline with corticosteroids from the adrenal gland. All these factors tend to lead to great fluctuation in blood sugar levels. Exhaustion of the pancreas and adrenal glands occur if this continues for a long period of time. The production of insulin declines leading to permanently raised blood sugar levels, i.e. diabetes mellitus.

The way to remedy this situation is by smoothing out the extremes of blood sugar levels. It is important to avoid refined carbohydrates, stimulant drugs and to live a relaxing life-style in order to reduce circulating levels of stress hormones. In this way, the peaks and troughs of blood sugar swings will be minimised. This, in itself, can radically affect health as people feel more energetic, less stressed and specific symptoms of a wide variety may be alleviated[13].

---

[12] Simple sugars, also known as monosaccharides, are single sugar molecules. Examples include glucose, fructose and galactose.

More complex sugars are disaccharides which are made up of double sugar molecules. Examples include sucrose, maltose and lactose.

Starches are polysaccharides where many sugar molecules are joined together. They are an important form of carbohydrate in the diet. Glycogen is also a polysaccharide and is a source of carbohydrate stores within the body. It is the equivalent of starch.

[13] There are many diets including Atkins, Pritikin and others which change blood sugar levels by advocating high protein, relatively low carbohydrate intakes. More healthy diets include the Hay diet

Such a life-style can be perceived as boring and lacking in interest. This is because Westerners live a roller coaster ride of uppers and downers. We become addicted to the extremes of experience and find it difficult to slow down. Nevertheless, such action will definitely lead to increased well-being. In the long-term there will be a greatly reduced chance of developing diabetes mellitus.

FACTORS DECREASING BLOOD SUGAR	FACTORS INCREASING BLOOD SUGAR
Exercise	Food (particularly carbohydrates but especially those of the refined type)
Relaxation (because less stress hormones released)	Lack of exercise
Insulin	Stressful situations (due to adrenaline and corticosteroid release)
Diet (reducing intake of carbohydrate but especially those of the refined type	Stimulant drugs, e.g. alcohol, nicotine, caffeine
	Glucagon

TABLE 15.6: FACTORS AFFECTING BLOOD SUGAR LEVELS

The disease of diabetes mellitus is when there are inadequate levels of insulin for the requirements of the body. Consequently, blood sugar levels start to rise. Conventionally, there are two types of diabetes mellitus. Insulin dependent diabetes mellitus (also known as IDDM or Type 1 diabetes) is due to almost total absence of insulin production by the pancreas. It requires the administration of insulin by injection to control sugar levels. The second type is non-insulin dependent diabetes mellitus (also known as NIDDM or Type 2 diabetes) and is due to a relative lack of insulin production. That is, there is insufficient production of insulin for the needs of the body. It is usually treated by diet with or without prescribed medication taken orally. The medication stimulates the pancreas to produce more insulin.

As with most diseases, these are a combination of constitutional and environmental factors. In insulin dependent diabetes, constitutional factors are more important. The presentation tends to be acute and occurs in childhood, particularly around 10 to 13 years. The incidence is currently rising in the West.

In non-insulin dependent diabetes, environmental factors are more important. The person may be overweight and have a long history of poor diet with excess refined carbohydrate intake.

Whatever the type of diabetes, it frequently develops in the weeks and months after a shock or injury. This may be physical as in cases of road traffic accident or emotional as with bereavement, separation, loss or some other kind of psychological stress. There is evidence to show that diabetes of both kinds is related to autoimmune factors. The suddenness of the onset is an indication of the rapidity of action of insulin. There may have been damage to pancreatic function by the immune system for some time prior to the appearance of symptoms.

The two types of diabetes mellitus are variations of the same disease process. I shall describe diabetes mellitus as a whole and where relevant point out distinctions between them.

Symptoms:

Diabetes mellitus may present in one of several ways. In mild cases, where symptoms may be absent or unnoticed, routine examination of the urine may reveal sugar (glucose). This, in most cases[14], indicates diabetes.

The two main presentations of diabetes reflect the insulin dependent and non-insulin dependent varieties discussed previously.

Insulin dependent diabetes occurs mainly in adolescents and children hence its other name of juvenile-onset diabetes. It is acute in onset and the main symptoms are caused by a high blood sugar

---

(also known as food combining) which takes the strain off the digestion and allows blood sugar levels and other homeostatic mechanisms to be more balanced.

[14] Sugar does not normally appear in the urine in health. It remains in the blood as its level is not high to spill over the *renal threshold*. About 1% of the population have a low renal threshold so that sugar appears in the urine. This is known as renal glycosuria and an inherited trait. It is not associated with any disease in conventional medicine.

level. As sugar levels in the blood rise, the sugar spills over into the urine. Extra water is excreted and so excess urination, dehydration and thirst are primary symptoms. Eventually there will be weight loss and toxic symptoms of vomiting, breathlessness. Over the course of a few days the child becomes rapidly and progressively ill. Coma and death intervene unless treatment with insulin is instituted. Before the use of insulin in the 1920's, all such people would die.

One of the main difficulties is the presence of ketones. Energy is normally obtained from sugar. If this is not possible fat is broken down as an energy source. By-products of fat breakdown are ketones. These are toxic, acidic and have the odour of pear-drops. Acetone is a related substance. Ketones are dangerous and are common in acute situations of hyperglycaemia. Other situations leading to ketone production are fasting and malnutrition. This is one of the dangers of very low carbohydrate diets as are proclaimed as helpful in weight loss. I remember when I worked in hospital practice that a woman was admitted for weight loss. She was put on a low (around 200 calories) carbohydrate diet. She started to lose weight but after 2 weeks had a heart attack and died. Whilst this may not entirely have been due to ketosis, such diets are potentially hazardous.

Non-insulin dependent diabetes is usually much slower in its onset. It occurs in older people hence it other name of maturity-onset diabetes. Overweight is a common precursor. There may be a relatively long history of raised blood sugar levels leading to tiredness and lethargy. Depending upon the height of blood sugar there may be thirst and excessive urination. These symptoms will be much milder than those of the insulin dependent type. Weight loss develops as the disease progresses. The development of ketones is unusual.

A common feature of the developing diabetic is a complaint of epigastric pain.

Complications:

These are many and varied and may be grouped into two. Firstly, there are the complications of the acute situation and these are commoner in insulin dependent diabetes at first presentation.

Secondly, there are long term consequences of diabetes mellitus. These arise because of the disruption in carbohydrate metabolism. Even with treatment, such metabolism does not return to normal. Most diabetics, therefore, have long-term problems with fat generation as the body cannot completely handle these basic energy sources correctly. The long-term complications are occasionally the way by which diabetes mellitus may present. This is the situation in some cases of the non-insulin dependent type where the symptoms of high blood sugar may be mild or unnoticed.

COMPLICATIONS	SYMPTOMS TO LOOK FOR
Short-term	
Hyperglycaemia	Tiredness, thirst, excess urination, dryness
Hyperglycaemic coma	Unconsciousness
Ketosis	Rapid respirations, pear-drop smell on breath or urine, nausea or vomiting, feels ill
Long-term	
Atherosclerosis	Cold limbs, pain in calves on walking, absent peripheral pulses
Diabetic neuropathy	Tingling and numbness especially in extremities. Feet more than hands
Retinal damage	Impaired vision
Glomerulonephritis	Oedema, loin pain, haematuria

TABLE 15.7: COMPLICATIONS OF DIABETES MELLITUS

Diagnosis:

This may be made clinically according to the precise symptom picture given above. Confirmation is by means of blood testing. Two fasting blood sugar levels above 6.7 mmol/l or random samples over 10 mmol/l are sufficient to diagnose diabetes mellitus. A glucose tolerance test[15] is only necessary in borderline cases.

---

[15] This is a sequence of blood sugar estimations performed over two and a half hours to check their response to the intake of sugar. In health, there is a normal response as the pancreatic secretion of

Sugar in the urine is not, in itself, adequate proof of diabetes mellitus and blood tests must be performed in such cases.

Other routine tests performed once the diagnosis has been established include urinalysis for protein, full blood count, urea and electrolytes, fasting blood sample for cholesterol and triglycerides. This last test is only valid once blood sugar levels have been controlled.

Treatment:

The main aim of conventional treatment is to maintain relatively normal levels of blood sugar throughout the day. This is done by two main methods. Dietary restrictions are placed on carbohydrate intake, particularly sugars. In addition, agents which reduce blood sugar may be required. These are of two types. Insulin itself may be administered in severe cases where other methods of blood sugar control would fail. This is given to those of young age with insulin dependent diabetes and some older people whose symptoms are too severe for control by other means. Oral hypoglycaemic drugs which stimulate pancreatic function are given to those older people where dietary restriction alone is inadequate but the case is not so severe that insulin is necessary.

Hypoglycaemic agents may reduce the level of blood sugar too much and lead to low blood sugar or hypoglycaemia. This situation is not of the same degree as that mentioned on Page 333. Here, the blood sugar may fall so low as to be life-threatening. There are similar symptoms of hunger, sweating, agitation and so forth. As the blood sugar level continues to fall there is the appearance of confusion. Eventually coma and death will occur. Some people think that hypoglycaemia develops as part of the disease. In fact, it is a result of the *treatment* of diabetes mellitus.

The optimal treatment of diabetes mellitus, therefore, is to thread a line between the extremes of hyperglycaemia and hypoglycaemia. The essence of good management is a restriction of diet, a regulated life-style in terms of exercise, stress levels and to monitor blood or urine sugar regularly. Nowadays, most diabetics use blood checks to monitor their diabetic balance. A level of between 6 and 8 mmol/l is about right. Tests performed before meals will give a good idea of what is happening to blood sugar levels throughout the day.

Urine testing is less commonly performed nowadays. Dipstick tests are used rather than the older tablet method. There are drawbacks to urine testing. These include:

- urine sugar is a reflection of the situation in the blood some time previously
- the level of sugar in the urine is a reflection of blood sugar but also of kidney function
- negative urine tests give no indication of blood sugar levels

Ketones may be tested by dipstick at the same time.

The diet of a person with diabetes mellitus is similar in many respects to that which is considered generally healthy. Carbohydrate intake needs to be based on unrefined, complex substances rather than simple sugars. Fat intake needs to be limited, particularly in diabetics who have a tendency to premature atherosclerosis. In terms of calories, 15% should be obtained from protein, 35% from fats and 50% from carbohydrate.

For those who take insulin, regular snacks between meals are required to prevent low blood sugar levels at that time. It is notoriously difficult for most of us to change our habits and particularly our eating habits. People with diabetes need information about their condition and how diet may affect it together with support to put necessary changes into action. In this way, the control of diabetes is managed by the person themselves and is not something which is prescribed from the outside.

The main methods of reducing blood sugar levels are insulin by injection and oral hypoglycaemic agents. In the case of insulin, there are several methods available. The common one is to give a long-acting insulin in the evening and 3 doses of short-acting insulin before each meal during the day. In this way a relatively smooth degree of control is attained in most people. The blood is tested before each meal and insulin given dependent upon the result.

---

insulin can respond adequately. In borderline and overt diabetics, there is an abnormal response shown as an excessive rise in blood sugar levels. This may only occur an hour or so after meals and so would not be revealed by a random test. Some people may require a five hour glucose tolerance test to note any abnormality. For this reason, conventional practitioners may not recognise latent diabetes.

Insulin, formerly, used to be obtained from the pancreases of pigs or cattle. Such pork and beef insulin have, to a large degree, been replaced by human insulin produced synthetically. The changeover to human insulin has led to various problems with sudden attacks of hypoglycaemia but no warning symptoms. As a result, deaths have occurred over the 10 years or so since human insulin has been introduced.

The injection of insulin is clearly not physiological and so control of blood sugar levels is not perfect. The absorption of injected insulin is variable, it is into the systemic rather than the digestive circulation, absorption is delayed and there are individual variations. The cases I describe below provide good examples of how diabetes can be controlled by such methods.

The second type of control is by means of oral hypoglycaemic agents. Essentially, these stimulate the pancreas to produce more insulin. They are only appropriate for those with milder diabetes mellitus. Certainly, almost all diabetics who develop the disease at a young age will require insulin. There are two main groups of drugs available. The sulphonylureas, such as tolbutamide and chlorpropamide, are commonly used. They are contraindicated in pregnancy and may damage the liver. Hypoglycaemia may be produced which can be severe and long-lasting.

Biguanides are the other group available. Metformin is the usual example and is reserved for those in middle and old age. It may induce anorexia, indigestion and diarrhoea. Some people develop an acidotic reaction which is potentially life-threatening. It is not licensed for use in the US.

Alternative management:

In terms of Chinese medicine, diabetes mellitus usually corresponds to 'thirsting and wasting disease'. It is the generation of Internal Heat due to the excessive intake of sweet and greasy food or emotional stagnation. The Heat damages the Yin leading to the classical symptoms. The condition is further divided into upper, middle and lower types depending upon the presence of thirst, hunger and frequent urination respectively. In clinical practice, there is a mixture of the three types seen.

Insulin, therefore, has an effect of cooling the Heat and moistening the Yin. This is why heat signs are not commonly seen in treated diabetics. The cooling effect will also damage the Spleen Qi further and lead to digestive symptoms, desire for sweet food, oedema and DampPhlegm Accumulation[16].

CASE

A man of 25 years came for treatment of his diabetes mellitus. He had first developed this at the age of 8 years when his grandmother died. He had been very close to her as she had mainly been responsible for his upbringing.

He generally felt exhausted. He had loose stools at least five times each day. His current insulin dosages were 26 units of long-acting at night and variable amounts of short-acting three times daily but usually around 8, 10 and 8 units. His blood sugar estimations were unstable.

- Fasting - 20 mmol/l or more
- Midday - 15 mmol/l
- Tea time - 15 mmol/l
- Evening - 15 mmol/l

These blood levels were an indication of his life-style which was quite irregular. He had a large intake of cigarettes, coffee and recreational drugs with late nights and stressful job. It is important to be careful with such cases at these blood levels of sugar. It is more worrying if there are ketones in the urine or strong symptoms of thirst and frequent urination.

In terms of Chinese medicine, his diagnosis was Spleen Yang Deficiency, Kidney Yang Deficiency, Liver Qi Stagnation and Heat in the Stomach. I decided to begin with improving his digestive energy and we discussed the effect of treatment on his blood sugars.

Some two days after treatment, he noticed that his blood sugars were more moderate and when he returned one week later they were much more stable.

---

[16] This corresponds to atherosclerosis and retinal damage which are common in treated diabetics.

Fasting - usually 10 but on one occasion 5 mmol/l
Midday - 5 mmol/l
Tea time - 5 mmol/l
Evening - 5 mmol/l

Over the course of the next few weeks, his blood sugars continued to regularise. He began to change his dietary and drug habits as he felt better and his energy returned. It is a common finding that people can change their lives when they have the energy to do so. It is rarely, if ever, beneficial to lecture people about their 'bad habits' in the hope that they will change. Such change only comes from within, certainly if it is to be long-lasting and effective.

In the next few months, he progressed to reducing his insulin dosage until he was taking 20 units of long-acting at night and about 6 units at each meal. He felt generally much better although his loose stools had not completely eased. His treatment will need to be long-term but you would expect him to remain well. In such a circumstance it is not realistic to expect him to be able to come off insulin completely.

- ADRENAL GLANDS -

The adrenal glands (also known as suprarenal glands) are situated on top of the kidney. They are made up of an inner medulla and an outer cortex. The medulla has connections with the sympathetic nervous system and produces the hormones, adrenaline and noradrenaline. These are involved in the flight and fight response. Clinically recognisable disorders of this area are extremely rare and I shall concentrate here on disorders of the adrenal cortex.

The adrenal cortex produces several hormones with differing functions as shown in Table 15.8. Each hormone has an effect in several areas but, with each, there will be an emphasis of one function over the others. For example, cortisone primarily has a glucocorticoid action but also some mineralocorticoid and androgenic effects.

ACTION	EFFECTS	EXAMPLE OF HORMONE
Glucocorticoid	Opposite to insulin Anti-inflammatory Convert protein to sugar	cortisone, cortisol (hydrocortisone). corticosterone[17]
Mineralocorticoid	Retains sodium Loses potassium	aldosterone
Androgenic	Masculinising	testosterone
Oestrogens	Feminising	oestrogen

TABLE 15.8: HORMONES SECRETED BY THE ADRENAL GLAND AND THEIR FUNCTIONS

There are some differences between these hormones and so I shall deal with them separately for the sake of clarity. Oestrogen is covered in detail in Chapter 18 - Gynaecology.

Cortisone and its relations have a primary glucocorticoid action. They have an effect which is opposite to that of insulin. That is, it raises blood sugar by activating glycogen stores in the liver.

It causes the breakdown of protein into carbohydrate, primarily sugar. This leads to depletion of protein structure such as the underlying substance of bone, collagen and connective tissue and muscle.

The anti-inflammatory effects are used clinically in diseases characterised by inflammation of non-infective origin. These include rheumatoid arthritis, Crohn's disease, ulcerative colitis, eczema, asthma, psoriasis and so forth. The function of inflammation is to localise a problem in a defined area. It does so by allowing plasma into the area and an outpouring of white cells to fight any infection or cell damage. The inhibition of this action is a primary role of cortisone.

The consequences of these functions, in cases of excessive production, lead to certain clinical features which are shown in Table 15.9.

---

[17] The hormones used in clinical practice for their anti-inflammatory effects are betamethasone, prednisolone, prednisone, triamcinolone, cortisol (hydrocortisone) and dexamethasone.

ACTION	EFFECTS	SYMPTOMS
Glucocorticoid	Opposite to those of insulin	Thirst, frequent urination, dehydration, increased susceptibility to infections[19]
	Anti-inflammatory	Risk of spreading infection and cell damage.
	Converts protein to sugar[18]	Weakening of bone[20], thinning of skin and mucous membranes, easy bruising, poor wound healing, ulceration of the stomach or duodenum
Mineralocorticoid	Retains sodium	Water retention manifesting as oedema and high blood pressure
	Loses potassium	Muscle weakness, palpitations and tiredness
Androgenic	Masculinising	In men there may be aggressive and violent behaviour In women there is deepening of the voice, male distribution of hair on the face, temporal recession hair, hair along the central line of the abdomen, enlargement of the clitoris, reduction in breast size, disturbance of menstruation with scanty or absent periods
Oestrogens	Feminising	Leads to female distribution of fat, breast enlargement, reduction in size of penis in men

TABLE 15.10: SYMPTOMS ASSOCIATED WITH OVERPRODUCTION OF ADRENAL CORTICAL HORMONES

OVERACTIVITY OF THE ADRENAL CORTEX

CUSHING'S SYNDROME

This is a syndrome due to excess corticosteroid production. It has many similarities with the clinical picture seen when corticosteroids are prescribed to treat disease. Cushing's syndrome itself may be due to overstimulation by adrenocorticotrophic hormone:

Symptoms:

These are primarily due to an increased glucocorticoid action. There is central obesity, that is, thin arms and legs with increased weight centrally on the trunk and face. The limbs are thin due to muscle wasting and the muscles are weak. There is oedema in the ankles or lower legs. The skin is thinned and bruises easily. Injury to the skin easily results in tears which are slow to heal. Infection is more likely and improves slowly. There is sugar in the urine The bones become weaker due to osteoporosis and fractures may develop. High blood pressure is common and the complexion is ruddy. Skin infections are common. The skin is stretched and purple striae are seen. There is male pattern baldness with a masculine distribution of hair.

These symptoms are also seen with corticosteroid use for diseases such as rheumatoid arthritis but without the masculinising effects since synthetic hormones are used.

Alternative management:

The use of corticosteroids is discussed fully in Chapter 10 - Musculoskeletal System.

---

[18] The ability to breakdown protein reveals the strength of these chemicals.

[19] These are the classical symptoms of raised blood sugar as described in the section on diabetes mellitus. There is a real possibility of this disease developing in such a circumstance.

[20] Osteoporosis.

UNDERACTIVITY OF THE ADRENAL CORTEX

Underactivity of the adrenal cortex is unusual in clinical practice. I describe it because it is similar to the effect of sudden withdrawal of corticosteroid drugs. With long-term corticosteroid use, the adrenal glands atrophy and decline in function. If the drugs are reduced suddenly, the adrenal glands cannot produce sufficient quantities and symptoms of underactivity are evident.

The disease state may be due to primary disease of the adrenal as in Addison's disease, congenital deficiency of enzymes required for the synthesis of adrenal hormones (congenital adrenal hyperplasia) or secondary to underactivity of the pituitary or hypothalamus.

ADDISON'S DISEASE

This is usually of an autoimmune nature. Occasionally, tuberculosis of the adrenal glands may lead to adrenal destruction. Women are affected twice as commonly as men. Antibodies to the adrenal gland are found in the blood.

There are frequently associated autoimmune disorders such as thyrotoxicosis, Hashimoto's thyroiditis, pernicious anaemia and insulin-dependent diabetes mellitus. The adrenals are atrophied and smaller than normal. The onset can be acute or chronic.

Symptoms:

There is weakness, weight loss, low blood pressure, gastrointestinal disorders including anorexia, nausea, constipation and diarrhoea. There is increasing mental and physical tiredness. Amenorrhoea is common in women. There is disturbance of pigmentation in long-standing cases with hyperpigmentation or vitiligo. The pigmentation disorder is often the first clinical sign. Increased melanin affects the area exposed to light and pressure and so is seen primarily on the face, neck, backs of hands, knuckles, elbows and knees. Scars present before the onset of symptoms are normal and those after become pigmented. Vitiligo develops in 10-20% of people especially in dark-skinned races.

Treatment:

This is by means of corticosteroids. The drugs usually given are cortisol with fludrocortisone.

Alternative management:

Cases of corticosteroid withdrawal are described in Chapter 10 - Musculoskeletal System and Chapter 13 - Gastrointestinal System. In terms of Chinese medicine, too rapid a reduction of corticosteroids may lead to Collapse of Yang.

- HOW TO RECOGNISE A SERIOUS CONDITION OF THE ENDOCRINE SYSTEM -

Most people who come to the clinic with endocrine disease will already have a conventional diagnosis. In cases of underactivity of a particular endocrine gland, they will be taking hormone supplementation. In such situations it is merely necessary to be sure of what would indicate an imbalance in their hormone control.

In those cases where diagnosis has not already been made, you can rely on symptoms as I have stated at the end of each Chapter dealing with a particular system. For example, in cases of diabetes mellitus with excessive urination you can refer to Chapter 9 - Urinary System. In cases of hyperthyroidism with palpitations you can refer to Chapter 7 - Cardiovascular System.

In Table 15.11 I list the endocrine disorders I have discussed in this Chapter with comments on how to recognise a situation of poor hormonal control.

DISEASE	SITUATION OF IMBALANCE	COMMENTS
Hyperthyroidism	Appearance of symptoms of overactivity	Review case. May be exacerbation due to too rapid drug withdrawal. Assess according to severity of symptoms
Hypothyroidism	Appearance of symptoms of underactivity	Review case. May be ineffective alternative treatment, too low a dosage of thyroxine
Diabetes insipidus	Excess urination, thirst	Is there too low a dosage of vasopressin?
Diabetes mellitus	Hyperglycaemia	Check factors such as diet, recent reduction in exercise, increased stress levels, use of stimulant drugs, excessive reduction of hypoglycaemic agents, infection. Assess according to severity of symptoms.
	Hypoglycaemia	Check diet, recent increase in exercise, relaxation, cessation of stimulant drugs, failure to reduce dosage of hypoglycaemic agents. If frequent then must adjust hypoglycaemic drug dosage as a matter of urgency

TABLE 15.11: DISEASES OF ENDOCRINE SYSTEM AND STATES OF IMBALANCE

- SUMMARY -

Diseases of the endocrine system are increasing in incidence in the West. This is in line with the general increase in chronic disease.

People with endocrine disease will be seen in the clinic but not always because of their original disease.

Monitoring of endocrine function is important when dealing with such cases.

It is important to have an understanding of the overall issues affecting function of a particular endocrine gland.

Alternative treatment shortly after conventional diagnosis and treatment may have a realistic chance of removing the need for hormone therapy in the long-term.

Alternative treatment after a long period of conventional treatment will generally lead to increased health and a reduced dosage of hormone replacement (hence the need for monitoring).

16 PSYCHOLOGICAL DISORDERS

OBJECTIVES:
At the end of this Chapter you will be able to:
State the philosophical differences of conventional and alternative medicine with respect to psychological disorders
Describe the conventional and alternative classifications of psychological disorders
Describe the clinical appearances of the main categories of psychological disorder
Differentiate between psychosis (mental disturbance) and neurosis (emotional disturbance)
Discuss how to manage people with such disturbances

- INTRODUCTION -

As I discussed in Chapter 2 - Philosophy, conventional medicine concentrates on physical matters. In most cases this is to the exclusion of everything else. There *is* a recognition that people have psychological symptoms but the conventional explanation is that they arise from a physical basis, usually the brain. There is also the important added factor that such symptoms are frequently seen as being unimportant. In extreme cases they may be ignored completely. This leads to a paradoxical situation where, on the face of it, psychological symptoms are taken seriously as indicating an imbalance in the central nervous system. However, there is frequently a hidden subtext where certain symptoms are disregarded.

There is, therefore, a common thread throughout much of conventional medical practice where psychological symptoms are ignored or seen as a secondary component of a 'real' or physical disease. In diseases where psychological symptoms predominate such as schizophrenia, there is an assumption that a physical basis will, at some time, be found. Research is directed either at biochemical abnormalities within the central nervous system or attempts made to discover a genetic abnormality. In themselves, such efforts are not particularly harmful. However, when an emphasis is placed on physical matters, people's psychological states are diminished. People are dismissed as being neurotic[1]. They may be given chemicals in an attempt to 'rebalance' supposed chemical abnormalities in the substance of the brain. Surgical procedures are performed on the brain in an attempt to correct these abnormalities. In my experience, these are rarely of benefit and frequently lead to more problems.

In conjunction with a general increase in the number of chronic diseases in the West, it is more common to see psychological disorders. Homoeopaths report that remedies are used now to affect deep mental and emotional levels which would hardly, if ever, be used 100 years ago. In the UK there has been a 65% in the number of children admitted to psychiatric wards in the past 5 years. The cost to national health budgets is extreme. In the UK, some £100 million per year is spent on drugs to affect mood. This is 25% of the national drug budget. There seems to be no end to this suffering and as each year passes, increasing numbers of people exhibit psychological symptoms. The use of conventional medical techniques merely deal with the symptoms - the effect - rather than the cause and so can only be suppressive.

The consequence of such attempts to deal with psychological disturbances is frequently to exacerbate the situation. Conventional medical techniques become part of the problem rather than the solution. Are there other ways of viewing these situations?

Oriental medicine has always sought to see all symptoms within the context of an integrated whole. This is true of those traditions with which I have had closest contact, Chinese and Tibetan medicine. Unfortunately, due to political developments in the People's Republic of China over the past 40 years or so, access to psychological aspects of Chinese medicine has been restricted. Nevertheless, the understanding, or at least its possibility exists. People have looked to related sources such as Tibetan medicine, sources in Korea, Taiwan, Vietnam and Japan for help in understanding how to apply energetic medicine to psychological disturbances. The discussion below is based upon my understanding of sources from Tibetan Buddhist[2] and Chinese medical thought.

From a Buddhist point of view, all suffering comes originally from the mind. It arises from our mental processes which see events, ourselves and others as fixed entities, unchanging and permanent. This is not the true nature of reality as we know from our understanding of energetic systems of medicine and the insights of modern physics. The whole of matter is merely a manifestation of a constantly changing energy. Nothing is static and permanent.

Since all suffering comes from the mind, we must affect this level to achieve any long-lasting change. It is considered that the true nature of the mind, its innermost essence[3] is inherently pure and unstainable. It is likened to the sky on a cloudless day. The usual thoughts and emotions of our everyday experience are likened to the clouds which appear from time to time. They are not the sky itself but merely obscure it. They come and go. It is when we are attached to the clouds of our thoughts and emotions that we begin to experience suffering.

The aim of any medical treatment is to allow people to see their mental and emotional processes as merely manifestations of their true nature. In this way, people can become less attached to their problems and suffering and so experience periods of comfort and ease.

It is possible to become confused about the role of medical treatment and spiritual progress. I do believe that there is a division here and that we have to be sure about the role we are fulfilling. Any progress on a spiritual path towards ultimate enlightenment requires the help of a qualified spiritual teacher. Someone who has already realised the true nature of their own mind. In this way, they are able to help others towards ultimate freedom from this cycle of suffering where we identify so strongly with our clouds of thoughts and emotions. At this level, we are all confused, neurotic beings who require such help to progress along a spiritual path.

At the level of treatment, we are dealing more directly with psychological states. This is done, hopefully, from the perspective of an overall view of the true nature of reality although this may be, currently, an intellectual understanding only. It is possible to help people with psychological disturbances and I described in Chapter 2 - Philosophy the aim of treatment. This is to achieve a

---

[1] The common usage of neurosis and neurotic is invariably pejorative. They are applied more readily to women than men.

[2] For more details of the Tibetan medical approach, I would recommend "The Healing Buddha" by Raoul Birnbaum (Rider, 1980) and "The Diamond Healing - Tibetan Buddhist Medicine and Psychiatry" by Terry Clifford (Crucible, 1984).

[3] "The Tibetan Book of Living of Dying" by Sogyal Rinpoche (Rider, 1993) provides a clear discussion of mind and its true nature. Chapters 4, 5 and 10 in particular deal with mind.

degree of freedom, to remove limitations to the expression of our mental and emotional levels. This can be described as dealing with problems on a relative level when compared to the absolute level of spiritual practice. However, I would emphasise that unless we have the overall perspective or view. any help will tend to be stuck in the relative level of thoughts and emotions. Problems then circulate around and around with no progress.

The division between these relative and absolute levels is important. It also explains why approaches which directly deal with inner, mental states are the most powerful methods of transformation. Visualisation and meditation are just some of the methods which can be used to transform states of mind.

- CLASSIFICATION OF PSYCHOLOGICAL DISORDERS -

The conventional classification of psychological disorders is fairly complex[4] and difficult to follow as there are many subcategories. The list in Table 16.1 is a simplified version. This is a somewhat confusing classification since the emphasis is on naming. There is little overall logic and it is of minimal use for practitioners who are not going to be using conventional methods of treatment. Another source of confusion is the use of the word, mental. In conventional medicine, this is applied loosely to any psychological disturbance[5]. I intend to use it as I did in Chapter 2 - Philosophy where I applied it to thought, cognition and perception[6]. I use the term 'emotion' to describe mood, feeling or affect[7].

A further difficulty is the use of the term, organic[8]. This means that symptoms are associated with physical, structural changes which are considered in conventional medicine to be the cause of any symptoms. This underlines the emphasis on physical matters.

---

[4] A common system of classification is the *Diagnostic and Statistical Manual of Mental Disorders (Third Edition (DSM-III)*. The latest edition is *DSM-III-R*. In common with all conventional labels, these tend to be rigid terms into which the person is forced, thus enabling a certain treatment to be given.

[5] Psychosis is defined by conventional medicine as "Severe mental illness in which the sufferer loses contact with reality. Delusions and hallucinations occur and so thought processes may be altered" - Concise Medical Dictionary, Oxford Medical Publications, 1981.

A neurosis is defined conventionally as "A mental illness in which insight is retained but there is a maladaptive way of behaving or thinking that causes suffering. A classification of neurosis is based on the symptoms which may be a pathological severe emotional state or physical complaints" - Concise Medical Dictionary, Oxford Medical Publications, 1981. Here we see the confusion of conventional medicine in that mental, emotional and physical are all included in the same definition.

[6] I, personally, restrict the term ' psychosis' to mean a disturbance of the mental level.

[7] I, personally, restrict the term 'neurosis' to mean a disturbance of the emotional level.

[8] Organic is another term for physical disturbance. It is a term which is frequently paired with functional which implies a non-physical, i.e. psychological, disturbance.

DISORDERS USUALLY FIRST EVIDENT IN INFANCY, CHILDHOOD OR ADOLESCENCE
Developmental disorders
      Mental retardation
      Pervasive developmental disorders, e.g. autism
      Specific developmental disorders, e.g. skills disorders, speech disorders
Disruptive behaviour disorders
Eating disorders
Gender identity disorders
Tic disorders
Elimination disorders, e.g. enuresis
Other disorders - those which cannot easily be categorised above
ORGANIC MENTAL DISORDERS
Dementias such as senile dementia, Alzheimer's disease
Psychoactive substance-induced, e.g. alcohol, amphetamines, caffeine, cannabis, cocaine, hallucinogens, nicotine, opiates and others
Those associated with physical disease
SCHIZOPHRENIA
MOOD DISORDERS
Major depressive illness. Other terms include bipolar disorders, cyclothymia, manic depression.
ANXIETY DISORDERS
Panic disorder
Phobias
Obsessive compulsive disorder
Post-traumatic stress disorder
Anxiety disorder
SOMATOFORM DISORDERS
Hypochondriasis
Somatisation disorder
DISSOCIATIVE DISORDERS
Multiple personality disorder
Psychogenic amnesia
SEXUAL DISORDERS
Several subcategories including exhibitionism, fetishism, paedophilia, sexual masochism, sexual sadism, voyeurism
SEXUAL DYSFUNCTIONS
Several subcategories including impotence, premature ejaculation, dyspareunia, vaginismus, sexual aversion disorder, sexual arousal disorder
SLEEP DISORDERS
Insomnia
Hypersomnia
IMPULSE CONTROL DISORDERS
Several subcategories including kleptomania, pathological gambling.

TABLE 16.1: CONVENTIONAL CLASSIFICATION OF PSYCHOLOGICAL DISORDERS

The alternative view of psychological disorders is that they are part of the whole picture of a person. A psychological disease, such as schizophrenia, would merely be a label applied to a disturbance which mainly manifests on the mental level. In terms of alternative medicine, the key to differentiation is to assess where is the emphasis of the symptoms. If they are primarily on the mental level, then one could say the person has a mental disturbance. The term, psychosis is appropriate here. If the symptoms are primarily emotional in nature then an emotional disturbance can be diagnosed. The term, neurosis is appropriate here. The significance for the person's health of these manifestations is discussed in Chapter 2 - Philosophy. Clearly these divisions are not rigid since most people develop symptoms on all three levels, mental, emotional and physical. The important factor is which level is *mainly* affected. Therefore, an alternative classification of psychological disorders can be summarised as in Table 16.2 The point here, therefore, is not the particular 'name' of the disorder, but the manifestation of the symptoms.

MILD DISEASE

NEUROSES[9] - Disturbances of mood/emotion
Anxiety, , phobias, depression, obsessions, hysteria

PSYCHOSES[10] - Disturbances of thought/perception

Acute	Delirium[11]
Chronic	Eating disorders
	Manic depression
	Schizophrenia
	Dementias

SEVERE DISEASE

TABLE 16.2: ALTERNATIVE CLASSIFICATION OF PSYCHOLOGICAL DISORDERS

The psychoses, thence, may be seen as being primarily disorders of thought. The neuroses, are primarily disorders of emotion.

- INVESTIGATION OF PSYCHOLOGICAL DISORDERS -

Generally, a psychological disorder is clearly diagnosed by the symptoms. However, individual people may have investigations if there is an underlying physical abnormality suspected. The relevant investigations which may be performed in any situation are detailed with the individual disorders.

- DISORDERS OF THE MENTAL LEVEL (PSYCHOSES) -

DELIRIUM

This can be defined as an acute disturbance of the mental level which accompanies a physical disease. It may also be known as acute brain syndrome, acute confusional state, toxic psychosis or metabolic encephalopathy. It is seen in the following situations:

- drug intoxication, e.g. alcohol, LSD
- drug withdrawal
- infectious disease particularly when associated with a fever
- metabolic disturbances, e.g. liver failure, kidney failure, hypoglycaemia
- vitamin deficiency, e.g. Vitamin B$_{12}$
- lack of oxygen supply to the brain, e.g. pneumonia, chronic bronchitis, cardiac failure.
- head injury[12]

---

[9] These may be termed, 'minor' disorders to differentiate them from the 'major' disorders of the psychoses. They are frequently treated by means of 'minor' tranquillisers, e.g. benzodiazepines.
[10] These may be termed, 'major' disorders to differentiate them from the 'minor' disorders of the neuroses. They are frequently treated by means of 'major' tranquillisers, e.g. phenothiazines.
[11] This correponds to subcategories of organic mental disorder in Table 16.1. It is the acute development of mental symptoms associated with other disease, e.g. respiratory or cardiac disease or with the use, abuse or withdrawal of intoxicating drugs.
[12] I have placed this here as head injury is an acute event although the resulting clinical picture has more in common with that of dementia described below.

Symptoms:

The onset of delirium is usually rapid with a short history and a speedy development of symptoms. There may be the symptoms of the associated physical disease together with disturbance on the mental level. These include mental restlessness, disorientation, poor memory, hallucinations particularly visual which may be fearful and, eventually, confusion. Insomnia is common and agitation may be more marked at night.

A particular syndrome is related to the withdrawal of excess alcohol intake. This is termed 'delirium tremens' (DTs).

Investigations:

Those done will depend upon the suspected underlying disease. Details of these can be found in their relevant section. For example, see Chapter 7 - Cardiovascular System for cardiac failure, Chapter 8 - Respiratory System for pneumonia, chronic bronchitis, etc.

Treatment

The treatment is of the preceding condition.

Alternative management:

In terms of alternative medicine, the occurrence of mental symptoms in association with physical disease means that the imbalance on an energetic level has passed much deeper into the person. It necessarily indicates a more worrying situation. Such situations are described at the end of relevant Chapters dealing with symptoms. For example, the occurrence of breathlessness associated with confusion indicates a serious underlying condition - see Page 162. You may need to refer such people for acute medical care.

DEMENTIA

This a chronic situation which becomes more common with increasing age. There are considered to be around 1 in 20 cases at the age of 70 years and 1 in 5 at the age of 80 years. In conventional medical thought, it is considered to be secondary to a chronic disease of the brain. These include cerebrovascular disease and Alzheimer's Disease[13].

Symptoms

The age of first development of symptoms is variable and partially dependent upon the associated condition. For example, Alzheimer's disease may first develop when aged 40 years or so. Cerebrovascular disease manifests at later ages. A distinction is sometimes made at the age of 60 years. Onset before this is denoted presenile dementia whilst the later development of symptoms is called senile dementia.

The onset is slow as would be expected with a chronic disease. The symptoms depend upon the previous personality and emotional state of the person. There is interference with judgement and reasoning. Memory becomes poor, particularly for recent events. There may be emotional instability and the emotions may fluctuate from euphoria or mania to depression.

Eventually the person affected may have difficulty with personal hygiene, dressing, eating and so forth. There can be increasing agitation, particularly at night, insomnia and eventually confusion. In severe cases, there is complete memory loss for even close relatives and the only events remembered may be several decades previously. Consequently, this can be distressing for relatives who are involved with care. There is a large part to be played here by voluntary organisations or

---

[13] Be careful not to confuse physical changes and mental symptoms. In terms of the classification of a disease, it depends upon where the symptoms manifest. If symptoms are primarily mental in nature then the disease is classified as mental. It does not matter whether there are physical changes. It is only the conventional view that physical changes lead to mental symptoms.

professional carers to help support the family.

In the most severe cases there is gradual deterioration until the person cannot leave the bed. At this stage there is a risk of respiratory problems and pneumonia may be the final life-threatening event.

Investigations:

Routine investigations may be performed to exclude treatable causes of such a clinical picture. These will include brain scan, thyroxine and Vitamin B_{12} level determination. It is important to review medication as there are many drugs which cause confusion as part of their side-effects especially in the elderly.

Treatment

The conventional treatment of psychotic disorders is summarised below.

SCHIZOPHRENIA

This condition can be described as a disintegration of the personality leading to detachment from the social environment. It can affect any age but usually first develops between the ages of 19 and 25. There are some 250,000 people with schizophrenia in the UK and 55 million world-wide. Schizophrenia affects 1% of the UK population at any one time but the diagnosis is ten times more common in young Afro-Caribbean men. The Irish are also more likely to so diagnosed. The reasons for these racial differences in *diagnosis* are discussed later.

Symptoms:

Schizophrenia is primarily a disorder of thought. In the classical case, thoughts are rambling and disjointed. The emotions may be inappropriate. Actions, as a consequence, may be impulsive. Hallucinations are a characteristic feature. There may be threatening or unfriendly voices. Bizarre delusions are common. It is usual for people with this condition to consider their actions are controlled from the outside. This leads to ideas that they are controlled by aliens from another world. Delusions tend to be culturally specific. In the latter part of the 20th century in the West, it is common to see them related to space travel, electronics and computers. In a more religious age they tended to be linked to devils and spirits.

Another perception is that other people place thoughts in their mind - or that they are removed. Paranoia may be a feature where the person thinks they are surrounded by people who watch them and want to do harm. This can lead to delusions that the CIA or KGB is plotting against them. There is little insight with this condition although this varies from person to person and may change with time.

The person's ability to function declines with little capacity for work. Social relations are disrupted and self-care may be poor. Abrupt inexplicable behaviour is seen which may be socially unacceptable to most. Compulsory hospital admission may be required in severely affected cases where there is disruption to the ability to care for oneself.

There may be worry about the safety of the person with schizophrenia or those who come into contact with them. This is frequently overstated and it is unusual that people need to be compulsorily admitted for their own or others 'good'.

Conventional treatment:

Here I shall summarise the treatment of any condition which is characterised by thought disorders, confusion and lack of insight. Even without such treatment, many cases of schizophrenia improve spontaneously within 3-9 months after the flare-up of symptoms. The conventional treatments of manic depression and eating disorders are detailed separately later.

Conventional treatment is invariably with drugs which suppress thoughts. They are essentially sedative in nature and are classified as the 'major' tranquillisers[14]. These are not to be confused with the 'minor' tranquillisers which are used to treat simple anxiety. There were nearly 4.5 million prescriptions for anti-psychotic drugs in the UK in 1987.

The main group of drugs is the phenothiazines of which chlorpromazine is a common example. Other groups include the butyrophenones, e.g. droperidol, benperidol, and the dibenzoxazepines, e.g. clozapine[15], loxapine.

There are many side-effects with these groups of drugs but the most severe is a Parkinson's disease-like disorder - tardive dyskinesia. It is a result of damage to the brain by prescribed drugs and is usually irreversible. Up to 65% of long-term users of anti-psychotic drugs develop tardive dyskinesia. Symptoms include tremor, slow movement, uncontrollable facial grimaces and lip smacking.

In acute situations, large doses of such drugs may be given and this can lead to fatal consequences. Professor Malcolm Lader, Professor of Clinical Psychopharmacology at the Institute of Psychiatry, estimates that one death per week in the UK occurs from reactions to anti-psychotics. The cause of death may often be attributed to a disease rather than the drug and so accurate figures are difficult to obtain. There are, however, regular occurrences of deaths in psychiatric hospitals after the administration of large doses of anti-psychotic drugs. A Channel 4 television programme, Dispatches, identified 52 cases in the UK in the period 1988-92.

The doses used may be in excess of those recommended in the literature. The drugs are used to immobilise people. Chlorpromazine (Trade name - Largactil) is known in prisons as the 'liquid cosh' for this reason. It is certainly a method of restricting activity and is quicker than more gentle methods which may require more staff and care.

Hydergine which may be used in Alzheimer's disease can accelerate the progression of the disease[16]. The newer formulations which manufacturers claim reach the brain in higher concentrations have been found to be no better than placebo.

Some people with psychotic illnesses are compulsorily admitted to hospital. There is much discussion about the need for and usefulness of such an action. Certainly, there have been notable critics of dealing with psychological problems in this way. Well known, at least in the UK, is R.D. Laing who questioned the right of any society to deem some of its members 'insane'[17]. Medical labels applied to groups of people may appear, on the surface, to be for the benefit of the patient. In reality, the reasons for such labels and subsequent treatment may be more to do with social control[18]

---

[14] In this text I use the terms 'major' tranquillisers, anti-psychotics and neuroleptics interchangeably to indicate groups of drugs which suppress thought disorders.

[15] All the antipsychotics have powerful side-effects and I mention some in this book. For more details see, "Prescribed Drugs and the Alternative Practitioner" by S. Gascoigne (Ashgrove Press, 1992).

In the case of clozapine, 2% of users develop a potentially lethal blood disorder. People who take it require weekly blood tests for early signs. The average yearly cost to prescribe and monitor clozapine is over £2000 per person.

[16] New England Journal of Medicine, Aug 16, 1990.

[17] "The Divided Self" by R.D. Laing (Penguin, 1990) This was first published in 1960 and continues to be a radical alternative to the suppressive actions of people who cannot bear to face mental and emotional states. As he quotes in his preface, "....psychiatry can so easily be a technique of brainwashing, of inducing behaviour that is adjusted, by (preferably) non-injurious torture. In the best places, where straitjackets are abolished, doors are unlocked, leucotomies largely forgone, these can be replaced by more subtle lobotomies and tranquillizers that place the bars of Bedlam and the locked doors *inside* the patient. Thus I would wish to emphasize that our 'normal' 'adjusted' state is too often the abdication of ecstasy, the betrayal of our true potentialities, that many of us are only too successful in acquiring a false self to adapt to false realities." Other books by Laing which pursue these themes are "The Politics of Experience", "The Bird of Paradise", "Sanity, Madness and the Family" with A. Esterson, "Self and Others".

[18] There are excellent sociological analyses of the impact of modern medical techniques and the reasons behind their application (rather than the oft-quoted superficial one that they are 'for your own good'). These include "Medical Nemesis" by Ivan Illich (Bantam, 1976) and "The Mirage of Health: Utopian Progress and Biological Change" by Rene Dubos (Anchor, 1959).

High rates of psychiatric admission are found amongst people from central urban areas of low social class and with a high concentration of immigrants. Although, in the UK, it may be true that West Indian immigrants are no more likely to become psychiatric in-patients, when they do so it is more likely to be on a compulsory basis. Those of West Indian origin are twice as likely as whites to have been admitted compulsorily. They were also more likely to be sent to hospital from prison or by police agencies with little GP involvement[19].

In one survey, out of 286 patients admitted by police to a psychiatric hospital, an excess of black admissions was recorded. Black men were younger, were more likely to be given antipsychotic drugs, to be put on compulsory orders and to be given an out-patient appointment when discharged from hospital. More black men were given a diagnosis of schizophrenia or drug-induced psychosis.[20]

In the UK, the numbers of compulsory admissions have been falling over recent years. In 1964 this was 32735 (21% of total admissions) and in 1977 had fallen to 19426 (10.5%). There is a general move in recent years away from hospital admission for psychiatric disturbances. It has been part of a much-advertised 'care in the community' scheme[21]. This is a euphemism for lack of care by the community and large numbers of vulnerable people have been left to fend for themselves. There has been some effort to replace hospital beds by sheltered housing or hostel accommodation. However, this has been generally inadequate and many people with severe mental problems wander the streets as best they can. Some have died as a result and others live a miserable existence.

In the UK, the Mental Health Act of 1983 regulates the compulsory admission and treatment of people with psychiatric illness. It is applied when a person has a named psychological disorder, their own or other's safety is at risk and unwilling to be hospitalised voluntarily. It clearly must not be applied without serious thought on the part of those applying since the individual is deprived of their liberty and certain legal rights.

The Act also deals with people's rights, appeals tribunals and the supervision of the use of compulsory powers. Despite these safeguards, many people find themselves in the difficult position of having to *prove* that they are sane within the meaning of conventional psychiatry. How many of us would find this easy or even possible! Therefore, it can be difficult for some people to obtain discharge from hospital or remove themselves from continual supervision.

Different sections of the Act deal with different situations. Table 16.3. is a summary.

SECTION	DETAILS	COMMENTS
2[22]	Valid for 28 days. Requires signatures of nearest relative or social worker plus two doctors one of whom must be an approved specialist psychiatrist	Used for assessment and treatment
3	Valid for 6 months. Requires signatures of nearest relative or social worker plus two doctors one of whom must be an approved specialist psychiatrist	Used for treatment
4	Valid for 72 hours. Requires signature of nearest relative or social worker plus one doctor	Emergency admission
5(2)	Valid for 72 hours. Requires signature of the doctor in charge of care	Emergency detention of person already in hospital
5(4)	Valid for 72 hours. Requires signature of registered mental nurse	Emergency detention of person already in hospital
136	Police officer	Assessment. Used in public places when person thought to be mentally ill and requiring place of safety

TABLE 16.3: MAIN SECTIONS OF THE MENTAL HEALTH ACT 1983.

[19] Psychiatric Hospital Admissions in Bristol. Ineichen, Harrison and Morgan : British Journal of Psychiatry 1984; 145: 600-611.
[20] Police Admissions to a Psychiatric Hospital. Dunn and Fahy: British Journal of Psychiatry 1990; 156: 373-378.
[21] Some 70,000 in-patient places have disappeared in the UK in the last 15 years.
[22] In 1989, there were 16,900 compusory admissions to hospital, 56% of these were under Section 2. In-patients formally detained under the Mental Health Act, 1984-90, Department of Health.

Operations on the brain, so-called psychosurgery, are not common but may be performed for a range of psychological conditions. Such treatment used to be more common for schizophrenia around 30 years ago but have reduced in popularity due to the use of drugs. Nowadays it is usually reserved for severe depression unresponsive to drugs, obsessional neurosis, anxiety neurosis and manic depression. There were 27 operations in the UK in 1990 comparing with 70 in 1979. Parts of the brain are surgically disconnected or destroyed by the implantation of radioactive materials. Those who perform such operations claim they are successful despite the fact that no trial of their usefulness has ever been performed. In addition, the understanding of the relationship between the emotions and the brain is tenuous to say the least. Noted effects include apathy, excessive weight gain, disinhibition and epilepsy. It has been known to be used in the UK to reduce aggression and anti-social behaviour.

Alternative management:

These disorders, in any terms, are difficult. As I discussed in Chapter 2 - Philosophy, disturbances of the mental level indicate some of the most severe disorders of health. A multiple approach is necessary preferably involving people experienced in dealing with serious mental disorders. The more severe the problem, the more it seems necessary to take complete care of someone[23]. There are several groups who look after and treat mentally disturbed people without recourse to drugs and conventional treatment. It is helpful to have access to these for those few people who seek your help.

I have rarely been approached for help with such disorders. I describe a case of manic depression below which is helpful in describing a general approach. You must be aware that prescribed drugs are heavily suppressive of thought disorders. Their removal may result in an acute flare-up of symptoms including loss of insight. This may only develop some weeks after total cessation of the medication with no or little prior warning. This is the reason why several approaches are necessary with facilities for care. In the context of out-patient practice it may well be impracticable to treat such people.

In terms of Chinese medicine, there are considered to be two main categories of schizophrenia although a similar diagnosis may be made in any similar mental disturbance. There is an active, manic (Yang) type where depression and anger transform to Fire in the Liver and Gall Bladder. This is accompanied by Phlegm which disrupts the Spirit in the Heart.

The quiet, depressive (Yin) type is where excessive anxiety impedes the circulation of Qi and causes fluids to congeal and form Phlegm. When Phlegm rises, the senses become obscured and consciousness is disrupted.

MANIC DEPRESSIVE DISORDER

There are several categories of mania and depression depending upon the particular manifestation. Classical manic depression is a swing between the extremes of mania (elevated mood), and depression (depressed mood). Some people exhibit only mania whilst others seem to develop only depression. This type of depression may also be known by the term 'endogenous' depression. The milder, 'reactive' form of depression is described below under depressive neurosis.

The conventional view at the moment is that these disorders are due to imbalances of chemical transmitter substances within the brain. In mania, they are in excess. In depression, they are lacking. This is seen very much as a justification for chemical methods of control. Psychological and psychotherapeutic models are not given credence at this time. Consequently, treatment is invariably by means of drugs.

Symptoms:

Mania is a persistent elevation in mood which may last for weeks or months. There is agitation, insomnia, restlessness. Thoughts arrive rapidly and usually involve grandiose yet unrealistic plans. The mood is essentially euphoric but with lack of insight. There is resultant behaviour which may be disruptive such as spending large amounts of money, travelling long distances and so forth. The

---

[23] 'In treating insanity, the physician should constantly stay with the patient....'. "Nei Ching and Nan Ching". Volume III, 22.1. Translation by Henry Lu.

person may become violent if their ideas are resisted. There may be associated hallucinations, delusions and other thought disorders resembling classical schizophrenia. Milder forms are known as hypomania.

Mania may alternate with depression. The use of the word depression is somewhat of a misnomer. The term can mean many different things to different people. It may be a state of sadness, a low mood, an apathy and so forth. In this condition, it is a gloominess or despair and is severe.

It is not the feeling of lowness that many people have from time to time and could be considered to be a variation of normal. It is the depths of a black despair where there may be severe associated symptoms of unworthiness, self blame, guilt and perhaps even suicidal thoughts or feelings. There may also be associated physical symptoms of constipation, poor appetite, weight loss, headaches, reduced libido and so forth. Suicide is a risk. In severe cases, the feelings of guilt, self-blame and futility may attain delusional levels.

Some people seem to only develop mania or only depression.

Treatment:

The florid phase may be life-threatening due to lack of insight. At this stage, compulsory hospitalisation may be necessary. Sedation by means of medication is the rule. This is primarily with lithium compounds. Lithium should only be used for manic depressive states. I have seen some people with simple depression treated with lithium and this is an example of inappropriate prescribing. The use of powerful drugs in such circumstances can only lead to more problems. The drug requires careful medical supervision as it can affect several organs including the thyroid, liver, kidney and central nervous system. It may also interfere with water and mineral homeostasis. The rationale behind the use of lithium is to attempt to correct a perceived chemical imbalance in the brain. Chemically, it is closely related to sodium and so lithium toxicity is a risk when sodium depletion occurs, e.g. excess sweating, hot climates.

Without treatment, manic depressive episodes may resolve over several months or a year or so. Treatment is often continued for life. Other treatments include electroconvulsive treatment and perhaps additional tranquillisation.

Alternative management:

Manic depression, in terms of Chinese medicine, corresponds to the syndromes listed under schizophrenia.

CASE

A woman of 28 years came for treatment with a past history of a 'breakdown'. She had been diagnosed as suffering from schizophrenia at the age of 16 years and was prescribed an antipsychotic together with an anti-Parkinsonian drug - a common combination. She stopped this after a few years and was fine until at the age of 22 years she had a recurrence. This was not so severe and was diagnosed as hypomania. She was prescribed lithium which she had remained on ever since.

This illustrates a common observation in conventional medicine that the diagnosis may change according to the drugs people are given. I have known people diagnosed as schizophrenic and given 'major' tranquillisers. When they have failed to respond, the diagnosis has been changed to manic depression and they are then given lithium. The diagnosis is more related to the drugs used rather than the symptom picture.

In a breakdown, she would have rapid thoughts, agitation, inability to sleep and great physical restlessness. She was currently taking lithium 400 mg twice daily and had blood tests every 6 months to check her liver function. With this dosage of lithium she felt fairly well but wanted help in coming off it as she wanted to start a family at some point in the future.

Her original symptoms developed after a broken love affair and the ingestion of large amounts of recreational drugs, namely cannabis and amphetamines. There is frequently a history, around puberty or in the teenage years of an emotional upset. In addition, with many psychological disturbances, there may be the ingestion of drugs which affect mood and thought.

In the case of the psychoses, any emotional disturbance which is unresolved may, if it worsens, then flip over into the mental level and lead to thought disturbances. Curative treatment, therefore, would almost inevitably see the arisal of emotional disturbances as part of improvement. As this process develops, it is important to support people and perhaps use psychological approaches such as counselling or psychotherapy to help resolve these issues.

Drug reduction must not take place until improvement in the person's underlying psychological state has begun. Otherwise, reduction will lead to a flare-up of symptoms which may overwhelm the person. Long-term treatment is necessary and it may take several years to resolve these problems.

EATING DISORDERS (ANOREXIA NERVOSA/BULIMIA NERVOSA)

Anorexia nervosa is a desire to lose weight associated with a perception of being overweight or 'the wrong shape'. Bulimia nervosa is a situation of overeating with changes in perception.

These conditions may be considered together as they are related and seem to be opposite sides of the same coin. They are associated with disturbances in perception and may be realistically labelled as psychoses. They may be categorised by the general term, 'eating disorders'.

95% of those who develop such disorders are female. Such conditions, therefore, cannot be separated from societal views of women and their shape. Women are bombarded from an early age with images of (supposedly) fit and healthy women. In my opinion, such images are the result of anorexic behaviour and certainly not to be considered a normal female shape. Females tend to be Yin which manifests as a rounded shape. Angular forms are a sign of malnutrition. It is interesting that almost all the speakers at international conferences on these conditions are men!

Symptoms:

There is a preoccupation with food. A variety of feelings and thoughts about appearance are invariable. The person frequently has feelings of disgust for food yet with uncontrollable urges to eat. There may be almost complete absence of desire for food. Eating to the point of vomiting or producing vomiting is common. Cathartics and laxatives may be taken in an effort to reduce weight.

There is a general lack of concern for any physical deterioration as weight, appearance, and food intake preoccupy the person. Extreme weight loss can be seen in some cases. Amenorrhoea is a common occurrence. Emotional and sexual immaturity is associated.

Treatment:

This is notoriously difficult and some people may die with anorexia nervosa. In-patient treatment may be required for severe cases where malnutrition is evident. The conventional medical approach is to combine regimes of forced feedings to achieve a certain rate of weight gain with behavioural approaches A 'carrot and 'stick' method may be applied. 'Counselling' may also be used but is impossible in an atmosphere of punitive feeding. Such treatments may be considered to be similar to the use of ECT and antipsychotic drugs in terms of their effectiveness and usefulness

Various approaches are attempted to help alleviate the mental symptoms. Psychotherapy is the best option to help attain emotional maturation.

Alternative management:

This is a condition which reflects a disturbance at deep levels. The person has difficulty in nourishing themselves. This is a consequence of a lack of nourishment on a mental and emotional level in the past. There are frequently disturbances in the family unit and these need to be addressed if possible. The desire for weight loss is an attempt not to grow and mature. Common associated events are the disappearance of menstruation together with emotional and sexual immaturity. There may be sexual or emotional difficulties between the parents which are resulting in this particular manifestation in the child.

In terms of Chinese medicine, it is common to see Spleen Qi deficiency as a result of irregular eating together with Liver Qi Stagnation as a result of long-term emotional suppression. It is important to take a general approach to treatment with support from several areas. A psychological approach is helpful as well as treatment to strengthen the digestion. The case below is a useful illustration of the course of treatment.

CASE

A woman of 30 years came for treatment who had a reaction to a bowel cleansing formula of oils and herbs. She felt 'hungover', weak and emotionally upset. She had a history of episodes of over-eating alternating with fasting. In terms of Chinese medicine, her diagnosis was Spleen Qi Deficiency of long-standing caused exacerbated by a history of irregular eating together with Liver Qi Stagnation.

In my experience, this is not the origin of the problem as the irregular eating is the result of earlier disturbances. This condition arises early in childhood due to a lack of nourishment within the family. This may not be, and often is not, a lack of physical nourishment. It is more related to a deprivation of emotional care together with the development of messages of guilt and responsibility. Feelings and thoughts of disgust and a poor self-image are universal. This is particularly common in women for reasons I discuss in the Introduction to Chapter 18 - Gynaecology. Also, women are bombarded with images in the media of women who, frankly, are anorexic themselves. The shapes of such women are abnormal and are reminiscent of pre-pubertal girls. This is not the shape of mature women. The attempt of women to attain and maintain such a shape is very destructive of their digestive health. A cycle of eating, fasting and excess exercise can only be depleting and this is discussed on Page 290 with an illustrative case.

I treated her by strengthening her Spleen and recommending a regular diet of warm food. Over the course of the next few months, she experienced feelings and dreams which were unpleasant as old memories surfaced. Gradually she became more positive and after 6 months of treatment she only occasionally would revert to her old eating patterns. Even so, the associated emotions and thoughts were not so strong and she felt a greater sense of non-attachment. Interestingly, her weight increased in this time by some 10 pounds. This was of some concern for her but it is important to reassure people that this is healthy and that internal levels are of prime importance. Any weight fluctuations will eventually settle although many women in this situation are underweight.

- DISORDERS OF THE EMOTIONAL LEVEL (NEUROSES) -

A useful working definition of neurosis is to say that it is an over-production of a normal emotional state. We all have emotions such as anxiety, depression, sadness, anger and so forth. When these become excessive or unbalanced in some way, then it may be possible to say that a neurosis exists. In one sense we may all be considered to be neurotic. What do I mean by this? We all, at some stage in our lives, exhibit symptoms associated with an emotional disturbance.

In conventional medicine, a diagnosis of neurosis is made according to certain criteria. There must be one of the typical syndromes with a recent setback, e.g. disturbance in a relationship. This is in order to exclude a physical cause and underlines the rigid line of division between aspects of the person. The setback may not be gross but may trigger off an association from the distant past.

ANXIETY NEUROSIS

This is a state of inner tension and anticipation which is perceived as unpleasant. There may also be feeling of fear and panic. There are, in addition, accompanying physical symptoms. It is the commonest form of neurosis. There are frequently symptoms in the immediate family. Some 15% of parents and siblings are affected compared with 5% of the general population. Women are diagnosed twice as commonly as men. There is often a past history of emotional disturbance and insecurity The overt symptom picture may be precipitated by bereavement, disappointment, work problems, or relationship difficulties.

Symptoms:

The main emphasis may be either on the emotional state or the associated physical symptoms. There may be anxiety and nervousness, a feeling of apprehension, anticipation or panic. In some, there may be preoccupation with fear of physical illness such as cancer or heart disease. There is poor concentration, indecision, restlessness and agitation. Sleep may be disturbed, either getting off or waking in the night. Shortness of breath with feeling of faintness may lead to confusion with heart attack or stroke. This latter presentation is usually termed 'hyperventilation'.

Accompanying physical symptoms include sweating, tremor and palpitations. Tiredness is common. Headache, frequent urination and loose stools may also be present.

Treatment:

The mainstay of conventional treatment is by means of drugs. Those commonly used are the 'minor' tranquillisers which are not to be confused with the 'major' tranquillisers used in the treatment of psychotic illnesses. Examples of 'minor' tranquillisers include the benzodiazepines, e.g. diazepam, chlordiazepoxide, and the barbiturates. All these drugs have a propensity for being rapidly addictive and there are well-described withdrawal syndromes.

In recent years, at least in the UK, there has been some recognition of this. However, this has, sadly, led to the increased prescription of 'major' tranquillisers, antidepressants or betablockers. Medical practitioners usually tell people that other drugs are safer and non-addictive. This is nonsense. No drug is non-addictive and it is dangerous to assume so. This is because people may stop their drugs thinking there will be no problems. Also, the prescription of drugs such as betablockers or antidepressants to replace tranquillisers are more likely to cause difficulties as they are more powerful. They have stronger side-effects particularly on the heart. Betablockers are described in detail in Chapter 7 - Cardiovascular System.

'Minor' tranquillisers are commonly used with almost 16 million prescriptions for benzodiazepines in the UK in 1992. Side-effects are extremely common with all drugs given to alter mood. This is more so with some than others but no drug is exempt. Triazolam, a benzodiazepine, has been linked with paranoia and aggression. Side-effects include amnesia, anxiety, depression and, more seriously, aggressive behaviour. Between 1984 and 1991, some 3555 adverse reactions were filed to the Food and Drug Administration (FDA) in the US compared to 833 with flurazepam since 1970 and 318 for temazepam since 1981. The FDA had received reports of 49 'homicides and attempted homicides' connected to use of the drug[24]. It was banned from use in the UK in 1991.

Alternative treatment:

The general alternative management of the neuroses is summarised below. In terms of Chinese medicine, the benzodiazepines are cooling and primarily affect the Heart. They can be likened to the group of Chinese herbs which Calm the Spirit. There are three main consequences of using single substances particularly for a long period of time. Firstly, the calming of the Spirit leads to depression. Secondly, long-term use damages other organs particularly the Spleen and Kidneys. Thirdly, in some people there is the generation of Heat as a result of their action and this manifests as violent outbursts, aggression and the like.

Withdrawal of these drugs leads to flaring up of Heart Fire such as anxiety, mania, hallucinations and, in severe cases, convulsions. Such withdrawal must be done slowly in conjunction with treatments which strengthen and support.

CASE

A woman of 37 years came for treatment of her headaches. She had received acupuncture 4 years previously which had helped but they had started to return in recent months. The headaches were at least once or twice per week and in the temples. They would last for at least 24 hours. There would be associated nausea

Her other symptoms were, to me, more important, however. She had a feeling of a lump in the throat all the time with a feeling of mucus stuck there. She was continually worried about her health and any symptom she developed. She would always think that she had cancer. This had been particularly severe since her husband died of cancer some years ago but had been present from childhood after a close relative died.

She had a past history of depression after childbirth and had taken antidepressants in the past. She would feel irritable before a period and this would be the time when a headache was particularly likely to develop. Her vision was weak with floaters.

---

[24] Article in Independent of Dec. 3rd, 1991.

In terms of Chinese medicine, her diagnosis was Heart and Liver Blood Deficiency, Liver Qi Stagnation and Kidney Yang Deficiency. Her energy was extremely low when she first came for treatment. A clue was the fact that in the past, she would develop a headache whenever she had acupuncture or reflexology treatment. This could be an aggravation as part of a curative response but for it to happen repeatedly suggests that the treatment is too strong for her. Certainly her pulses were extremely weak in all positions but particularly those of the Heart and Liver.

I treated her with herbs and acupuncture to strengthen her Blood and Kidney Yang. The process was slow yet continued and after 2 years of treatment she felt strong enough to begin counselling. Psychological approaches such as counselling and psychotherapy require a lot of energy. If people are too weak they may find it difficult. In recent months she has been well with much reduced symptoms.

These problems arise from deep levels and long-term treatment is necessary. Support is required as people experience symptoms which they find difficult to cope with, let alone understand. Nevertheless, with help and appropriate treatment, real transformations take place. I have no doubt that this woman will remain well and now has the understanding as well as tools of relaxation and meditation to help her in the future.

PHOBIC NEUROSIS

This is a fear of an object, situation or activity. It is described as irrational in conventional texts although every event must have a preceding cause. It may not be known but this does not make it irrational. The fear may be non-specific as when people feel generally afraid. On the other hand it may be directed towards a specific situation. A common manifestation is fear of open spaces - agoraphobia. This may also be an inability to leave home or be in situations which the person finds stressful. The person may avoid such situations entirely and live their life in a restricted manner. In less severe cases, the situation may be tolerated but with marked feelings of fear. The number and variety of foci for phobias are limitless and each case must be dealt with on an individual basis.

Symptoms:

These are similar to those of anxiety neurosis described above. They are particularly severe when a specific trigger is present. Otherwise, there is a general feeling of tension and apprehension.

Treatment:

This is frequently by means of prescribed drugs. This is usually with antidepressants of which the tricyclic, imipramine is the commonest used. Benzodiazepines, usually alprazolam, may also be employed. Drugs are less effective where the fear is non-specific.

Psychotherapy with or without behaviour therapy may also be used. Some people are treated by graduall increased exposure to the phobic situation as a type of desensitisation.

HYSTERICAL NEUROSIS

This is the production of physical symptoms as a result of a psychological disturbance. The appearance of the physical symptoms, e.g. paralysis, numbness, blackouts, memory loss, leads to relief of the psychological symptoms. Challenge and confrontation lead to a return of the psychological disturbance and the physical symptoms may improve or disappear only for them to return in the same or a different form some time later.

This so-called 'conversion' hysteria is not so common now. It may occasionally be associated with compensation awards after an accident. It is usually anatomically incorrect. Such symptoms may be viewed by the conventional profession with disdain and an unvoiced accusation that the person has deliberately and wilfully developed them.

The term 'dissociative' hysteria is used to describe a similar process which manifests as altered states of awareness. These may be faints, fits or trances.

The diagnosis is made by excluding structural disease whilst considering the actual symptom picture. There will be a precipitating event.

Treatment:

This is difficult as the person finds some comfort with their situation.

OBSESSIONAL NEUROSIS

This term is applied to those people who perform activities on a repetitive and compulsive basis. There are constantly recurring thoughts or feelings but the person has insight and recognises these as their own. In the classical psychoses, the person thinks that such thoughts are placed in their mind from the outside. Some 1% of the population is considered as obsessive but the true incidence is certainly higher.

There is an element of anguish with such symptoms and people seek to perform repetitive actions as a way of relieving them. Resisting the urge to perform actions leads to exacerbation of the symptoms.

It is important in the assessment of such people to determine whether the issue is *primarily* with thoughts or feelings. This distinction may not be made conventionally. However, for our purposes this would greatly affect the meaning. Obsessions of thought indicate a more serious disturbance than those of emotions. In some cases, it leads to a particular behaviour consequent upon the particular thought process and belief system. This would classify the disorder as being psychotic in nature. Other cases are where the compulsive action relieves a particular emotional state. This can be classified as being truly neurotic in nature[25].

Symptoms:

There are usually three forms of this condition. There may be merely ideas and thoughts in the mind. There may be impulses to perform a particular action or the fear that they may develop such an impulse. Lastly, there may be the constant churning of things over in the mind. The performance of an action relieves such symptoms. The thoughts are frequently of an aggressive or sexual nature.

There may be combinations of these and may be so severe that they take over a person's life. Typical actions include hand-washing or constantly checking that doors and windows are closed.

Treatment:

This is notoriously difficult conventionally. Reassurance and behaviour therapy are employed. People are frequently treated with tricyclic antidepressants, usually clomipramine.

DEPRESSIVE NEUROSIS

It may come on at any age, with women twice as likely to be diagnosed than men. Around 10% of people develop such symptoms at some time in their life.

It is usual to classify depression as being 'major' or 'minor' in type. 'Major' depression, so-called endogenous depression, is the type described under manic depressive illness. 'Minor' depression, so-called reactive depression, is the type discussed here.

It occurs after a personal setback, e.g. loss such as divorce or bereavement. There is not always a clear line between this and the depression described in manic depression above. Depression, as a low mood, is a common feeling and all of us develop this from time to time. When it becomes excessive, it may be diagnosed as clinical depression. Women are more likely to be so diagnosed than men. Recurrences are common although the first presentation is usually as a young adult.

Symptoms:

The term depression is a loose one which is often applied to mean low mood. It may be used to mean sadness, weeping, unhappiness, dissatisfaction and so forth. When clinically diagnosed there are several criteria to be fulfilled:

---

[25] The differentiation in this paragraph into psychotic and neurotic is my own. You would not hear these ideas voiced by conventional practitioners.

- personal setback
- pre-disposing situation of vulnerability or emotional difficulties
- fluctuating situation which responds to changes in the environment

The distinction between this type and that of 'major' depressive illness is that the latter has more severe symptoms. There are strong feelings of negativity and self-blame along with associated physical symptoms. However, even in this type there may be physical symptoms such as sleep disturbances, loss of libido and tiredness. Occasionally, suicidal thoughts or feelings may be seen in severe cases.

Treatment:

This is commonly by means of prescribed drugs - the antidepressants. They are commonly given and there were 8.5 million prescriptions for antidepressants in the UK in 1989. There are two main groups of antidepressants - the tricyclics and the mono-amine oxidase inhibitors. They aim to affect the chemical balance in the brain and are evidence, if such were needed, that the conventional belief is that psychological disturbances originate from physical structures.

A newer antidepressant, fluoxetine hydrochloride (Prozac) is much in vogue at the moment. It is advertised as helping clinical states of depression as well as relieving some of the minor irritations and dissatisfactions of life. It is currently taken by four and a half million Americans and half a million Britons. 70% of users in the US are women.

It has many side-effects which are shared by the other antidepressants. They include anorexia, weight loss[26], anxiety, nervousness, mania, hypomania, insomnia, fatigue, tremor, dizziness, convulsions, reduced libido, excess sweating and rash. All the antidepressants have a similar action reminiscent of 'speed' (amphetamine). This lifts the mood of depression but, of course, does nothing to remedy the underlying cause. They can only, therefore, lead to more emotional confusion as the person loses any insight as the true nature of their problem.

The disturbing danger is that Prozac is being marketed as much more than an anti-depressant. The approach is similar to that taken with the benzodiazepine, diazepam when it was launched. Officially there are no or very few serious side-effects but there is an increasing level of anecdotal evidence. These range from mild paranoia to murders.

The 'non-pathological' trend of prescribing is increasing as Prozac is touted as the answer to all psychological ills. Doctors in the US are giving the drug to people who wish to overcome perceived personality deficiencies. There are people who take Prozac to boost their confidence for a job interview, to be more 'successful' with relationships and as a recreational drug to "feel good".

Many people, however, feel that the personality produced is not a real or useful one, as it has not been learned or earned. It also has the effect of making people who take it develop the same personality, 'shiny, happy people' as Professor David Rothman[27] has described them. He sees a danger of it being used as a method of pharmacologically-induced social control. I would say here that there is no *danger* of this occurring as this is what is already happening now.

Conventional psychiatric treatment is an example of how one group of the population seeks to remove or control the feelings, thoughts and experience of another, more vulnerable, section of the population. It happened with the benzodiazepine tranquillisers, it happens daily with powerful anti-psychotic agents and electroconvulsive treatment and it is beginning to happen with Prozac. This is not to say that people with psychological disturbances do not have real problems. Of course they do. However, once one group of society starts to label such disturbances and prescribe mind-altering drugs, the result can only be dependence and powerlessness.

The main advocate of Prozac is Dr Peter Kramer, author of "Listening to Prozac" which is a best seller in the US and due to be launched in the UK in the Spring of 1994. In the book he suggests that people are largely biologically determined and so Prozac can be used to replace psychoanalysis. The suggestion is that all people should be outgoing, extrovert and confident and that if they are not then taking this drug will make them 'normal'. This is a flourishing of the Yang aspect as that term is understood by Chinese medicine. It is inherently unbalanced and can only lead to more disease. It

---

[26] For this reason, it may be used to 'treat' bulimia nervosa.
[27] Article in Guardian newspaper Dec. 4th, 1994.

is the result of a false view of reality where there is a belief that people can be in one state all the time. This state of permanence, besides the fact that it is philosophically impossible to be unchanging, can only lead to a rigidity and brittleness of mind. Although depression may not be evident, other more severe imbalances of mind are likely.

Kramer describes such effects as 'cosmetic psychopharmacology'. He also described Prozac as a 'feminist drug, liberating and empowering'. He states that some 20-30% of users are not just returned to the state they were in before they became ill but become 'better than well'. Because the side-effects are regarded as minor, doctors are much more willing to prescribe Prozac to mildly depressive people they would not have given the older anti-depressants.

Symptoms of panic and anxiety will be treated with tranquillisers. These are discussed in detail in their relevant section. It is interesting that the side-effects of tranquillisers include depression and those of anti-depressants include anxiety. It is common, therefore, to see both prescribed to the same person. This combination of 'uppers' and 'downers' is similar to the recreational use of amphetamines with barbiturates.

Electroconvulsive treatment (ECT) is the administration of electric shocks to the brain. It is performed under general anaesthesia[28] and is a related to earlier methods of inducing epileptic attacks. An example was was insulin shock treatment where doses of insulin were given to induce hypoglycaemic coma[29]. These and similar treatments are described in an interesting book based upon real-life experiences in the 1940's[30].

Some 20,000 people in the UK have ECT each year. There are differences according to area as psychiatrists have different preferences. If you live in the West of England, you are twice as likely to receive ECT than if you live in Oxford. At least 600 children have had ECT over the past decade which is particularly worrying as consent is hardly informed and their development is still taking place. About 70% of recipients of ECT are women. This is not surprising since depression is twice as likely to be diagnosed in women as in men. ECT is relatively overused in people from ethnic minorities but this reflects the more common diagnosis of psychological disturbance in these groups.

A series of 5 treatments is usually given with follow-up administration of anti-depressants.

It is claimed that improvement in depression can result from ECT[31]. Short-term side-effects include confusion, headache, disorientation, muscle ache, physical weakness, dizziness and memory loss. Longer lasting side-effects which may be permanent include memory loss[32], apathy, learning difficulties and loss of creative drive and energy. If people have such treatment as an out-patient they have to be taken to their house rather than dropped off at the end of the road. It may be that the confusion and loss of memory loss are the methods by which improvement is claimed. ECT advocate, Max Fink, ascribes the damaging effect to the substance of the brain as the reason for improvement. He states, "it is similar to that of craniocerebral trauma or head injury"[33]. The person no longer knows or can remember how they feel[34]! And this is a system of medicine?

---

[28] The death rate from ECT is similar to that from general anaesthesia.

[29] All these treatments (ECT, insulin shock treatment, drugs) have one thing in common. They produce brain damage. Post-mortem examinations reveal evidence of the death of nervous tissue. This is how they produce their effect. They replace one group of symptoms by another. This can scarcely be described as treatment, cure or even relief of symptoms.

[30] "Savage Sleep" by Millen Brand (Crown, 1968).

[31] Studies in the UK at Leicester, Northwick Park and Nottingham have revealed that ECT produces short term improvement in depression for some people but that this is not sustained beyond four weeks. In contradiction, Dr Richard Weiner, a psychiatrist who specialises in treating people with ECT at Duke University, puts the success rate at 75% in people with complications and 80-90% in those without. These are amazing claims, to say the least, for a complex condition such as depression. If I thought there were any truth in them I might consider ECT myself!

[32] It has been stated in one study that "some husbands used their wives memory loss to establish their own definitions of past situations in the marital relationship". Electroconvulsive Therapy, the Self and Family Relations by C.A.B. Warren, 1988.

[33] Euphoria is common after any neurological damage and this could be the source of any lift in mood.

[34] "It is easier to numb people and induce forgetfulness than to try ot eradicate poverty, provide worthwhile jobs and deal with people's demands to be listened to, understood, loved and valued as part of the community." See "ECT - Effective but for whom?" by J Wallcraft.

In the US there is a lobby group of 500 people who have experienced memory loss for up to 2 years. Psychiatrists reveal their innermost thoughts by their reactions to various groups. They state that the memory loss of ECT is temporary when describing housewives but still express caution over treating "patients whose occupation requires intellectual ability"[35].

A further issue is that ECT, as is the case with all conventional medical treatments, gives the message that psychological distress is a mechanical process. This denies a person's experience and feelings and is necessarily depersonalising. It is also depowering as it leaves the doctor with the responsibility for relief. This continues dependency and an uneven sharing of power within the doctor-patient relationship. Compulsory treatment is clearly more disempowering and may be experienced as a form of punishment[36] or torture.

A muscle relaxant is used during treatment to prevent muscle contraction due to the passage of electric current through the brain. It renders the person unable to breathe independently and necessitates respiratory support (essentially a general anaesthetic). This leads to further feelings of lack of control.

Depression is frequently accompanied by despair and worthlessness. Any reinforcement of these by disempowering treatments can only be harmful.

ECT is banned in California and Italy with restrictions on its use compulsorily in Canada and the Netherlands.

Counselling and psychotherapy tend to be utilised more with this type of depression than with the 'major' type described above. This tends to be more difficult if the mood is severely affected. There are many schools and techniques of such therapies and this is discussed below.

Alternative management:

The general alternative management of the neuroses is described below. In terms of Chinese medicine, the antidepressants are heating and primarily affect the Heart and Liver. They move the Qi by warming and dispersing. This causes weakening of Qi and damage to Blood and Yin. Long-term there will be syndromes of Heart and Liver Blood and Yin Deficiency with ultimately Kidney Yin Deficiency. Withdrawal of antidepressants leads to a flare-up of Yin manifest as Stagnation syndromes such as Stagnant Liver Qi, weeping and emotional releases, depression and so forth. Withdrawal of such drugs must be slow with appropriate support and treatment at the same time.

CASE

A woman of 42 years came for treatment. She had been taking Prozac for over 2 years after suffering from depression for some time. She was taking 3 tablets per week. She had been on courses of antidepressants in the past. She had low energy, frequent urination with leaking and lumbar pain. The diagnosis in terms of Chinese medicine was Kidney Yang Deficiency and Heart Blood Deficiency.

I treated her with herbs and acupuncture to primarily strengthen her Kidney Yang. Her energy slowly improved and her urinary symptoms lessened. It is important in such cases not to attempt a dosage reduction of such powerful drugs too early or too quickly.

After several months of treatment, we discussed the possibility of drug reduction. She decided that she would try to do so. She found that reducing the dose gradually made her feel quite ill and she decided to stop completely. She began to develop some depression with negative feelings, sensitivity and critical thoughts. This was not as severe as she had experienced previously. They began to subside after two to three weeks.

Her treatment continues but she finds that she is coping without the drug and not descending into depression. She was worried that this would happen as it had in the past. The point here is that people can change their responses when they have support. It is difficult to stop a drug without the help of balancing and curative health care. This time she had that help and the outcome is markedly different.

---

[35] Herskovitz, 1943.

[36] Atonement was given as an explanation of how ECT worked. "Fifty Shock Therapy Theories" by L Gordon, Military Surgeon 1948; 103.

– GENERAL COMMENTS ABOUT ALTERNATIVE MANAGEMENT OF THE NEUROSES –

As stated previously, alternative medicine does not seek to divide and separate the levels of a human being. Therefore, physical, emotional and mental aspects are considered as a whole. In terms of Chinese medicine, each of the five major organs, Liver, Heart, Kidney, Spleen and Lung have aspects which correspond to these three levels. Details of these are included in the relevant Chapters. Here, I shall concentrate on their mental and emotional aspects as well as their paired organs. These are listed in Table 16.4.

ORGAN	MENTAL ASPECT	EMOTIONAL ASPECT
Liver	Kindly and giving attitude, sharing	Anger, assertiveness, jealousy, resentment, guilt
Gall Bladder	Decision making	Timidity, lack of courage
Heart	Responsibility, gratitude, appreciation, politeness, humility	Joy, happiness
Small Intestine	Awareness, sensitivity, discernment	
Kidney	Intellect, intelligence, wisdom, insight, will power, ambition	Fear
Urinary Bladder		Jealousy, resentment
Spleen	Belief, faith, confidence, trust	Sympathy
Stomach	Endurance, stamina, ability to keep going	
Lung	Sensibility, sensitiveness, compassion, attitude, vulnerability	Grief, sadness
Large Intestine	Forgiveness, letting go	

TABLE 16.4: MENTAL AND EMOTIONAL ASPECTS OF ORGANS[37]

It can be seen from this Table, that emotions such as depression may arise from several sources. It may be sadness and grief due to a Lung imbalance or a lack of joy from the Heart. It may be the apathy due to lack of ambition with the Kidney. There may be a lack of free-flowing of Qi due to a Liver imbalance or a churning, rumination from the Spleen. It is essential, therefore, whatever the prime, presenting symptom, to individualise the case and give appropriate treatment. What is not helpful is to give every person the same thing as in conventional prescribing of tranquillisers or antidepressants.

It is helpful to summarise the help which can be offered people with psychological disorders. A specific treatment such as homoeopathy, acupuncture or herbs is of inestimable value in supporting people and correcting energetic imbalances. It is not enough, however, to think that this is the complete story. In the West, particularly, psychological disturbances are deep-seated. They frequently arise out of infancy and childhood. We are often brought up in environments which, more or less, may be emotionally deprived and conflictual. They expose us at early ages to inappropriate influences.

A common 'inappropriate' influence is abuse. This may be sexual and is frequently emotional. It is probable that at least one third of adult women and half as many men have had sexual contact with an older person as a child. 20% of women who had been sexually abused as a child have mental health problems, as opposed to 6.3% of the non-abused population. Almost half of psychiatric in-patients had histories of sexual/physical abuse.

These issues are not going to be completely remedied by the application of alternative medicine over some weeks or even months. Although we all have our remarkable success stories where genuine transformations have taken place rapidly, for most people, the process is more gradual[38].

---

[37] I would remind you that these organs are energetic rather than the narrow physical understanding of conventional medicine.

[38] It is difficult, on occasions, to see the benefits of a particular course of action. This is particularly true when dealing with energetic matters. Our relatively gross minds may not be able to perceive subtle changes. This does not, of course, mean that there is no effect from a particular treatment or

Psychological approaches are valuable in giving people extra help. My own view is that sometimes this may be counterproductive if it is too cathartic, too confrontational, too invasive. I discussed, in the Introduction to this Chapter, the importance of seeing psychological states in the context of a complete view of the mind. Because the mind is so complex, its neuroses so rich and varied, we can dig for ever and come up with a problem or difficulty to be analysed. This is not the point. The important issue, for me, is how to facilitate people to recognise their own wisdom and clarity. As the Tibetans say, "If the shit's dry, do not stir it." Gentle methods of transformation are usually more helpful than constant identification with the problem. Identification with the solution is more beneficial. There are too many individual therapies to list here and it is, in any case, the approach of the therapist which the key. "It is not what you do but the way you do it". It is helpful for us as practitioners to know such therapists in our area to whom we can refer people.

- CLASSIFICATIONS OF THE PERSONALITY -

The idea of personality groups arose from the view that a number of people do not conform to the prevailing norm. This has led to a late recognition of personality disorders. It was noted that certain personality types tended to develop particular patterns of behaviour and psychological states, e.g. obsessional neurosis in people with obsessional personality disorder. The precise classification and description depend upon the source[39].

The concept of 'disordered personality' is a tricky one and certainly a source of potential abuse. It is difficult to see the rationale behind labelling some people as 'sick' whilst society at large is hardly 'sane'. These ideas have been discussed at length and remain a dilemma for conventional psychiatry which is usually not addressed.

Any classification of personalities may be used in a judgemental way. It is more helpful to use personality classifications as a way of trying to understand how different people may respond to different situations. Eventually, it is for each individual to come to terms with their own 'neurosis' and find the ways in which they can function most effectively.

In the clinical setting, such issues arise because the person is dissatisfied with themselves most of the time, there is a limitation to their everyday life and relationships or there is difficulty in achieving goals and ambitions.

OBSESSIONAL PERSONALITY

This person has little regard for the emotional aspects of a situation. There is rigidity and attention to detail. Such people prefer order and predictability. They are methodical and punctual. There are psychological disturbances if routines are upset.

The desire for order and perfection may lead to interference with other aspects of life. The energy and emotions may suffer as a result. Blind faith and reliance on others in authority is common.

---

action. The following story was told by Christine Longaker at a workshop on death and dying at Rigpa Buddhist Centre, London in 1993.

There was a multiple car pile-up on the M4 motorway in England. A woman about 10 cars from the front of the crash, was unhurt but couldn't get out of her car because of other vehicles. She knew that some people had probably been injured or killed and she began to pray.

About a year later, a man came to see her at her home who she had never met. He had been in the same crash on the motorway but had been seriously injured. He had an out-of-body experience which is not unusual as part of a near death experience. He remembered passing over smashed cars and injured people and then seeing a woman praying. He felt the powerful effects of this and felt drawn back towards his body. He spent some time in hospital but very much felt that the power of her prayers had an important influence on his recovery. He had managed to trace her through the number plates of her car which had seen during his out-of-body experience.

This story reveals that our actions can have effects in areas which we may not be aware of. This is important to remember when treating people as we may not see any short-term or obvious result.

[39] There are many and varied ways of labelling personality. A clear description is contained in "Body Centred Psychotherapy: The Hakomi Method" by Ron Kurtz (Hakomi Institute, 1988). Also see "Personality Types - Jung's Model of Typology" by Daryl Sharp (Inner City Books, 1987).

There may be 'tightness' with money. It is difficult for such people to share with others or to delegate of responsibility.

SCHIZOID PERSONALITY

This type of person is solitary, detached and distant from other people. They may be the classical 'introvert'. They are frequently shy, solitary workers and have little empathy with other people. There may be strong emotions which are hard to express. There may be suspiciousness and sensitivity.

There is a lack of lightness of mood. Vulnerability, warmth and the ability to relate to others feelings is difficult.

Such people may become fixated on matters which assume great importance. They may take up campaigns and crusades with fervour.

It is considered by some that such traits arise because of an upbringing where anger is dominant, obvious and inappropriate.

HYSTERICAL PERSONALITY

This group is liable to excessive displays of emotion. They crave attention and seek to please and influence others. They are frequently the result of emotional deprivation in childhood. It is a type which tends to be overdiagnosed in women[40]. Such people are showy and histrionic in behaviour. Long-term relationships are difficult due to the lack of emotional maturity.

The extremes of emotion may be manifest quickly and fluctuate as easily. There may be a history of failed relationships.

Personality theorists have indicated that such a style stems from a dependency with associated feelings of inadequacy and lack of confidence.

SOCIOPATHY

Such people are described as 'affectionless'. It is the most severe of all the personality disorders. There is a lack of conscience. They are loveless, indifferent and may be destructive. There is impulsive behaviour which may be manifest as socially unacceptable, e.g. stealing, excessive gambling, physical assaults. There is a noted lack of regard for the consequences of actions. There are frequently legal problems as a result and management is difficult.

- HOW TO RECOGNISE A SERIOUS PSYCHOLOGICAL DISORDER -

Psychological disorders are common and particularly so in the alternative medical clinic. They are frequently neurotic in nature and mild. Occasionally, they can be severe and limiting. Rarely, they may be psychotic in form. It is important for you to know the significance of psychotic symptoms and the differences in management between neurosis and psychosis. Table 16.5 is a list of the symptoms which would indicate cause for concern. Such people may require hospitalisation or other place of safety.

SYMPTOMS	WHEN TO WORRY
Suicidal thoughts	Always
Suicidal feelings	Always
Hallucinations	Always
Delusions	Always
Thought disorders	If severe
Emotional symptoms, e.g. anxiety, fear, depression	If severe
Disturbance in body image	If associated with weight loss, amenorrhoea

TABLE 16.5: HOW TO RECOGNISE A SERIOUS PSYCHOLOGICAL DISORDER

---

[40] The word hysteria, is derived from *hysterus*, the Latin for womb. It was believed, and probably still is in many areas, that such states could only exist in women and hysterectomy would cure them.

- SUMMARY -

Psychological disorders are extremely common in the West.

It is important in your management of the case to be able to determine the emphasis of the symptoms - mental or emotional.

People with these disorders need help and support from several areas.

Counselling and psychotherapy, of an appropriate nature, are extremely beneficial in helping people resolve psychological issues.

It is essential for the practitioner to understand mind and its functioning. This is so that the person's psychological state can be viewed within the whole perspective of human experience and its possibilities.

17 PREGNANCY AND CHILDBIRTH

OBJECTIVES:

At the end of this Chapter you will be able to:
State the normal stages of pregnancy and labour
Describe the changes which occur at each of these stages and the abnormalities which may arise
Describe the conventional medical management of pregnancy and labour
Describe the management of these by an alternative medical practitioner

- INTRODUCTION -

Obstetrics is the term used to indicate the management of women who are pregnant or giving birth. There is some relationship with gynaecology which is discussed in Chapter 18. Although the application of alternative medical techniques to pregnant women is not well advanced, this will change in the future. I have, therefore, spent some time discussing common problems of pregnancy, labour and childbirth.

There are essentially two types of difficulties which may face pregnant women. The first, and sadly the commonest situation nowadays, is medical interference in normal processes[1]. The second, are those seen due to abnormalities of these normal processes. In this Chapter, I describe the normal events of each stage of pregnancy, labour and delivery followed by difficulties which may occur and how they may be addressed.

The usual method of classification is according to the stage at which they occur. This is summarised in Table 17.1.

First trimester[2]
      Morning sickness
      Miscarriage
      Large-for-dates
Second trimester
Third trimester
      Pre-eclampsia
      Antepartum haemorrhage
         Abruptio placentae
         Placenta praevia
First stage of labour[3]
      Difficult labour
      Disproportion
      Malposition
      Malpresentation
      Multiple pregnancy
Second stage of labour
      Difficult labour
      Disproportion
      Malposition
      Malpresentation
      Multiple pregnancy
Third stage of labour
      Retained placenta
      Post-partum haemorrhage
Post-natal period

TABLE 17.1: CLASSIFICATION OF OBSTETRIC DISORDERS

---

[1] "A Savage Enquiry" by Wendy Savage (Virago, 1986) is an account of attempts to suspend a woman gynaecologist who tries to offer mother's choices in childbirth.

"The American Way of Birth" by Jessica Mitford (Gollancz, 1992) is an excellent account of the pressures of conventional obstetrics.

[2] Trimester is any one of the three-monthly stages of pregnancy.

[3] Labour is defined as 'the sequence of actions by which a baby and afterbirth are expelled from the uterus at childbirth. "Concise Medical Dictionary (Oxford Medical Publications, 1980). In normal obstetric practice, the definition may be made of regular uterine contractions with progressive cervical dilatation. This, however, leads to fixed ideas of what is the normal duration of labour and the need for frequent vaginal examinations.

- BASIC ANATOMY AND PHYSIOLOGY -

The knowledge of anatomy and physiology which is required for the study of gynaecology is also useful here. This is the baseline from which any changes during pregnancy can be noted. I have listed the objectives which I consider useful to achieve as a preliminary to study of pregnancy and childbirth. These are detailed in Table 17.2.

As a preliminary to study of pregnancy and childbirth you are able to:
List the structures which develop after fertilisation of the egg
Describe the subsequent changes in hormone release and control
Explain the changing anatomy and physiology of the pregnant woman divided into the three trimesters
Describe the process of labour
List the stages which occur during childbirth
Describe the puerperium[4]

TABLE 17.2: OBJECTIVES FOR ANATOMY AND PHYSIOLOGY AS PREREQUISITE FOR STUDY OF PREGNANCY AND CHILDBIRTH

In common with gynaecology, conventional medicine sees the processes of pregnancy and childbirth as being essentially mechanical. Abnormalities are seen as being inevitable if not inherent. Manipulations to the function by hormones or to the structure by physical interferences during pregnancy and childbirth are common.

- ALTERNATIVE VIEW OF PREGNANCY AND CHILDBIRTH -

The ideas I express in this section are mainly gathered from texts of Chinese medicine and provide an energetic explanation of the events which occur at conception and pregnancy. They are necessarily holistic in nature. They provide a model which can be easily understood so that people can learn how to optimise their health and that of the baby.

In YinYang theory, it is the interaction of Yin and Yang which creates everything. A human being is but one aspect of this. Immaterial Yin and Yang[5] transform into material Yin and Yang. One consequence is the formation of a new life, the baby.

Conception occurs when the Yang sperm meets with the Yin egg. The best time for this is considered to be at about the time of the first cock-crow - about 4 or 5 a.m. This is when the energies are balanced with the Yang energy beginning to flourish. The Yang energy, in this context, is the life-force itself.

It is well recognised by Oriental philosophies that life begins with conception. As the Yang of the father and the Yin of the mother come together, this provides the material basis for Mind to enter. Mind does not enter later at some artificially determined date dependent upon political, conventional medical or financial factors.

Thus, conception is the starting point and all follows from this. If this idea was accepted and acknowledged by conventional medicine, many of the techniques of obstetrics and gynaecology would remain unused. Interferences with life at such an early stage have long-lasting effects which may be detrimental to health - physical and psychological. Methods include in-vitro fertilisation, freezing of embryos, experimentation on embryos and termination of pregnancy.

Techniques of termination, for example, have consequences far beyond this life as they end the life-force of a sentient being. They also have effects *in* this life as they disrupt the intimate connection between the foetus and the mother. Long-term problems of menstrual abnormalities and psychological disturbances are common. They can be relieved by treatment, perhaps with the help of counselling, but need to be addressed if they are to be resolved. Meditation and spiritual practices are of inestimable value in transforming such effects.

Health arises from supporting, in a natural way, the processes of conception and foetal development. In the Orient, the tradition is that people take care of their children whilst they are still

---

[4] The period up to 6 weeks after childbirth.

[5] All material aspects must arise from the immaterial. This is a fundamental principle of all energetic philosophies.

in an immaterial form and whilst they are still in the uterus. So, preconceptual and antenatal care are of paramount importance.

The material aspect develops into the foetus in the uterus. The uterus is known as the Envelope of Yin and is intimately connected with the three Yin organs of the Liver, Spleen and Kidney. The foetus develops from the Yin and Blood of the mother. In order for the foetus to remain in the uterus and develop there need to be several associated changes.

There has to be some degree of Liver Qi Stagnation[6] to prevent the energy moving and the foetus being lost. There has to be some degree of Spleen Qi Deficiency[7] to prevent the developing foetus being transformed and transported. There has to be some degree of Kidney deficiency[8] to allow the development within the uterus. These statements explain why certain acupuncture points and herbs are proscribed during pregnancy. It is important not to move Liver Qi too strongly or tonify the Spleen or Kidney too much.

In this way, the foetus continues to develop throughout the nine months of pregnancy (ten lunar months). At the end of this time, labour will begin as the energies begin to descend. This is a normal and natural process which becomes abnormal either because of some specific energetic imbalance or because of outside interference.

The delivery of the baby is the culmination of the whole process of pregnancy. It is to be interfered with as little as possible to maximise the health of the baby. There is no need, in most cases, for interfering, invasive techniques at birth. These include sucking out the mouth of the baby and injecting with Vitamin K. The baby must not be taken from the mother unless in a life-threatening situation.

The baby can be taken directly to the breast for feeding or lain in close contact with the mother to allow an early connection to be made. Bright lights and loud noises can be avoided. Delivery in water is much in vogue now amongst some mothers and of great effectiveness in reducing pain[9]. Labour seems to go more smoothly and is much enjoyed by mother, partner and baby. There is no danger with giving birth in water as the baby has been in water for nine months already! The baby obtains nourishment through the umbilical cord and this continues to pulsate for several minutes after delivery. Whilst the baby is under water it does not breathe. It only breathes on first contact with air.

There have been various scare stories about babies born in water and these are used by conventional doctors as excuses to ban such deliveries. There is no evidence that this is true and if performed correctly is perfectly safe. I had the opportunity to observe a woman in labour who used a birthing pool and she found it a pleasurable, helpful experience. It was her first pregnancy and labour was prolonged over about 15 hours. She had chosen to deliver at home and had a supportive independent midwife. She delivered a healthy baby boy by face presentation[10] which in hospital would have been an automatic Caesarian section.

The delivery of the placenta is the final stage of childbirth. The placenta is an integral part of the baby as it develops from the embryo. It may be eaten by the mother in some cases where it is an excellent preventative for post-natal depression. It is a rich source of Qi and Blood. It may be dried and powdered or turned into a jelly to be given to the child at major times of progress such as birthdays and attending school. It is very strengthening on many levels.

The post-partum time is an opportunity for the body to cleanse itself and the lochial discharge is its manifestation. This is one of the reasons why women live longer than men. They have opportunities at childbirth and menstruation to remove toxins. This time must not be interfered with and the process allowed to complete normally. Treatment can be given if necessary but care must be

---

[6] The energetic functions of the Liver are described in Chapter 14 - Central Nervous System. It has several functions but the important one of relevance here is its role in the free-flowing of Qi.

[7] The energetic function of the Spleen are described in Chapter 13 - Gastrointestinal System. It has several functions but the important one of relevance here is its role in transforming and transporting. This usually refers to food but not exclusively.

[8] The energetic functions of the Kidney are described in Chapter 9 - Urinary System. It has several functions but the important one of relevance here is its role in governing the function of the pelvic area.

[9] "Waterbirth" by Janet Balaskas and Yehudi Gordon (Unwin, 1990 and Thorsons, 1992).

[10] Presentation is that part of the baby which is lowermost during labour. A face presentation is difficult to deliver because the presenting part is of a large diameter. A further discussion of presentations, normal and abnormal, can be found later in this Chapter.

taken not to strengthen energies inappropriately in this time of release. Care needs to be taken that the mother does not become overtired or exposed to extremes of climate. The Chinese texts state that the mother is best attending only to herself and the baby for the first four weeks after delivery.

- HOW TO HAVE A HEALTHY PREGNANCY[11] -

At the moment, the vast majority of women deliver in hospital (around 95%). Pregnancy and particularly labour, are seen by the conventional profession as inherently dangerous and certainly life-threatening events. At all costs the mother and baby must be protected from these 'dreadful risks'. So, intervention by highly trained professionals is conventionally seen as the only way to ensure a healthy live infant. This thinking is, of course, only one aspect of a medical system which sees disease as unchanging external happenings and people as mechanical victims to be 'repaired' if they should fall ill. Hormone replacement therapy at the menopause is merely another example of the technological manipulation of a normal phase in women's lives.

The current movement towards home deliveries and natural childbirth is a reflection of the desire to find alternative methods. Ancient texts of Chinese medicine describe pregnancy as a spiritual practice which lasts for the nine months of child-bearing. The mother is encouraged to spend time in prayer and contemplation surrounded by pleasant things - mental, emotional and physical. This is not only an opportunity for the mother to benefit from such actions but also for the baby to begin life with a solid foundation of spiritual education. There are direct connections between the mother's mind and that of the developing baby[12].

If this is true, that pregnancy is an opportunity for the development of spirituality and emotional well-being, I would suggest that delivery is of at least equal importance. Many problems are caused by current practices of induction, inappropriate use of epidural anaesthesia and subsequent forceps delivery. Anxious staff may want to rush the whole process quickly as well as the application of a whole range of invasive techniques brought to bear in hospital.

There are, of course, some women for whom these techniques may be necessary. Vaginal delivery is not possible in every woman and it would be foolish to suggest otherwise. However, the vast majority of women could deliver at home given adequate support and preparation. It is simply not true that normal pregnancy must end in hospital delivery as the safest option. Remember that 98% of the people currently alive in the world were born at home - not in hospital. In Holland where more than two-thirds of deliveries are in the home there is no evidence of more problems and there may be less. Intervention leads to difficulties - ask any farmer or veterinary surgeon.

How can women prepare themselves for delivery at home in a safe environment? Intervention at the time of health problems is the crudest form of care and attention should be paid to prevention. In this way, difficulties are minimised or do not occur.

The mother's diet needs to be well balanced and most people nowadays understand what this means. Regular gentle exercise moves the energy of the body and benefits mother and baby although strenuous activity should be avoided in later months as the joints and ligaments start to loosen in preparation for childbirth. Specific yoga exercises are of benefit and if done regularly prepare the mother for the time of delivery.

Attention to the emotional and mental aspects are of supreme importance as the Chinese texts observe and relaxation techniques are a good grounding in this. A spiritual practice can play a larger part of the mother's life during the pregnancy but, at the least, relaxation sessions and an avoidance of unpleasant situations and stimulation would be of benefit. The Chinese classic, Admonitions to Ladies says, "A pregnant woman carries with her the finest piece of jade. She should enjoy all things, look at fine pictures and be attended by handsome servants". Whilst some of this advice may not be possible the meaning is clear.

Drugs are harmful to life and should be avoided unless they are necessary to maintain or preserve the life of the mother. Massage during pregnancy also helps to prepare mother and baby for delivery. For the baby it can be one of the first contacts with the outside world. During delivery, massage can help with pain relief and the progress of labour. It may be that, despite all these

---

[11] An excellent book, "The Path of Pregnancy" by Bob Flaws (Blue Poppy Press, 1982) outlines the Chinese philosophical view of pregnancy. This was my main source text for this section.
[12] The Chong channel. See discussion in "The Path of Pregnancy" by Bob Flaws (Blue Poppy Press, 1982) on Page 12.

preparatory measures, a health problem arises. Perhaps this was a condition present before conception or a result of the pregnancy. Whatever the origin it is preferable to seek out any required treatment perhaps with Chinese medicine or homoeopathy both of which have proven track records of safety and effectiveness.

Acupuncture is helpful at the end of the third and the sixth month to treat the mother's kidney energy and thereby strengthen the baby. This aims to help the mother and minimise problems for the baby. Chinese medical treatments exist to help ease the pain of labour, regulate contractions and help prevent problems such as retained placenta.

Essentially the choice for the mother will depend on what she wants. Whatever the mother's decision, this should be supported and conflict avoided. There is little benefit in creating argument since this only disturbs the mother and the baby. If a home birth is chosen then pressure may be put on the mother by conventional practitioners. Avoidance may be the wise option at this vulnerable time.

Despite all this discussion of what to do when pregnancy has arrived the ideal situation would be one of planning where the woman and her partner prepare themselves before conception. Attention to diet, exercise, relaxation and any specific health condition at this stage will go a long way to minimising problems in pregnancy.

So, if pregnancy is expected or has already happened, think of a plan of action:

- Look at diet, exercise and relaxation to maximise health.
- Seek advice and information about place of delivery and when selected search out supportive help.
- Obtain treatment for specific health problems.
- Think about homoeopathic, Chinese medical or other options to minimise difficulties during delivery and afterwards.
- Who will you want at the actual birth? I would suggest a maximum of partner or helper, midwife and perhaps one other. You don't have to invite the whole neighbourhood or sell tickets!
- Arrange for at least a month of rest and recuperation afterwards so that you can be involved solely with the new baby (or as far as possible given your home situation).
- Relax and enjoy the experience. Pregnancy and delivery are a normal, human event.

- INVESTIGATIONS -

Most people were surprised when it was announced in 1978 by the US Office of Technology that, "It has been estimated that only 10 to 20 percent of all procedures currently used in medical practice have been shown to be efficacious in controlled trial."

There have been two results of this statement. Firstly, there have been many reassessments of long-established procedures since 1978. Secondly, and unfortunately, the reporting of a procedure's overuse, obsolescence or uselessness has little effect on the practice of medicine.

Two procedures commonly used in labour are included in the many medical techniques which are irrelevant to producing a healthy baby, if not downright dangerous. Electronic foetal monitoring leads to high rates of Caesarean section and surgically assisted childbirth. A new study has revealed that when premature infants are given such monitoring, the rate of cerebral palsy is increased by three times. In the case of episiotomy, no evidence could be found to support the various reasons which doctors give for performing the surgery[13].

There are several investigations performed in pregnancy and these are listed in Table 17.3 on Page 374 along with an assessment of their invasiveness according to criteria discussed in Chapter 4 - Investigations. I would remind you that a medical practitioner will request a particular investigation for a different reason from the person having it. A doctor is looking for an abnormality whilst the mother will be looking for reassurance that all is well. This dichotomy is more important than it may appear since a doctor cannot possibly detect normality from an investigation, only the absence of an abnormality. This provides the basis for, at the very least, disappointment on the part of the mother.

---

[13] HealthFacts, August 1990 v15 n135 p1(2).

ULTRASOUND

This information is supplemental to that in Chapter 4 - Investigations. It is a commonly performed procedure. It is used with 85% of pregnant women in England, between 15 and 40% in US and 100% in Germany.

When I trained in medicine in the mid-1970's, it was performed for specific indications in early pregnancy. Now, it is almost universal with, in some centres, two or more ultrasounds during pregnancy.

There are several reasons for concern which we can consider. It may not be of any value in changing outcome. Routine ultrasound scanning during pregnancy does not result in an increase in the number of live births or reduce the chances of infant illness in the 28 days following birth. Scanning can detect foetal growth retardation and multiple pregnancies but early detection does not affect the management of these conditions[14].

It is easy to misinterpret results and there are cases of women told of abnormalities detected only to find later that the foetus is normal. Conversely, some women are told that their baby is normal only to find later that it is not. This fallibility, of course, is true of all investigations.

Experiments into the safety of ultrasound are usually done with continuous wave or high intensity pulse lengths. The ultrasound used in clinical practice is not of these types. Finally, it is difficult to relate tests in animals to those in humans. The tragedy of thalidomide and other drug effects confirm this[15]

The adverse effects of ultrasound are thought to be caused by the generation of heat or by mechanical effects. It is stated conventionally that ultrasound does not cause damage to the foetus but the truth is that it is not known. The possibility exists, however, and there is some disturbing evidence[16 17 18 19 20 21 22 23 24 25 26 27 28 29 30 31]. It would seem that the potential for harm is greater at the earlier stages of development.

---

[14] Bucher, Heiner C. et al: British Medical Journal, July 3, 1993 v307 n6895 p13(5).

[15] Animal tests may show no effect but this does not mean that the same will be true in humans.

[16] Flynn 1982, Edmonds and Sancier 1983

[17] Suppression of immune response in mice after spleen exposed to diagnostic ultrasound (Anderson and Barrett, 1970).

[18] Disruption of platelets by use of continuous wave ultrasound. No effect on human platelets has been identified (Zarod and Williams, 1977).

[19] Increase in foetal abnormalities (exencephaly and skeletal abnormalities) in mice when exposed to continuous ultrasound at day 9 of gestation (Shoji et al, 1971 and Shimizu and Shoji, 1973).

[20] Weight reduction of foetus following exposure to ultrasound in utero (O'Brien, 1976, 1983, Fry et al, 1977, 1978, Stolzenberg et al, 1980).

[21] Affect on cell division of rat's liver (Kremkau and Witcowski, 1974).

[22] Increased chromosome fracturing after exposing human lymphocytes to diagnostic levels of ultrasound (MacIntosh and Davey, 1970).

[23] DNA changes in human lymphocytes exposed to diagnostic ultrasound (Liebeskind et al, 1979, Haupt, 1981)

[24] Alterations in reflexes and emotional and cognitive behaviour after continuous wave ultrasound (Murai et al, 1975).

[25] A survey of 10,000 in Canada showed some to be underweight (Bolsen, 1982).

[26] Comparison of 426 children who had prenatal ultrasound against control group of 381 from 1966 to 1972 revealed a higher rate of dyslexia in the ultrasound group. This was considered to be statistically 'insignificant' by the researchers.

[27] According the Royal College of Obstetricians and Gynaecologists there are no studies to suggest an effect on the incidence of cancer. However, Dr Alice Stewart is currently conducting a study on 234,764 children who died of cancer between 1953 and 1981. She states "an early examination of the data indicated that children above the age of 6 who were examined in utero by ultrasound have an increased risk of childhood cancer."

Certainly the information above indicates effects on the immune system.

[28] An Australian study in 1993 showed that pregnant women who had frequent ultrasounds were more likely to give birth to underweight babies.

There are several stated aims for performing ultrasound scans in early pregnancy. These are:

- determine age of foetus
- diagnose multiple pregnancy
- diagnose foetal abnormalities
- localise placenta - determine if possibility of placenta praevia.

The age of the foetus and the possibility of multiple pregnancy can be determined by clinical examination. If the foetus is 'large-for-dates', that is, the size of the uterus is larger than expected, it may indicate that the foetal age is not that expected or that more than one foetus is present.

The detection of foetal abnormalities is only necessary if the mother is contemplating termination of the pregnancy. If this is not the case, and there are moral and religious beliefs to be considered here, there seems little point in performing potentially hazardous investigations just for information. It also important to consider the possibility of error as investigations are not infallible. There are several court cases currently pending where terminations were performed only to discover that the foetus was normal.

It may be important in later pregnancy to determine the site of the placenta where there may be a possibility of placenta praevia. This is the presence of the placenta near the cervix and is discussed later. It is impossible for the baby to be born vaginally and a Caesarian section is necessary. This condition can be suspected if the head of the baby does not go down into the pelvis in late pregnancy. It would seem sensible to reserve ultrasound for those cases and at that stage. In this way, the foetus is not exposed at early stages of its development. In any event, diagnosis by ultrasound of placenta praevia in early pregnancy is unreliable and, conventionally, is always followed by a repeat examination in the final months.

I would consider the following to be reasonable considerations for the use of ultrasound in pregnancy:

- confirmation of life or death of the foetus after threatened miscarriage (to detect missed or incomplete miscarriage)
- localisation of placenta in those cases where the foetal head does not engage

OTHER INVESTIGATIONS

Those such as amniocentesis and chorionic villus sampling are described in detail in Chapter 4 - Investigations. These are specific tests to determine foetal abnormality but carry a marked risk of miscarriage.

Chorionic villus sampling during the first nine weeks of pregnancy has a risk of causing limb deformities[32]. This is because the crucial time of limb development is nine weeks. No-one knows what damage is done to the placenta by this procedure. It has been recommended that it is not done until after 9½ weeks[33]. As a consequence there is a move to bring amniocentesis forward from 16 weeks' gestation to 14 weeks or before. The result will be that a significant proportion of amniotic fluid will be removed at a critical stage of foetal lung development.

All current methods of determining the appearances of foetal cells are invasive and carry a definite risk to the foetus.

There are currently three routine ways of obtaining foetal tissue. These are amniocentesis at 15 to 20 weeks' gestation, chorionic villus sampling at 10 to 12 weeks and umbilical blood sampling after 18 weeks. In addition, experimental invasive foetal sampling methods such as early

---

[29] A Norwegian trial showed that by the age of 8 or 9, children who had received prenatal ultrasound had a higher frequency of left-handedness.

[30] A study of 2600 women at Queen Charlotte's Hospital, Chelsea found that those who received routine ultrasound were more likely to have miscarriages - 17 deaths compared to 7 in the control group. Lancet 28th November, 1992.

[31] Ovarian ultrasound may precipitate premature ovulation. Testart et al, British Journal of Obstetrics and Gynaecology, 1982.

[32] Saul, Helen. : New Scientist, April 10, 1993 v138 n1868 p12(2).

[33] The Lancet, Vol 341, p 468.

amniocentesis, late transabdominal chorionic villus sampling, skin biopsy, liver biopsy, and muscle biopsy are being used. Research is currently being carried out to develop possible tests for non-invasive diagnosis by identifying foetal cells in the mother's blood[34] but is not yet at the clinical stage.

There are blood tests available which measure levels of substances which may indicate foetal abnormality[35]. They are performed in the second-trimester and may detect conditions such as open spina bifida[36], Down's syndrome, trisomy 18, multiple pregnancy and adverse pregnancy outcome. The investigations measure levels of alpha-foetoprotein, human chorionic gonadotrophin and unconjugated oestriol[37]. Such blood tests may be used as a screening for those who can be offered ultrasound examinations, amniocentesis or other intervention.

The blood testing of alpha-foetoprotein is most accurate when done between 16 and 18 weeks. When time is allowed for the return of the results it can be seen that any subsequent termination of pregnancy is late. In some cases it may be approaching the stage where survival is possible when born by premature labour.

Neural tube defects can be prevented by the administration of vitamin supplements and especially folic acid[38].

Foetal blood sampling involves the removal of blood from the umbilical cord under ultrasound guidance. Complications that can occur include bleeding, local collection of blood, transient decrease in foetal heart rate, premature labour, abruptio placentae, or premature detachment of the placenta[39].

I know of a woman of 25 years who had these blood tests at an early stage of pregnancy. She was unsure whether they were necessary but the expectation was to have them. She would clearly be considered unusual if she had declined and gave into the pressure from the hospital. The tests were abnormal and she was told that an amniocentesis was necessary. She was unsure because of the risk of death to the baby but decided she had to know. She spent several weeks of worry and anxiety before the amniocentesis result came back showing no abnormality. It was only at the stage of the amniocentesis that the hospital discussed the possibility of termination with her.

There are several points to make here. Women are put under intolerable pressure by hospital and medical staff to conform to a standard approach. They are made to feel that *they* have a problem if they decline such an approach. Women are not counselled about the management and treatment of abnormal results *before* an investigation. Hospitals and medical staff often rely upon persuading people to have investigations and treatment because of fear rather than a rational decision made in an informed way. The consequences of this are emotional difficulties for the mother and these will be passed to the baby.

---

[34] Chueh, Jane; et al. :The Western Journal of Medicine, Sept 1993 v159 n3 p308(4).

[35] Tests may give false-negative results. That is, they suggest normality when the foetus is abnormal. Effects in this direction include foetus older than expected, multiple pregnancy, low weight of the mother (less than 90 lb.) and race. Women of African extraction have normally higher levels.

False-positive results may also be found in about 5% of cases. That is, abnormality is suggested when the foetus is normal. Effects in this direction include foetus younger than expected, insulin-dependent diabetes mellitus in the mother and overweight.

[36] This is one of several conditions which are known as neural tube defects. The others are acrania (anencephaly) and encephalocele.

In the United States, the incidence of neural tube defects is 1 to 2 per 1,000 births.

[37] See Rose, Nancy C. et al. : The Western Journal of Medicine, Sept 1993 v159 n3 p312(6) for a discussion of their uses.

[38] Results of the Medical Research Council Vitamin Study. Lancet 1991; 338:131-137.

[39] Ghidini, Alessandro, et al. : American Journal of Obstetrics and Gynecology, May 1993 v168 n5 p1339(6).

INVESTIGATION	COMMENTS	INVASIVENESS
Weight measurement	Done regularly for early detection of pre-eclampsia	1
Blood pressure	Done regularly for early detection of pre-eclampsia	1
Full blood count	Done regularly for early detection of anaemia	1
Urine test	Done regularly for early detection of pre-eclampsia	1
Maternal blood tests	Screening test for foetal abnormalities. May lead onto invasive procedures of amniocentesis and chorionic villus sampling	1
Ultrasound	Used at least once in most pregnancies. Best to delay to the third trimester	2
Amniocentesis	Threatens the life of the foetus. Only to be risked in those who are contemplating termination	3
Chorionic villus sampling	See comments for amniocentesis. Risk of foetal abnormalities	3
Foetal blood sampling	See comments for amniocentesis	3

TABLE 17.3: INVESTIGATIONS PERFORMED IN PREGNANCY

- DISORDERS IN THE FIRST TRIMESTER -

GENERAL OVERVIEW

The first trimester is considered to begin at conception and end at 12 weeks. Most of the disorders listed here may occur during this time and some, e.g. morning sickness, may continue through to about 14 weeks or so. The first three months is the time of greatest foetal development. This is the time when the foetus is particularly vulnerable to the toxic effects of drugs and chemicals. It would seem that to perform routine ultrasound at this time is at the least, foolish and, at worst, hazardous.

MORNING SICKNESS

This occurs in about a third of pregnancies. It is important to remember that a pregnant woman may also develop other causes of nausea and vomiting. These symptoms are considered in Chapter 13 - Gastrointestinal System. In terms of conventional medicine, morning sickness is associated with rising levels of chorionic gonadotrophin. These reduce around weeks' 12-14 of pregnancy when the symptoms usually start to subside.

Symptoms:

There is nausea and sometimes vomiting which begins at about the 6th week of pregnancy. It usually subsides at around the 14th week. It is frequently only present in the morning, hence its name, but may occur at any time of day.

In some women, the vomiting may be severe and continue beyond the 14th week of pregnancy. It may then be called hyperemesis gravidarum. Occasionally, dehydration may occur and require hospital care.

Treatment:

This is by reassurance and simple dietary measures. Drug treatment with antihistamines such as promethazine may be used. If symptoms are severe and require hospitalisation, rehydration with intravenous fluids may be required.

Alternative management:

In terms of Chinese medicine, there are two main syndromes represented by morning sickness. Firstly, Fire in the Stomach and Liver may pass upwards together with thickened fluids. Secondly, Phlegm and Dampness may interfere with the normal descent of Stomach Qi so that it rises leading to nausea and vomiting.

Treatment of these conditions by specific treatment and dietary changes are effective at providing relief. The general advice of dietary management discussed in Chapter 13 - Gastrointestinal System is applicable here. It is clearly helpful to avoid cold, sweet and greasy food. Food should be taken at regular intervals throughout the day.

It may be helpful to consider such symptoms from a psychological perspective. Nausea and vomiting are a result of an inability to 'stomach' a situation. The developing foetus is a new life within the mother and this may produce a state of conflict. Nausea may be the consequence as the mother tries to 'vomit up' the foetus. The strength of symptoms may be a reflection of the strength of the foetus. Some women have strong symptoms as a result of a strong life within them. This is not to say that absence of nausea or vomiting indicates a weak foetus! The symptoms subside as the mother becomes more comfortable with the situation.

BLEEDING IN THE FIRST TRIMESTER

This is always abnormal although it is a relatively common symptom. There are considered to be several causes:

- miscarriage[40]
- ectopic pregnancy
- gynaecological conditions

I want to concentrate here on miscarriage. The other conditions are discussed fully in Chapter 18 - Gynaecology. The majority of cases of miscarriage are due to unknown causes. There are various theories but it is unusual for there to be a specific reason:

- foetal abnormality - over a third of miscarriages reveal chromosomal abnormality in the foetus
- immune system defect leading to maternal antibodies attacking the developing foetus
- structural abnormalities of the uterus (rare)
- maternal illness, e.g. fever, diabetes mellitus, kidney disease
- drugs, e.g. ergotamine, quinine, cancer chemotherapy agents, lead
- hormone deficiency

Symptoms of miscarriage:

There are considered to several categories of miscarriage. I shall describe these in turn.

A threatened miscarriage is one which subsides and results in continuation of the pregnancy. There is slight vaginal bleeding which is frequently brownish or dark red in colour. There may be backache and dragging pains in the lower abdomen.

An inevitable miscarriage is one which ends with death of the foetus. Vaginal bleeding occurs which is heavier than with a threatened miscarriage. It is often red in colour. Pain may be greater depending upon the duration of the pregnancy. After 10 weeks or so, cramping pains are marked. If the foetus and uterine contents are expelled, this is classified as a complete miscarriage.

An incomplete miscarriage is when there is any placental tissue or foetal parts remaining within the uterus. There is a danger of infection in these cases.

---

[40] Abortion is a medical term meaning loss of the foetus from the uterus up to 28 weeks of pregnancy. I use the term miscarriage in this text as, colloquially, abortion is used to indicate termination of pregnancy.

Investigations:

These are only performed in more severe cases. Ultrasound will determine if the foetus is alive.

Complications:

COMPLICATION	SYMPTOMS TO LOOK FOR
Infection	Fever, offensive vaginal discharge, malaise
Toxic shock	Low blood pressure, rapid pulse rate, pallor, sweating
Missed miscarriage	Missed periods, slight vaginal bleeding, foetus dies but is not expelled, uterus does not enlarge, pregnancy tests may still be positive. Spontaneous labour is the rule.

TABLE 17.4: COMPLICATIONS OF MISCARRIAGE

Treatment:

Rest is essential for threatened miscarriage. This should be absolute until vaginal bleeding has stopped. Hormonal supplementation with progesterone may be given with little evidence that it makes any difference to the outcome. This is a routine prescription in cases of several miscarriages (habitual miscarriage).

Inevitable miscarriage is treated by administration of ergometrine to empty the uterus.

Dilatation and curettage may be carried out to ensure that all tissue has been removed from the uterus.

Alternative management:

Specific treatment is helpful in treating such symptoms. In terms of Chinese medicine, miscarriage is usually seen as part of a condition known as 'Motion of the Foetus'. There are six categories of this which are:

- Qi Deficiency
- Blood Deficiency
- Kidney Deficiency
- Hot Blood
- Liver Qi Stagnation
- Injury or accident

Treatment is helpful during the pregnancy after the bleeding has settled. This is important so that any underlying cause is addressed. If the miscarriage is complete, it is helpful to also have treatment so that the woman's health can be helped. She may wish for another pregnancy and treatment will help her prepare for this.

LARGE-FOR-DATES

This is the detection of a uterine size which is larger than expected for the duration of the pregnancy. It may be found at any stage of pregnancy but, with good antenatal care, will be spotted relatively early. There are considered to be several reasons:

- multiple pregnancy
- excess amniotic fluid, e.g. foetal abnormality, unknown cause
- maternal diabetes mellitus - leads to large foetus and placenta

Symptoms:

There may be none at early stages of pregnancy but the unexpected uterine size may be detected at routine antenatal visit. After about the 30th week of pregnancy, the enlarged uterus may cause pressure symptoms such as abdominal discomfort and, in severe cases, breathlessness.

Pre-eclampsia is more common in cases of multiple pregnancy and symptoms of this may be present.

It is useful to know the normal stages of development in pregnancy so that comparisons can be made with women in the clinic. Before the 12th week, uterine size can only be determined by vaginal examination (or by ultrasound).

By the 13th week or so the uterus becomes palpable above the symphysis pubis. The top of the uterus (fundus) reaches the umbilicus by the 24th week and the xiphoid cartilage by the 36th. It may descend a little if the baby's head engages in the pelvis.

Foetal movements may be felt at 19 or 20 weeks if a first baby and at about 17 or 18 weeks in subsequent pregnancies. Foetal heart sounds may be heard with a stethoscope at about the 24th week.

Management:

This lies in detecting the cause of being large-for-dates. The management of each condition is detailed in the relevant section.

- DISORDERS IN THE SECOND TRIMESTER -

It is unusual for women to have difficulties during the second trimester. Miscarriage may occur due the reasons discussed above. The foetus gradually grows in size, most development having taken place in the first trimester.

Monitoring is done of weight, blood pressure and urine as well as uterine enlargement. The aim is to detect early any evidence of pre-eclampsia (see below).

- DISORDERS IN THE THIRD TRIMESTER -

GENERAL OVERVIEW

The third trimester is the final stage of pregnancy and when the body prepares for the labour to come. There are several problems which may arise during this time. It is now that the benefits of any preparation will be experienced. The healthier the woman, the less will be any difficulties.

It is beneficial if the mother can sleep and rest with her legs straight on a small soft pillow as this helps the head of the baby to engage. The temperature of the room should be neither too hot nor too cold. Gentle walks after meals are helpful and the avoidance of hard or heavy work. It is important to avoid cold, raw food and emotional stress and worry. Emotional upsets deplete the Qi and Blood and may lead to difficulties during labour. Strengthening of Qi and Blood is very helpful from about 32 weeks as this helps to ensure that labour is easy and smooth.

PRE-ECLAMPSIA

This is the appearance of high blood pressure, oedema and proteinuria in the last three months of pregnancy. It is labelled pre-eclampsia as a small number of women will progress to full blown eclampsia with convulsions. It may also be known as toxaemia of pregnancy.

It is differentiated from other causes of such symptoms, e.g. essential hypertension, glomerulonephritis, systemic lupus erythematosus.

It is more common in teenage women, women over 35 years and in multiple pregnancies. The symptoms quickly resolve after delivery or if the foetus dies.

Symptoms:

These usually only develop after the 28th week of pregnancy. The blood pressure rises with an increase of at least 20 mm Hg in the systolic and 10 mm diastolic. Oedema, which may be slight in 'normal' pregnancy, is marked particularly in the ankles, face and hands. Weight increases normally in pregnancy but a gain of more than 1 KG (2 lb.) per week may indicate the collection of oedema fluid. Proteinuria is found in severe cases.

Headaches and vomiting develop if the diastolic pressure rises over 100 mm. There may be blurred vision. Epigastric pain and jaundice arise in severe cases due to liver damage.

The problem with pre-eclampsia for the foetus is that placental function is diminished. The foetus is underweight and in severe cases may die in utero.

If the symptoms progress, eclampsia may supervene. This is the occurrence of repeated convulsions, unconsciousness and the development of spontaneous labour. Maternal and foetal death rates are high.

Investigations:

These are performed to exclude other causes of these symptoms. Urinalysis reveals only proteinuria with no blood or casts. In pre-eclampsia there will be no evidence of bacterial infection. Blood tests reveal raised uric acid but normal urea and creatinine.

Treatment:

Ante-natal care is recommended for every pregnant woman as a means of early detection. There is no means of prevention according to conventional medicine. All women with such symptoms will be admitted to hospital for bed rest, observation and investigation. There is no specific treatment although tranquillisation may be used to reduce the blood pressure. When I worked on an obstetric unit, the antipsychotic promazine was frequently used to sedate women with pre-eclampsia. Diuretics may be given for the oedema. Hypotensive drugs such as hydralazine or methyldopa are used for high blood pressure.

The foetus is monitored by means of ultrasound and placental function tests[41]. Labour may be induced if symptoms are severe, foetal growth is greatly affected or the pregnancy is at or near term.

Eclampsia is an obstetric emergency which is treated by anticonvulsants and hypotensive agents. If labour has not already begun, it is induced. Caesarian section is performed if labour may be prolonged for whatever reason. The urgency here is to deliver the baby as symptoms subside soon afterwards. In eclampsia, the maternal mortality rate may be 5%. Foetal mortality in established pre-eclampsia is about 3% but 30% in eclampsia.

---

[41] Placental function tests are blood tests which give some indication of its efficiency. Serum oestriol measurement is the prime example of these.

Alternative management:

The main issue for alternative medicine is to ensure that the health of the mother is as good as possible. Treatment before conception will minimise any risk of such a condition developing. The maximisation of health during pregnancy is discussed at the beginning of this Chapter.

In terms of Chinese medicine, oedema in pregnancy is seen as being due to Spleen Deficiency, Kidney Deficiency or Qi Stagnation. Pre-eclampsia, specifically, often corresponds to Blood Deficiency, Heat in the Liver or WindCold Invasion.

BLEEDING IN THE THIRD TRIMESTER

This is always abnormal and can indicate several possibilities. It should always be viewed seriously. If bleeding is seen after the 28th week of pregnancy, it is denoted an antepartum haemorrhage. This term usually excludes non-pregnancy related causes of bleeding. There are several causes of vaginal bleeding in the third trimester which include:

- abruptio placentae
- placenta praevia
- gynaecological conditions, e.g. cervical erosion, cervical polyp, cervical cancer

ABRUPTIO PLACENTAE

This is bleeding from a normally situated placental site. It may (revealed haemorrhage) or may not (concealed haemorrhage) manifest as vaginal bleeding. The placenta partially separates from the uterine wall. The cause is not fully understood in conventional medicine. High blood pressure is seen in about a third of cases. It is commoner in women whose diet and social conditions are poor. Occasionally, injury[42] may precipitate bleeding.

Symptoms:

In a revealed haemorrhage, there is vaginal bleeding. There is pain and localised tenderness over the uterus. The uterus feels hard and may be distended. Labour may begin spontaneously.

A concealed haemorrhage will only be evidenced by the abdominal symptoms. A measure of knowledge of this condition will help in coming to a diagnosis.

Investigations:

Vaginal examination is absolutely contraindicated in all cases of vaginal bleeding at this stage of pregnancy because of the possibility of placenta praevia. An ultrasound scan will show placental position and any blood clot due to the placental separation.

Complications:

COMPLICATIONS	SYMPTOMS TO LOOK FOR
Shock	Rapid pulse rate, low blood pressure, pale, sweating
Foetal death	Absent movements, absent heart sounds

TABLE 17.5: COMPLICATIONS OF ABRUPTIO PLACENTAE

---

[42] External version of a breech presentation may be such a cause.

Treatment:

This is mainly supportive in hospital. Pain relief is given and blood transfusion may be required where blood loss is marked. Labour is induced or Caesarian section performed in severe cases.

If the symptoms are mild and there is no evidence of placenta praevia on ultrasound examination, bed rest is the only thing which is necessary.

Alternative management:

It is important that you understand the significance of bleeding in the third trimester (see also placenta praevia). Most women will be hospitalised as this is an obstetric emergency.

PLACENTA PRAEVIA

This is a placenta which is situated over or near the cervix. It occurs in about 0.5% of pregnancies. The placenta may overlie the internal opening of the cervix completely or only be situated on the uterine wall nearby. For all practical purposes, these slightly different cases are dealt with in the same way.

Symptoms:

There is vaginal bleeding which occurs late in pregnancy or in labour. It may be initiated by intercourse or vaginal examination. The bleeding is painless and may be recurrent. The head of the foetus cannot engage[43] and so the presence of placenta praevia may be suspected.

If bleeding is severe, there may be rapid pulse rate, low blood pressure, pallor and sweating.

Investigations:

Vaginal examination is absolutely contraindicated in all cases of vaginal bleeding in the later months of pregnancy. If placenta praevia is present there is torrential haemorrhage as the examining fingers damage the placenta.

Ultrasound examination reveals the placental position.

Treatment:

In cases of placenta praevia, there is clearly no treatment which can alter the placental position. Delivery by Caesarian section is the only option and this is done at about 39 weeks. If vaginal bleeding is heavy, an emergency section is performed with supportive treatment such as blood transfusion if necessary.

Alternative management:

It is important that you understand the significance of bleeding in the third trimester (see also abruptio placentae). Most women will be hospitalised as this is an obstetric emergency.

---

[43] The presenting part of the foetus is said to have engaged when its widest diameter has entered the brim of the pelvis.

PREMATURE LABOUR

This is the onset of labour before 40 weeks. There are several associated circumstances and these include:

- multiple pregnancy
- excess amniotic fluid
- smoking
- urinary tract infection
- rupture of membranes, e.g. multiple pregnancy, excess amniotic fluid, weakened cervix
- foetal abnormality
- foetal death

Symptoms:

There is the onset of the symptoms of labour but before 40 weeks' gestation. The consequences for the foetus are directly dependent upon its maturity. Birth after 34 weeks suggests a good chance of survival although increasingly premature babies are living.

Treatment:

It may be possible to stop some cases of premature labour with drugs which relax uterine muscle. These include isoxsuprine and salbutamol. Corticosteroids may be given, e.g. dexamethasone in an attempt to reduce the severity of respiratory distress syndrome[44].

POSTMATURITY

This is prolongation of the pregnancy beyond the accepted normal of 40 weeks. About 10% of pregnancies do not start until the 42nd week. There are some risks attached to this situation although they tend to be overstated by the conventional profession in an attempt to get every woman to deliver according to an accepted norm. Placental insufficiency may develop leading to a reduced growth rate of the foetus. Also, the foetal head may not mould during labour so well and so prolong delivery.

A consideration is that the 40 week gestation may not be as fixed or 'normal' as we think. There is no reason why there cannot be a range of normality with some pregnancies lasting 40 weeks, some less and some more. The danger with the conventional approach is that induction of labour, of whatever duration pregnancy, may lead to the delivery of a baby with immature lungs. This can occur at any stage of pregnancy although it is more a risk at earlier stages. I remember working in an obstetric unit where induction was performed on virtually all women who did not spontaneously begin labour at 40 weeks. There were a number of babies born with respiratory difficulties.

In my opinion, it is preferable to wait until there is clear evidence of problems requiring induction. Routine procedures lead to routine difficulties.

---

[44] This is a condition due to immaturity of the lungs where a sticky secretion may obstruct the smaller airways. In severe cases there is cyanosis and breathlessness.

- LABOUR -

INTRODUCTION

It is important for me to emphasise here that labour is usually a normal process with a healthy, normal baby at the end. Difficulties occur because of a health problem with the mother, a disproportion between the size of the baby and the size of the mother's pelvis or due to interference with this normal process. The latter case is common now as many women in the West deliver their babies in hospital. There are increasing moves towards technological management of birth. Despite this, women are becoming more vociferous in their requests for humane methods of childbirth. In the past few years, groups of women, midwives and health professionals have come together to offer help. Such methods, often labelled natural childbirth[45], are gaining ground albeit with little support or perhaps the outright hostility of conventional practitioners. This movement is gaining ground and increasing numbers of women are choosing to deliver at home or perhaps in hospital in a manner which suits them. It is still early days but as each year passes the movement of power shifts more towards women. This can only be beneficial and soon the days of passive childbirth and unnecessary intervention will be no more.

STAGES OF LABOUR

Labour is divided into three stages. Painless contractions occur throughout pregnancy. When the first stage of labour begins, they become painful and the cervix starts to dilate as the baby is gradually advanced down the pelvic canal. When labour begins there may be a 'show'. This is the discharge of blood-stained mucus from the cervix. The membranes may rupture at this stage or later.

The duration of the first stage depends upon the individual case. Conventional medicine frequently lays down quite rigid ideas about how long each stage and part of a stage should last. The degree of cervical dilatation is taken as the guide to progress. This is only a rigid labelling of a natural process and has no inherent truth of its own. Each case must be assessed on its merits. Consider factors such as number and strength of contractions, condition of the mother and condition of the baby. The reliance on the state of the cervix subjects women to repeated vaginal examinations during labour. This is unnecessary and invasive. If all is progressing, there is no need to interfere. Medical voyeurism is not a healthy aspect of pregnancy and labour.

The second stage of labour begins when the cervix is fully dilated and ends with the delivery of the baby. Full dilatation is heralded by a desire to bear downwards. This is the stage when the mother actively pushes the baby down the vaginal canal to help uterine contractions. The membranes usually rupture at this time.

The third stage ends when the placenta (afterbirth) is delivered. There is some bleeding as this occurs but eases as the uterus contracts. Putting the baby to the breast immediately after delivery stimulates contraction of the uterus.

The practice of shaving the pubic hair and giving women enemas in preparation for labour is, fortunately, dying out. There is no evidence of need for these procedures.

In the vast majority of women, labour progresses normally with no requirement for the paraphernalia of modern hospital obstetrics. The use of foetal monitoring, epidural anaesthesia and so forth tend to delay labour and make it more painful.

Induction of labour due to some perceived difficulty about delay also leads to painful labour and an increased incidence of intervention later. There is no need for induction if the mother is healthy and the baby is active and growing. It may be helpful to check the placental function tests but use these only as a guide, not as an absolute indication of what to do.

---

[45] Natural childbirth and active childbirth are two terms in common usage. They are gaining in popularity due to the benefit they offer to mother and baby. Excellent source books include "The Active Birth Partners Handbook" by Janet Balaskas (Sidgewick and Jackson, 1984), "The Encyclopaedia of Pregnancy and Birth" by Janet Balaskas and Yehudi Gordon (Little, Brown, 1992)and "Preparing for Birth with Yoga" by Janet Balaskas (Element, 1994).

INTERVENTION/INVESTIGATION	WHEN	COMMENTS
Shaving pubic hair, enema	Before or at start of labour	Not common now. Unnecessary
Urine test	Before or at start of labour	Check for sugar or protein
Blood pressure	Before or at start of labour and regularly throughout	Check for pre-eclampsia
Surgical rupture of membranes	To induce labour	Done via vaginal examination. Danger of placental separation or presentation of foetal hand or leg
Induction of labour	To induce labour	Dangerous if baby's lungs are not fully mature. Labour tends to be more painful and more likely to require intervention
Abdominal examination	Throughout labour	Check on engagement, strength and regularity of contractions
Foetal heart measurements	Throughout labour	Check on foetal heart rate - normal is 120-160 per minute. It may increase (or decrease) in cases of foetal distress[46]
Vaginal examination	Throughout labour - at least three hourly	Check on cervical dilatation and confirm presenting part of the baby. Frequently overused
Foetal scalp monitor	During first stage of labour	Electrode attached to scalp of baby. Painful and intrusive
Foetal blood sampling	During first stage of labour	Obtained from foetal scalp. Painful and intrusive
Pethidine injections	During first stage of labour	For pain relief. Suppresses the baby's respiration
Epidural anaesthesia	During first stage of labour	For pain relief. High risk of back pain for months afterwards
Forceps, Ventouse extraction	During second stage of labour	To assist delivery
Episiotomy	During second stage of labour	Cutting of the perineum to assist delivery. Can be prevented by adequate preparation and by experienced midwife
Oxytocin injection	At end of second stage of labour	To cause the uterus to contract in bid to prevent post-partum haemorrhage. Unnecessary in well-managed delivery where baby is put to breast immediately

TABLE 17.6: INTERVENTIONS AND INVESTIGATIONS DURING LABOUR

[46] Foetal distress is the oft-quoted reason for intervention in labour. You should not forget that 'obstetrician's distress' may also be a reason for such intervention.

DIFFICULT LABOUR

This is labour which progresses slowly or with difficulty. There are considered to be several causes in conventional medicine which include:

- foetus - malposition, malpresentation
- mother - small pelvis, pelvic tumours
- weak uterine action
- uncoordinated uterine action

Symptoms:

There will be a lack of cervical dilatation with continuing painful contractions of the uterus. The contractions may increase in strength and painfulness.

Treatment:

This depends upon the cause and the condition of the mother and baby. If there is evidence of maternal exhaustion or foetal distress, obstetric intervention may be necessary. If the cervix is not fully dilated, a Caesarian section will be performed with either general anaesthesia or an epidural. If the cervix is fully dilated, it may be possible to use forceps to help deliver the baby. This is done with local anaesthesia or an epidural. An episiotomy is necessary.

Alternative management:

In terms of Chinese medicine, there are two main situations of delayed labour. They are Deficiency of Qi and Blood and Stagnation of Qi and Blood. Deficient conditions can be prevented or minimised by tonifying treatments before and during pregnancy. Treatment can be instituted during labour by means of acupuncture, herbs, homoeopathic remedies or massage to help maintain uterine contractions and support the woman.

MALPOSITION

Normally, the vertex of the head is the presenting part. That is, the part which enters the pelvis first and leads into the vaginal canal in the second stage of labour. The occiput is towards the front (respective to the mother). Any variation from this with vertex presentation is known as malposition.

In 15% of deliveries, the occiput is to the back (respective to the mother). This is known as occipito-posterior position. In about 1 in 4 of these cases there are difficulties in labour because the head does not flex to reduce the diameter of the presenting part. Labour is likely to be prolonged and perhaps more painful. Backache is common in such situations.

The management of malposition is included in that of difficult labour described above.

MALPRESENTATION

Presentation of the head is the normal situation. Malpresentation is the presentation of any other part of the baby. All malpresentations tend to delay labour and the comments I made under difficult labour are relevant here.

The presentations which are possible are:

- face
- brow
- breech
- shoulder

Caesarian section will be employed if labour is unduly difficult or delayed and in cases of foetal distress or maternal exhaustion. Most face, all brow and all shoulder presentations have to be delivered by this method. Breech delivery is possible vaginally with care. It has always been stated that such deliveries must be done in hospital but home delivery is fine with competent midwifery support.

It is possible to turn a foetus so that it presents correctly. This is termed external version. It is used in the case of a transverse foetus or a breech presentation. It is performed after the 35th week or the baby merely turns back. There is a risk of placental separation or premature labour and for this reason is not so favoured.

There is an excellent method available in Chinese medicine which has no side-effects and is virtually 100% effective. The application of heat provided by burning moxa to the acupuncture point Urinary Bladder 67 will invert the foetus in almost every case. Merely warming this point is adequate.

In terms of Chinese medicine, malpresentation indicates that the Qi of the Kidney and Spleen is chaotic.

DISPROPORTION

This is the situation where the presenting part of the baby is too large for the size of the pelvis. It is a relative situation and depends on several factors such as movement of pelvic bones due to ligamentous softening in later pregnancy and moulding[47] of the baby's head. The size of the pelvis is assessed at about the 36th week of pregnancy although a previous delivery will be a definitive assessment of what is possible. Lack of engagement of the head may indicate a small pelvis. It normally engages at about 37 weeks in first pregnancies and not until labour in those who have previously delivered.

The results of assessment govern the management of these cases. In those situations where the outcome is unsure, a *trial labour* may be conducted. This is the monitoring of labour with preparation for Caesarian section if progress does not happen or stops.

If vaginal delivery seems to be impossible, an *elective* Caesarian section is performed at about 38 or 39 weeks. There is support amongst some obstetricians for such women to begin labour anyway as there are psychological benefits. There is less chance of feelings of failure and women may prefer to attempt even if Caesarian section will be the option for delivery.

---

[47] This occurs because of the pressures exerted during delivery. It is a normal event and allows for easier passage during labour.

MULTIPLE PREGNANCY

This is the occurrence of more than one foetus. Twins occur in 1 in 80 pregnancies, triplets in 1 in 1000 and quadruplets in 1 in 500,000. There is an increased chance of multiple pregnancy if there is a family history of such, with the use of ovulation stimulants in the treatment of infertility and when pregnancy is the result of IVF or GIFT treatment as several fertilised ova are replaced together.

The diagnosis is suggested by the finding of a large-for-dates uterus. Ultrasound will confirm diagnosis. When I worked in an obstetrics unit, a woman was expecting to deliver two babies, confirmed by ultrasound. Everyone was surprised when three appeared! No investigation is infallible, of course.

The symptoms of morning sickness are stronger with multiple pregnancy. Pre-eclampsia and premature labour are more likely. Most women are admitted to hospital routinely for rest from the 32nd week for the remainder of the pregnancy.

INDUCTION OF LABOUR

This is the artificial initiation of labour by means of drugs or surgical procedures. It is commonly performed in some hospitals but less than in the 1970's when it was routinely employed. Induction rates vary between 1 in 2 to 1 in 10 deliveries in the UK. It was originally employed as a way of preventing postmaturity but quickly became a way of trying to get all women to deliver between 9 a.m. and 5 p.m. on weekdays.

It tends to lead to more painful labour and therefore is intimately connected with epidural anaesthesia and other aspects of technological obstetrics. Intervention is more common with forceps and Caesarian section. This is either because labour is more problematic or because the woman finds it difficult to push a baby out when anaesthetised from the waist downwards.

The obstetric indications for induction include:

- hypertension
- chronic nephritis
- abruptio placentae
- unstable presentation
- postmaturity
- diabetes mellitus
- foetal abnormalities
- foetal death

Induction is likely to fail if there is no engagement of the presenting part, if the cervix is long, firm and tightly closed and it is before the 36th week.

There are various methods of induction. Prostaglandin pessaries inserted into the vagina stimulate the uterus to begin contractions. If contractions do not begin, the membranes are ruptured surgically by means of a metal hook during vaginal examination. Intravenous infusion of synthetic oxytocin is either given at the same time or if contractions fail to begin. The rate of infusion must be closely monitored and adjusted according to the rate and strength of the contractions. Overvigorous contractions produced by this method may lead to foetal death or uterine rupture. Monitoring of the foetus by means of foetal scalp monitors, monitors to the mother's abdomen to measure foetal heart rate and contractions and epidural anaesthesia are, therefore, integral parts of induction.

The American College of Obstetricians and Gynaecologists concluded that, "There is no clinical value to continuous electronic foetal monitoring." Listening with a stethoscope is of the same effectiveness.

DELIVERY

This is the second stage where the woman pushes downward to aid the uterine contractions. It occurs when the cervix is fully dilated (10 cm) and the woman has the urge to push downwards. It lasts for up to two hours but most are much shorter than this. An hour of the second stage with no progress indicates a serious problem.

A relatively high percentage of deliveries are the subject of medical intervention. Such intervention is usually the culmination of a series of invasive procedures where there is interference with natural processes.

The standard method of delivery was invariably with the woman lying flat on her back. It is not physiological and may lead to more foetal distress as the circulation is obstructed by the pregnant uterus.

Nowadays, women are more often requesting different positions with which they feel comfortable. The standard advice is changing slowly[48] but delivery at home with a sympathetic midwife[49] remains the best way to ensure the woman's wishes are respected.

There is ample evidence available to show that home delivery of the baby is at least as safe as that of hospital delivery[50]. Nothing is risk-free but it is helpful to consider how to ensure, as far as is possible, that a home delivery is problem-free. These are listed in Table 17.7

Good nutrition and adequate weight gain.
Abstain from smoking, drinking alcohol
Getting good prenatal care and avoiding high blood pressure and other complications which can be helped through nutrition.
Find a competent midwife who is skilled, confident and experienced in deliveries at home
Information through reading, classes, videos, and getting supplies together.
Ensure the baby presents head down - or that the midwife is skilled in breech deliveries, twins[51] and so on
Have adequate support during labour and postpartum.
Have a plan for emergencies, phone numbers easily available
Alternative medical practitioner to assist in case of specific difficulties

TABLE 17.7: HOW TO PREPARE FOR HOME DELIVERY[52]

The baby descends the birth canal with each contraction helped by voluntary efforts of the mother. The head (assuming a vertex presentation) is delivered first followed by the shoulders. Tearing of the perineum may occur if the delivery is rapid and episiotomy may be performed to prevent this. It is the cutting of the perineum so that any tear will not pass posteriorly to affect the anal sphincter. This risk is much overstated and episiotomy is unnecessary in all uncomplicated deliveries. Competent midwifery and care of the perineum in pregnancy will prevent any problems.

Throughout North America, the episiotomy rate is about 70 to 80 per cent of first-time vaginal deliveries. It would seem that at least as effective and infinitely preferable is the use of pelvic floor exercises throughout pregnancy and perineal massage before birth. Neither of these techniques, of course, involve doctors.

---

[48] The conventional attitude can be ascertained from the following quote. The italics are mine. "There a few patients who *demand* to be delivered in 'natural' positions, standing, crouching, or on their hands and knees. While their right of choice cannot be denied, it must be explained to them that there is a danger to the child if the foetal heart rate is not regularly observed, and that care of the perineum is hardly possible in such positions." "Obstetrics and Gynaecology" by Clayton and Newton (Churchill Livingstone, 1988).

[49] There are several groups of midwifes in the UK who now offer alternatives to obstetric interventions in hospital. They work in the community and are known as independent midwives or radical midwives.

[50] British Medical Journal, December 14, 1991, vol. 303, p. 1517.

[51] The delivery of twins at home after a previous Caesarian section may also be possible with care. An account of such an event is an article by Cronk, Mary. : Nursing Times, Nov 18, 1992 v88 n47 p54(2).

[52] Source text: Special Delivery, Spring 1992 p4(1).

Episiotomy is, paradoxically, likely to make tearing worse. A study of 241 births in the Albert Einstein Hospital in New York found that this practice, especially if the woman had her legs in stirrups (lithotomy position), led to more harm[53].

Researchers at the Jewish General Hospital and McGill University in Montreal, Canada studied women who had an episiotomy and compared them with a group who did not. There was no difference in the outcome as all had healthy babies. The second stage of labour was reduced in time by only nine minutes on average. There was the risk of sexual difficulties after birth[54].

In this study, 46 out of 47 women receiving episiotomies had the tear extend into the rectum which is the most serious complication. Researchers noted that doctors are so programmed to perform surgery that those in the part of the study where women did not have episiotomies, "... were unwilling or unable to reduce their episiotomy rate."

Intramuscular oxytocin is routinely given in hospitals when the baby's shoulders are delivered to contract the uterus and minimise the risk of post-partum haemorrhage. This, again, is very much overstated and the immediate placing of the baby at the breast will produce natural secretion of oxytocin.

The baby should be given to the mother immediately after delivery for eye and skin contact to be made. No attempt needs to be made to suck out the baby's mouth, rub it with a rough towel, spank it to make it cry and any of the other treatments meted out to new-born babies. Inappropriate intervention at this stage is grossly invasive and leads to psychological problems in the child. A baby is completely vulnerable and open. The last thing he or she needs is for a hard, plastic tube to be pushed into the mouth.

Vitamin K has been given to new-born babies since the 1940's and 1950's. It is given to prevent haemorrhagic disease of the new-born which may present at about 10 weeks of age. Cerebral haemorrhage is a possibility which may be fatal.

Babies are born with a slight vitamin K deficiency which may be a protective mechanism. The injectable medication contains phenol as well as Vitamin K. By 1958, about 5% of babies received it, 25% by 1970 and 98.5% by 1977-87. In the UK at the current time, 58% of babies have the injection form, 30% the oral form, and 12% nothing.

Two studies have shown a connection between Vitamin K injection and the development of childhood cancer. The first was published in 1990 and the second in 1992[55].

The risk of any child developing leukaemia by the age of 10 is about 1 in 1000 and that for all childhood cancers about 1 in 500. The results of these studies reveal that Vitamin K could increase this risk to about 1 in 200. Regarding Great Britain, there are about 700,000 births a year. The excess number of cancers caused by giving intramuscular vitamin K to all babies could range from 400 to 2000. By contrast, the risk of haemorrhagic disease of the new-born if no vitamin K is given is about 1 in 10000 which would work out as 70 cases a year in Britain. There was no association, however, between cancer and oral vitamin K[56].

The cord can be left alone until it has stopped pulsating and then cut. Early clamping and cutting of the cord leads to feelings of forced separation and loss. It is important to allow natural processes to run their course. In this way, long-term problems are minimised particularly on a psychological level. For years we have been delivering babies in a way which is harsh and unfeeling. It is time we took more care of these processes.

The delivery of the baby ends the second stage of labour.

If there is a delay in labour, signs of maternal or foetal distress delivery may be aided. Forceps delivery may be performed under local anaesthesia. It is more common in epidural

---

[53] 28% of those who had episiotomy and lithotomy had serious vaginal tearing. This rate dropped to 19 percent for women who had just the episiotomy and 1% of those who had neither. The Edell Health Letter, June 1989 v8 n6 p6(1).

[54] Mothering, Spring 1993 n66 p28(1).

[55] The conclusions of this study may be summarised. The figures relate to the UK. If no one received any vitamin K then there would be about 30-60 cases of late haemorrhagic disease and no extra cancers. If all received oral vitamin K there would be about 10 cases of late haemorrhagic disease and no extra cancers. If all received intramuscular vitamin K there would be one case of late haemorrhagic disease and 980 extra cancers. Golding, Jean. et al: British Medical Journal, August 8, 1992 v305 n6849 p341(6).

[56] Kingman, Sharon. : British Medical Journal, May 16, 1992 v304 n6837 p1264(2).

anaesthesia as the woman cannot push so well and she has little or no sensation of her perineum. The complications of forceps include:

- death or brain injury of the foetus
- skull fractures
- facial paralysis - usually completely recovers
- vaginal or cervical lacerations

An alternative to forceps delivery is the use of Ventouse extraction. This is the application of a metal cup to the head of the baby. It is attached to a vacuum pump so that the pressure exerted allows the cup to remain firmly fixed to the head. Traction on the cup can aid delivery. A large bruise develops over the site of the cup which fades in the next few days. Application of the cup for over 30 minutes may lead to serious injury to the scalp[57].

Epidural anaesthesia is commonly applied nowadays. It involves the passage of a tube into the epidural space in the lumbar spine. Local anaesthesia is injected so that there is numbness of the lower parts of the body. Complications include low blood pressure, temporary respiratory paralysis if the injection enters the theca, poor voluntary effort in the second stage leading to forceps or vacuum extraction.

The use of epidural anaesthesia during labour leads to the development of several long-term symptoms in women. These include backache, frequent headaches, neckache, pins and needles in the hands or fingers, numbness or tingling in the lower back, buttocks or legs. Backache is almost twice as common in women who have received epidural anaesthesia[58][59].

Some cases of epidural anaesthesia are complicated by dural puncture. This is puncture of the dura mater and arachnoid mater, which are the membranes surrounding the spinal cord and brain. Dural headache often affects the neck and shoulders as well, and symptoms usually arise within two days of the procedure. The headache is typically frontal, severe, throbbing and better for laying flat. The discomfort frequently affects the neck and shoulders and may be associated with auditory or visual symptoms or nausea. The headache can last for up to six days. There may be muzziness of the head for another day or so[60].

Caesarian section is the delivery of the baby through an abdominal incision. It may be performed under general or epidural anaesthesia. The indications for Caesarian section are similar to those of any aided delivery. That is, there has to be maternal or foetal distress usually with some degree of delayed labour. Elective Caesarian sections are performed in cases of known disproportion.

According to figures in 1993, about 25% of births in the USA and nearly 20% of those in Canada were by Caesarean section. This compared with 6-7% in the Netherlands, Japan, Slovenia, and the former Czechoslovak Republic. Rates for other 'developed' countries range from 10 to 15%. In the UK, it is difficult to obtain accurate figures. They seem to show an increase in the Caesarean section rate from 10% in 1988-89 to 12% in 1989-90 and 13% in 1990-91[61].

This operation has become increasingly common over the years as obstetricians become more interventionist[62]. The common justification is that of worry of litigation. It seems somewhat paradoxical that obstetricians will practise a *more* hazardous method of delivery just to prevent litigation. I would have thought that the most appropriate method of treatment is the one indicated rather than the one preferred by the medical defence company. Fear of litigation is considered to be the main reason why Caesarian rates are so high in the US. However, there are similar rates in Canada where litigation is not so widespread. Most deliveries in Canada and the US are supervised by doctors rather than midwives and this is more likely to be responsible. Countries where midwives are mainly responsible for delivery have consistently low rates of Caesarian section delivery.

---

[57] Cranial osteopathic treatment is invaluable for dealing with problems experienced after operative delivery. It is to be considered in any newborn or young baby with symptoms attributable to delivery.
[58] MacArthur, C. et al: British Medical Journal, May 16, 1992 v304 n6837 p1279(4).
[59] MacArthur C. et al: British Medical Journal 1990;301:9-12.
[60] MacArthur, C. et al: British Medical Journal, April 3, 1993 v306 n6882 p883(3).
[61] Macfarlane, Alison; et al. : The Lancet, Oct 23, 1993 v342 n8878 p1005(2).
[62] Some 1 in 8 babies in the UK are born by Caesarean section which is a doubling in the last 15 years. In some parts of S America, 80% of babies are delivered by this method.

High rates of Caesarian section are also observed where women receive private medical treatment[63]. Item-of-service payments also play a role here[64].

The complications of Caesarian section are those of any anaesthesia and abdominal operation. These are outlined on Pages 42 and 43. In particular, there are problems with anaesthesia if applied in an emergency. Other complications include haemorrhage, infection, pulmonary embolism and rupture of the scar in a subsequent pregnancy or labour.

There is no evidence that elective operative delivery leads to a better outcome for term breech or for very small babies. Despite this, Caesarean rates for these indications have increased in 'developed' countries[65].

A programme was developed with the intention of reducing the Caesarian delivery rate without harm to the mother or baby[66]. A target was set of between 11 and 12% Caesarian section delivery rate after two years of the programme. At the end of the pregnancy, 70% of women who had a previous section delivered vaginally. The reduction in Caesarean deliveries was not associated with a rise in forceps and other operative deliveries. The rate of operative vaginal deliveries fell during the study, from 10.4 to 4.3 per cent. The proportion of spontaneous vaginal deliveries increased during the study. There were no changes to the health of the new-born baby or foetal and neonatal mortality rates

RETAINED PLACENTA

This may occur with post-partum haemorrhage which is described below. Frequently, there is no excessive bleeding and the placenta does not deliver. It may be due to abnormal adhesion to the uterine wall or spasm of the lower part of the uterus. This latter may be caused by the injection of oxytocin as the baby is delivered.

Symptoms:

There will be no sign of placental delivery. It may have separated from the uterine wall. This is evidenced by a hardness of the top of the uterus, mobility of this area from side to side, lengthening of the umbilical cord and a small gush of blood.

Treatment:

Manual removal is performed under general anaesthesia if it cannot be removed by pulling on the umbilical cord.

Alternative management:

In terms of Chinese medicine, this may be due to either Deficiency of Qi and Blood or to Cold Invasion leading to Stagnation of Blood. It is helpful to massage acupuncture points such as Gall Bladder 21, Urinary Bladder 60, Large Intestine 4 and Spleen 6. These descend the energy and help the uterus expel the placenta. Most cases will be alleviated by such methods. There are herbal and homoeopathic treatments also. In extreme cases with haemorrhage, surgical intervention may be necessary.

---

[63] Macfarlane AJ. : British Medical Journal 1988; 297: 852.
[64] Stafford RS. Caesarean section use and source of payment: an analysis of Canadian hospital discharge abstracts. Am J Publ Health 1990;80: 313-15.
[65] Enkin MW. et al eds. : Pregnancy and childbirth module. Cochrane database of systematic reviews published through Cochrane updates on disk. Oxford: Update Software, 1993.
[66] American Family Physician, June 1989 v39 n6 p258(1).

POST-PARTUM HAEMORRHAGE

This is heavy blood loss after delivery of the baby. It may occur just after delivery or a day or so later. It is arbitrarily defined as blood loss in excess of 500 ml.

There are various causes which include:

- failure of uterus to contract adequately
- retention of placenta
- lacerations - due to delivery of the head and shoulders or to obstetric intervention

Symptoms:

The blood loss will be self-evident. In severe cases there will be pallor, rapid pulse rate, low blood pressure, sweating and light-headedness. Symptoms are more likely to occur in those women who were already anaemic.

Treatment:

It is fear of this condition which has led to the practice of oxytocin injection as the baby is delivered. If the placenta has not been delivered, manual removal under general anaesthesia is done immediately. If the placenta has been delivered, an injection of ergometrine is given to cause the uterus to contract.

Replacement of blood by transfusion may be necessary. Later iron supplementation is given.

Alternative management:

The treatment of women before and during pregnancy will go a long way to reducing the risk of such a complication. There are emergency acupuncture, herbal and homoeopathic treatments available. The stimulation of oxytocin production naturally by breast-feeding is helpful in prevention.

- POST-NATAL CARE -

The main issue in the post-natal period is the replenishing of Blood and care of the mother and baby. Supportive helpers to minimise the amount of work and worry are invaluable. It is preferable for 4 weeks after delivery. This may be an ideal which cannot be attained but perhaps something at which to aim.

Breast milk is a product of Yin and Blood and this places further demands upon the mother. Therefore, diet needs to be nutritious and similar to that described at the beginning of Chapter 13 - Gastrointestinal System. Cold food is depleting of digestive energy and may lead to the appearance of symptoms due to Cold in those with low energy.

The lochia is the loss from the uterus after delivery. It is red for the first few days and becomes pinker and less heavy with time. It is excessive if placental tissue remains in the uterus. It is offensive in cases of infection.

Care of the breasts is important to minimise problems with breast feeding. Engorgement or even overt mastitis may occur from about the fourth day as breast milk secretion increases. It is preferable to allow the baby to control the number and amount of feeds rather than keep to a rigid schedule. In this way, the baby is happy and there will be more harmony between baby and mother.

In terms of Chinese medicine, no lactation is due to Qi Stagnation in the Middle Jiao or to Qi and Blood Deficiency. Milk leaking continuously from the breasts is due to Kidney and Spleen Qi Deficiency so the milk is not held. Mastitis is due to weakness of the Ren and Chong channels, DampHeat Accumulation in the channels or disharmony of the Liver and Stomach with underlying Blood Deficiency. There are effective treatments available in homoeopathy and herbal medicine.

Breast feeding is more likely to be successful when the mother is in a supportive environment. The most preferred is at home. Hospitals can directly influence the number of women who breast-feed successfully with their policies of providing commercial milk formulae at discharge[67].

Post-natal exercises are helpful, particularly those which strengthen the pelvic floor. These can help reduce the frequency of urinary problems later.

There is a routine post-natal examination performed at six weeks after delivery. A cervical smear may be performed at the same time. Cervical erosions are commonly seen and do not require conventional treatment. Most resolve of their own accord.

- HOW TO RECOGNISE A SERIOUS CONDITION IN PREGNANCY OR CHILDBIRTH -

Most pregnancies are normal and those which are not rarely reach the stage of seriousness. It is important, however, to recognise those symptoms which may indicate a potentially serious problem for mother or baby.

SYMPTOM	WHEN TO WORRY
Bleeding	Always
Uterine pain	Always unless at normal time for labour
Vaginal discharge	Heavy, blood-stained
Vomiting	Severe, prolonged, evidence of dehydration
High blood pressure	If severe especially if associated with oedema and proteinuria
Oedema	If severe and especially if associated with high blood pressure and proteinuria
Proteinuria	With dysuria and backache, with high blood pressure and proteinuria
Delayed onset to labour	If more than two weeks overdue
Prolonged labour	If cervix not dilating, with exhaustion, with changes to foetal heart rate
Bleeding after delivery	If heavy
Retention of placenta	If with heavy bleeding, if prolonged (over an hour)

TABLE 17.8: HOW TO RECOGNISE A SERIOUS CONDITION OF PREGNANCY AND CHILDBIRTH

---

[67] "Commercial discharge pack studies indicated that the packs had a negative effect on total breast-feeding at one month and any breast feeding at one and four months. The packs were linked to poor lactation among women during their first delivery and poor women in developing countries. Rooming-in accompanied by breast-feeding guidance had a greater positive effect on lactation success than did either procedure alone. Other programs including early mother-infant contact after birth, breast-feeding on demand and removal of in-hospital commercial formula supplementation had significant beneficial effects on breast-feeding." Perez-Escamilla, Rafael. et al :The American Journal of Public Health, Jan 1994 v84 n1 p89(9).

- SUMMARY -

Pregnancy and childbirth are normal processes.

Difficulties appear either because of problems with mother and baby or because of inappropriate medical intervention.

You should know the symptoms which would indicate a potentially serious condition of pregnancy and childbirth.

Ensure you have treatment options which can be used when pregnancy or labour does not follow the normal processes.

Appropriate treatment of women in pregnancy, during labour and of the baby at delivery will greatly help future generations to regain their health[68].

---

[68] In my opinion, the major contributions to disease in this century have been mass vaccination, routine use of antibiotics and the medicalisation of normal processes.

18 GYNAECOLOGY

OBJECTIVES:
At the end of this Chapter you will be able to:
Describe the differences between the alternative and conventional views of women's health
List the symptoms attributable to disturbances of the female reproductive system
State when a symptom(s) would indicate a serious underlying condition
Describe the main symptoms of diseases covered in this Chapter
Explain the relevant management by an alternative practitioner of each disorder

---

- INTRODUCTION -

The word 'gynaecology' means the study of women. I have used this term since it is the one with which people are most familiar. I considered a term like 'Womens Health' since there are many negative associations with the term 'gynaecology'. Each group of students I teach has many and varied responses to gynaecology and the gynaecological treatment of women. They frequently revolve around the feelings of violation, of not being taken seriously, of mutilating operations such as hysterectomies, issues around fertility and contraception, termination of pregnancy and so forth. This is an emotionally charged subject. It is important to bear in mind when you are treating a woman that there may be a whole history of conventional gynaecological treatment to be considered. This is in addition to the original complaint and leads to another dimension which has to be addressed as well as clouding of the original symptoms or case.

In my opinion, the treatment of women by gynaecologists is a reflection of the current attitudes towards women in Western society. Therefore, sexist attitudes in society are reflected in the gynaecology clinic. Most gynaecologists are men and female gynaecologists frequently reflect the same male-centred attitudes. There is an underlying agenda that there is something inherently dysfunctional about female physiology. This idea is prevalent in Western society as a result of various religious and social ideas about women.

It is a Judaeo-Christian belief that woman as Eve is responsible for the initiation of a 'fall from grace'. Since menstruation is the symbol of being female, it must be a pathological discharge which is inherently abnormal or unclean. Women themselves take on this belief. Colloquially, there are terms for menstruation such as 'the curse'. There are negative associations with the pre-menstrual and menstrual times, with sexual activity, with pregnancy and childbirth. These are deeply ingrained and cover the whole treatment of women both in gynaecology and in obstetrics[1].

Certainly female physiology is poorly understood and this may be a reflection of Western philosophical thought which regards physical matters as all important. Women are considered to be mechanical objects and the use of female sex hormones, e.g. oral contraception, hormone replacement therapy, is a crude attempt to manipulate hormonal states in order to control menstruation and ovulation. The word 'manipulate', of course, can be used on many levels and I do not think that these drugs are used solely for their physical effects. Any study of the list of side-effects of these hormones makes it difficult to see the justification for taking these drugs. Following on from the above discussion, there is a subconscious view that as women are abnormal to begin with it is reasonable to take any means to try and 'make them better'.

Women just before, at and after the menopause are given large doses of female sex hormones in an attempt to treat the 'disease of menopause'. There is no end to the 'need' for treatment according to these views of conventional medicine. Women grow up and manifest symptoms and receive treatment in an atmosphere of negativity which teaches women not to express their thoughts and feelings. This energy then becomes blocked and causes pathology in the neck and throat area giving rise to thyroid dysfunction or in the pelvis giving rise to menstrual symptoms. Normal events such as menstruation, ovulation and the menopause are frequently seen as abnormal and require treatment. Symptoms are viewed negatively and removed by chemicals or surgery. Women feel negatively about themselves with feelings of shame, resentment, guilt, excessive responsibility and so forth.

---

[1] There are numerous books dealing with these issues. I mention "Changing of the Gods" by Naomi Goldenberg (Beacon Press, 1979), "Goddesses in EveryWoman" by Jean Shinoda Bolen (Harper and Row, 1985) and "The Paradise Papers" by Merlin Stone (Virago, 1976).

The alternative view of women's health is somewhat different and necessarily more positive. Chinese medicine, for example, is based upon an energetic anatomy and physiology and describes the importance of energetic channels in women. There is an energetic channel which directly connects the uterus with the heart[2]. The Heart in Chinese medicine, if I can remind you of Chapter 7 - Cardiovascular system is considered to house the Mind. This direct connection is important in that it explains why psychological factors frequently affect menstruation and why gynaecological interference can have such a dramatic effect on the psyche. It is of relevance in pregnancy since this allows for a direct connection between the mind of the baby and the mind of the mother. Some authors have named the uterus as the second heart and it is clearly an important organ. In conventional medicine, the uterus is seen as being unnecessary after women have their quota of children and so hysterectomy is frequently performed. The indications for hysterectomy in these situations may be slight indeed. It can be seen from this energetic connection that such treatment can lead to emotional and mental disturbances. In addition, the prescription of female sex hormones can themselves disturb mental and emotional states.

In Chinese medicine it is considered that in healthy females, menstruation begins on a regular monthly cycle at around the age of 14. This is because females go through cycles of 7 years[3]. The menstrual cycle continues regularly until the age of menopause which normally occurs at the age of 49 years. The menstrual cycle, which in health is 28 days in length, corresponds with the lunar cycle.

Everything can be divided into Yin and Yang. The first half of the cycle, beginning with menstruation, is related to Yin and ends at ovulation. Ovulation is the time when conception would occur, that is reception of the sperm and this is the most receptive time of the month. It corresponds to the new moon which is the most Yin time of the lunar cycle - difficult to be seen, hidden and a dark sky. At ovulation, the Yang phase of the cycle begins. The energy gathers to push the blood out at the time of menstruation. This occurs, ideally, at the full moon which is the time of greatest flow, both in terms of menstruation but also in terms of ocean tides.

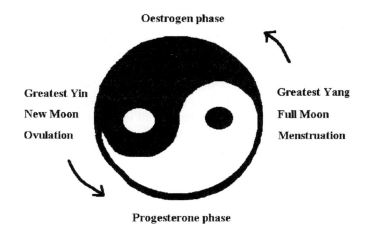

FIGURE 18.1: DIAGRAM OF YINYANG SYMBOL RELATED TO MENSTRUAL CYCLE

As there are changes physically, there are also changes mentally and emotionally. We live in a society where it is considered normal to be involved in some of routine and not take account of natural cycles. Nevertheless, it clear to most women that they feel differently through the month. These cycles are not so clear in men. This is partly because they are not so sensitive to natural cycles (they are Yang in relation to the Yin of nature and the earth) and menstruation is clear external evidence of such changes.

---

[2] The Chong channel. See discussion in "The Path of Pregnancy" by Bob Flaws (Blue Poppy Press, 1982) on Page 12.

[3] "Essentials of Chinese Acupuncture" compiled by Colleges of Traditional Chinese Medicine in People's Republic of China (Foreign Languages Press, Beijing, 1980).

The Yang phase, the second half of the cycle, is where the energy gathers to push out the Blood. At this time, the energy may stagnate and not move. This is why pre-menstrual symptoms of painful breasts, headaches, bloating, irritability and anger may manifest at this time. As menstruation begins, and this is the changeover to the Yin part of the cycle, the energy moves down and out as evidenced by menstrual flow and the whole cycle begins again.

Frequently, at or around the time of menstruation, women may have feelings of wanting to be quiet and separate. Historically, and in traditional cultures, this is a time when women in the community withdraw and spend time with themselves rather than taking part in the hurly-burly of community life. It is a time when women perhaps feel more in touch with spiritual matters, the artistic, receptive side and so is an indication of the power of femaleness. This, of course, is the reason why menstruation in modern society is regarded so negatively since recognition of this power would place women on an equal basis with men. Most trends in the modern world are designed to undermine women so there is a vested interest in undervaluing menstruation.

The absolute definition of normal menstruation I take from Chinese views of physiology. The normal cycle is of 28 days. This includes 5 days of menstruation. In health, the discharge of blood during menstruation is not too heavy or too light, it is painless with no clots, it begins clearly with a red flow, being heavier for the first day or so and then tailing off and it ends clearly. I would consider any cycle less than 26 days or more than 30 days as a symptom to be included in the case. If menstruation lasts less than four days or more than six days, this also indicates an imbalance. Pre-menstrually, women may have feelings of changing psychological state. Symptoms such as irritability, depression, tiredness and headache indicate an imbalance to be considered as part of the case.

As can be seen from this description, symptoms are very common at or around menstruation.. Unfortunately, there is an acceptance by many people that these symptoms are 'normal'. Education by the practitioner is clearly an important of our work in women regaining health.

The menopause which normally occurs around the age of 49 is also a normal event and is associated with the cessation of menstruation. The commonest occurrence is the gradual increase in the interval between periods with decreasing loss at each menstrual period. Sometimes menstruation stops suddenly. Marked emotional changes, heavy periods, intermittent bleeding, sweats and hot flushes are abnormal although common in Western society and where women are considered to be of less value after the end of child-bearing years. This is a reason why female sex hormones will be given after the menopause since this continues the occurrence of bleeding every month, together with feelings of social attractability and attractiveness. This illusion, or indeed delusion, is a major driving force in the prescription of hormone replacement treatment.

- BASIC ANATOMY AND PHYSIOLOGY -

It is important to have a basic understanding of the structure and function of the female reproductive system. I have listed the objectives which I consider useful to achieve as a preliminary to study of gynaecology. These are detailed in Table 18.1.

As a preliminary to study of gynaecology you are able to:
Identify the structures of the female reproductive system
Describe the functions of these structures
Explain the connections between the female reproductive system and the endocrine system
Describe the phases of the menstrual cycle
Describe the changes in the female reproductive system which occur at puberty and menopause
Describe the function of the breast and its relationship to the female sex hormones

TABLE 18.1: OBJECTIVES FOR ANATOMY AND PHYSIOLOGY AS PREREQUISITE FOR STUDY OF GYNAECOLOGY

It can be seen from a knowledge of anatomy and physiology that there are certain common symptoms which arise from disturbances. Table 18.2 lists the symptoms which may arise from gynaecological disease.

No periods (amenorrhoea)
Irregular periods
Late periods
Early periods
Heavy periods
Painful periods (dysmenorrhoea)
Abnormal vaginal bleeding
Vaginal discharge
Abdominal pain
Infertility

TABLE 18.2: SYMPTOMS OF GYNAECOLOGICAL DISEASE

- CLASSIFICATION OF GYNAECOLOGICAL DISORDERS -

The most useful classification of gynaecological disorders is to follow the pattern I have set throughout the book. That is, to take account of acuteness and level within the body. Such a classification is shown in Table 18.3. The conventional classification mainly centres on pathological processes, e.g. infective, inflammatory, tumours, hormonal.

MILD DISEASE

Dysmenorrhoea
Pre-menstrual syndrome
Vaginal discharge
Pelvic inflammatory disease
Menstrual abnormalities
Endometriosis
Cancer of the cervix of the uterus
Cancer of the body of the uterus

SEVERE DISEASE

TABLE 18.3: CLASSIFICATION OF GYNAECOLOGICAL DISORDERS

- GYNAECOLOGICAL DISORDERS -

INTRODUCTION

The disorders which are primarily considered in this Chapter are those which Chinese medicine lists for study. These are fourteen in number and may be divided into gynaecological and obstetric problems. They are mainly symptoms rather than conventional disease labels. They are discussed in detail in this Chapter in one form or another. The gynaecological disorders are:

- irregular menstruation
- amenorrhoea
- dysmenorrhoea
- infertility
- pre-menstrual syndrome
- abnormal vaginal bleeding
- leucorrhoea (this means vaginal discharge)
- menopausal symptoms
- uterine prolapse

The obstetric disorders will be discussed in Chapter 17 - Pregnancy and Childbirth and they complete the 14 listed in Chinese medicine. These are:

- morning sickness
- malposition of the foetus
- threatened miscarriage
- postmaturity and/or difficult and painful labour
- insufficient lactation.

- VAGINAL DISCHARGE -

Vaginal discharge can be an important pointer to gynaecological problems. It is important to specifically enquire about this. Sometimes a vaginal discharge is normal, particularly in the second half of the cycle, so avoid labelling all discharges as abnormal. It is important to enquire about the heaviness of the discharge, time of day, changes with menstrual cycle, colour of the discharge and any associated symptoms. It is also essential to enquire about the use of douches, tampons, sprays and drugs, particularly the contraceptive pill and antibiotics.

In Chinese medicine, the categorisation of vaginal discharges is in terms of colour. These are white, red, yellow, black, green and five-coloured. I use this terminology here as a basis for discussion

Black and five-coloured vaginal discharges are uncommon, particularly in out-patient practice. They usually occur in association with advanced cancer. I would refer you here to the sections dealing with cancer of the cervix of the uterus and cancer of the body of the uterus.

WHITE VAGINAL DISCHARGE

White discharge is known as leucorrhoea although in some Chinese medical textbooks the term is used to indicate any vaginal discharge. This is a misconception as the prefix 'leuco-' means white.

Not all white vaginal discharges are abnormal. You should consider situations of pregnancy, sexual stimulation, ovulation, pre-menstrually and post-partum as events which are associated with a normal white discharge. It is normal when it is not heavy and there is no associated smell, itching or discomfort.

In terms of conventional medicine, white vaginal discharge may be associated with several disorders including:

- cervical erosion
- cervical polyp
- fungal infection - Candida albicans (also known as thrush or monilia)

Symptoms:

Classically, fungal infection causes profuse vaginal discharge of a thick or curdy nature where patches of white are seen on the vulva or vagina. Scraping of the white patches reveals a raw, bleeding surface. This accounts for the symptoms of severe itching, soreness and discomfort. It commonly occurs after treatment with the oral contraceptive or antibiotics since these drugs alter the normal bacterial and fungal content of the body. After antibiotics, 80% of women have evidence of Candida whilst around one third of those will have symptoms.

In women who have not received treatment with antibiotics, up to 60% have evidence of candida. The appearance of symptoms is associated with various factors. These include:

- pregnancy
- sugar intake, tight clothes, synthetic materials, allergic reactions,
- prescribed drugs, e.g. antibiotics, corticosteroids, female sex hormones, immunosuppressant drugs
- diabetes mellitus, AIDS, herpes simplex

Some 50% of cases have no such factors.

Treatment

Treatment of white vaginal discharge is usually considered unnecessary by conventional medicine unless there is evidence of thrush. This is invariably with anti-fungal agents which may be locally or systemically given. Systemic anti-fungal agents have a predilection for causing liver disease such as hepatitis. 10-20% of women treated develop recurrent vaginal symptoms and this can be a major difficulty.

Alternative management:

In terms of Chinese medicine, white vaginal discharge infers deficiency of Spleen energy with the abnormal passage downwards of Dampness (mucus). There are mainly four variants seen which are Kidney deficiency, Spleen deficiency, PhlegmDampness and DampHeat.

The main point for alternative practitioners is that the occurrence of an abnormal white discharge implies an internal organ imbalance. This is not merely a disturbance of the vagina. It is important to enquire about any precipitating or maintaining cause such as those listed above. Of particular importance are the oral contraceptive, antibiotics and the use of irritant sprays and douches which frequently cause allergic reactions. If these are avoided and constitutional treatment begun, then improvement can be expected.

I would refer you to Chapter 9 - Urinary System and Chapter 13 - Gastrointestinal System for discussions about the Kidney and Spleen respectively.

CASE

A woman of 45 years came for treatment. Her main complaint was constipation. She would open her bowels for several days and then nothing for up to five days. She had leaking urine which was worse on exercise and straining. This was despite a surgical repair for prolapse some years earlier. She also had a vaginal discharge which had been continued from childhood. It was white, heavy but with no itching or smell. Other symptoms included tiredness, low back ache and general cold feelings.

Her diagnosis in terms of Chinese medicine was Kidney Yang Deficiency. I treated her with acupuncture and herbs. I gave her advice about eating warm food with ginger and cinnamon to increase her Yang energy. Within a few weeks of beginning treatment her energy had improved. Her urinary symptoms lessened and her vaginal discharge had disappeared.

In this type of case, the discharge, and indeed the urinary symptoms, are an example of fluids leaking because the energy is weak. Strengthening the energy will lead to retention of the fluids. Her constipation improved as she became stronger and her intestines were efficient.

She continues to receive treatment and now feels very well. Recently she has had mild flare-ups of some symptoms which she had as a child. This 'return of old symptoms' is a curative response and reflects her much increased levels of health.

YELLOW VAGINAL DISCHARGE

In conventional medicine, the appearance of any yellow or green vaginal discharge is considered to reveal the existence of bacterial infection. The causes of such a discharge are considered to be inflammation of the cervix (cervicitis), retained pessary, inflammation of the vagina or endometrium and pelvic inflammatory disease. Cervicitis is the term used to describe an inflammation of the cervix. It may be, but not necessarily, of infective origin, Any yellow discharge will automatically be treated with antibiotics.

Symptoms:

The precise symptoms associated with yellow vaginal discharge are dependent upon the site of the condition. In the case of vaginitis (vaginal inflammation) there will be soreness and discomfort in the vagina. Cervicitis (inflammation of the cervix) is associated with frequency of urination, tenderness of the cervix on pressure and painful intercourse. The symptoms of pelvic inflammatory disease are discussed in detail below.

Treatment

As stated above, this condition is invariably treated with antibiotics which lead to further problems with vaginal discharge as described in relation to white vaginal discharge. If there is disease of the cervix such as cervicitis or an associated condition, cervical erosion, then there may be cauterisation by heat or lasers.

Cervical erosion is considered to be secondary to cervical discharge in conventional medicine. It is not in itself a primary inflammatory condition, nor is it an ulcer, despite its name. This can lead to confusion and women can be very worried about the term unless it is properly explained. It is the growth of cells from inside the cervical canal over the surface of the cervix.

An erosion is seen as a bright red velvety area extending from the external opening of the cervix over the vaginal surface. The surface bleeds easily, especially on contact and postcoital bleeding is a common symptom. Erosions are common in women on the pill. They commonly occur in pregnancy and in the postnatal period and usually disappear with no treatment. They seem to be related to high hormonal levels.

Alternative Management

In terms of Chinese medicine, yellow vaginal discharge is again due to Dampness as in white vaginal discharge. There is associated Heat causing the yellow colour. This usually implies some Stagnation of Liver energy.

CASE

A woman of 33 years came for treatment because she had not been well since glandular fever some 4 years previously. She had particularly been ill for the past six months. Her main complaints were extreme fatigue, occasional fever with sore throat. She had diarrhoea four or five times each day with undigested food in the stools, nausea, palpitations and general muscle weakness.

In terms of conventional medicine, this could be diagnosed as myalgic encephalomyelitis (ME) although no-one had ever made that diagnosis. In terms of Chinese medicine, this was a case of Heart Blood Deficiency and Spleen Yang Deficiency with Damp Accumulation.

After some weeks treatment, her bowels became normal and she began to feel more energetic. Her treatment continued for some five months. At the end of this time, she felt generally well with good energy. She then developed a vaginal discharge with lower abdominal pain. It was yellow in colour and occasionally blood-streaked. It was particularly heavy after menstruation.

She had a history of inflammation of the cervix which had been discovered by cervical smear investigation. She was somewhat worried about her symptoms and had a repeat cervical smear. This showed normal cells. A vaginal swab showed evidence of 'thrush'. Despite this, her doctor gave her antibiotics. This is a common reaction when medical practitioners see a yellow discharge.

During and after the course of antibiotics she felt tired and depressed with diarrhoea and a bloated abdomen. As noted in Chapter 5 - Infectious Disease, the energetic qualities of antibiotics are Coldness and Dampness. Her Spleen energy was clearly still depleted and so the antibiotics caused a recurrence of her original symptoms. If she had further courses of antibiotics, these would worsen and she would develop a clinical picture similar to that of ME discussed on Page 60.

Her vaginal discharge was the passage of mucus out of the body and, in that sense, is a curative response. Mucus collects in the intestines and this may be evident in the stools or, in women, as vaginal discharge as the uterus is often involved also. The mucus had begun to move out of her body as her energy had been improving.

It is important in such cases to continue the process so that the movement towards health can be maintained.

GREEN VAGINAL DISCHARGE

This is a more severe condition than yellow vaginal discharge and in conventional medicine is usually associated with infection by Trichomonas vaginalis. This is an organism classified as a protozoon. A related organism is Giardia which is associated with bowel symptoms.

Symptoms:

There is the appearance of a green vaginal discharge containing tiny bubbles. There may be small red erosions over the surface of the vagina with severe inflammation. There is marked pain and discomfort in the area. There is frequently evidence of the organism in sexual partners and so sexual transmission is an issue in this condition.

Treatment

This is by means of the antiprotozoal agent, metronidazole, for around 7 days and the sexual partner is treated in the same way. Sexual intercourse should be abstained from during this time.

Alternative Management

This is a more severe type of yellow vaginal discharge and therefore in terms of Chinese medicine there is much more Heat, as evidenced by the green colour and the degree of pain. There are similarities energetically between this condition and the description of cystitis in Chapter 9 - Urinary System.

RED VAGINAL DISCHARGE

This is, clearly, bleeding and must always be taken seriously. In terms of conventional medicine it may occur with conditions such as:

- cervical erosion
- tumour, benign or malignant of uterine cervix or uterine body
- inflammation of the vagina
- inflammation of the endometrium[4]
- retained pessary
- associated with pregnancy.

The latter case is considered in Chapter 17 - Pregnancy and Childbirth.

Such bleeding from the vagina, other than around the time of the menses, may be of serious significance. In the case of cervical cancer there may be an association with intercourse and in cases of uterine cancer there may be intermenstrual bleeding.

Alternative Management

It is important to bear in mind the significance of the possible diagnosis in terms of conventional medicine. In Chinese medicine, red discharge is seen as a consequence of DampHeat or Blood and Yin deficiency where there may be signs of Deficient Heat

- PELVIC INFLAMMATORY DISEASE -

This is a term which indicates inflammation in the pelvis usually involving the fallopian tubes and ovaries. This may also be known as salpingitis or salpingo-oophoritis. It is considered to be associated with infection. This used to be of the gonococcal type but is now usually associated with organisms such as chlamydia. The relationship between these two organisms was discussed in Chapter 9 - Urinary System - Page 169.

Symptoms:

There are a wide variety of presentations here but in the severe acute case there may be confusion with other causes of acute abdominal pain. The differential diagnosis of acute lower abdominal pain is shown in Table 18.4.

In the case of pelvic inflammatory disease, there is sharp, lower abdominal pain which is usually felt in both iliac fossae. If the pain is only on the right side then the possibility of appendicitis must be considered. There is disturbance of menstruation with spotting around the period, heavy and painful periods. There is a yellowish discharge and frequent urination. There may be associated nausea and vomiting. Painful intercourse is common. There is a fever of around 39°C (102°F) with lower abdominal tenderness and guarding.

---

[4] Inflammation of the vagina and endometrium may occur at or after the menopause due to the reduction in oestrogen secretion.

Pelvic inflammatory disease is more common when there is vaginal douching and frequent sexual intercourse particularly with different partners. With any vaginal discharge it is helpful to think about whether there are associated symptoms developing in pelvic inflammatory disease. It is useful to enquire of previous medical history which may reveal:

- gonorrhoea
- non-specific urethritis
- genital herpes
- genital warts
- trichomonal infection
- recent change of sexual partner
- urethral symptoms in a partner
- use of intra-uterine contraceptive device (the 'coil')
- gynaecological or pelvic surgery

Chronic pelvic inflammatory disease is usually characterised by recurrent attacks of lesser severity than the acute picture. There are persisting pelvic pain and back ache. Painful periods are common and intercourse may be painful. Periods may be heavy. There is an associated yellow vaginal discharge. The recurrence of continuing pain, discomfort and heavy menstruation may cause general symptoms of ill health. Blockage of the fallopian tubes causes infertility. Fever may be absent.

DISEASE	SYMPTOMS	COMMENTS
Appendicitis	Pain central abdomen which migrates to right iliac fossa. Vomiting, fever	Classical cause of pain in right iliac fossa. Short history
Ectopic pregnancy	History of amenorrhoea in the sexually active, vaginal bleeding usually brownish or dark	Symptoms worsen over days and possibly weeks. Surgical emergency
Pyelonephritis	Dysuria, haematuria, loin pain, fever	Pain mainly in the loin but may be referred down the ureter on the affected side to give iliac fossa pain
Torsion[5] of ovarian cyst	Pain in the iliac fossa, vomiting, rapid pulse and low blood pressure if severe, slight fever, uterine bleeding (occasionally)	More likely during pregnancy or after childbirth
Rupture of ovarian cyst	Severe abdominal pain but of short duration	

TABLE 18.4: DIFFERENTIAL DIAGNOSIS OF ACUTE LOWER ABDOMINAL PAIN

Investigations:

This is by means of vaginal swabs to isolate any organism associated with the symptoms. Green vaginal discharge may occur in several situations. Table 18.5 itemises how to differentiate its causes.

SYMPTOM	VAGINITIS	CERVICITIS	PELVIC INFLAMMATORY DISEASE
Vaginal discharge	green	green	green
Menstrual abnormalities	no	no	yes
Painful intercourse	superficial	deep	deep
Frequent urination	no	yes	yes
Fever	no	no	yes

TABLE 18.5: COMPARISON OF CONDITIONS ASSOCIATED WITH GREEN VAGINAL DISCHARGE

---

[5] This is twisting of a cyst on its stalk.

Treatment

Conventionally this is a combination of several antibiotics such as metronidazole and tetracycline. Non-steroidal anti-inflammatory agents may also be prescribed but the condition often becomes chronic.

Alternative management:

It may be considered as a more internal problem than the causes of vaginal discharges we have considered above, particularly the white and yellow types. This comparison can be seen in Table 18.5.

There are increasing numbers of women with these symptoms over the past few decades. It is almost certainly related to changes in sexual habits together with the increasing use of drugs such as female sex hormones and antibiotics.

In terms of Chinese medicine, the usual diagnoses include DampHeat in the Lower Jiao, Stagnation of Blood in the Lower Jiao and Deficiency of Spleen and Kidney Qi. The occurrence of the symptoms in women indicates a chronic constitutional imbalance and treatment may need to be prolonged. Complicating factors such as the use of antibiotics or female sexual hormones need to be stopped. Advice about stress, sexual activity and diet is helpful. These factors were discussed on Page 176 in relation to cystitis. Those comments are relevant here.

- MENSTRUAL ABNORMALITIES -

Before considering whether a particular pattern of menstruation is normal or abnormal, I would refer you to the beginning of this Chapter when normal situations were discussed. Any variation from this implies abnormality. I will describe several conditions in turn so that the major symptom pictures are described..

DYSMENORRHOEA

This is painful menstruation. It is generally considered that about 5% of women have sufficient pain to seek treatment but this is probably an underestimate. The number of women who have painful periods is far in excess of this figure. It is stated that about half of these women are too ill to work when symptoms are present.

Symptoms

The pain may begin before menstruation, at the onset of menstruation or towards the end of the period. These are important questions to ask together with information about the menstrual loss and associated symptoms.

In terms of conventional medicine, painful menstruation is divided into two categories. So-called primary dysmenorrhoea usually starts after puberty. There are colicky pains in the lower abdomen due to uterine contractions (spasmodic dysmenorrhoea). It may cease after childbirth, hence the old advice 'to have a baby'.

Secondary dysmenorrhoea is the appearance of menstrual pain after several years of painless periods. This is considered to be due to the development of conditions such as uterine fibroids, endometriosis or pelvic inflammatory disease. The pain tends to be prolonged throughout the period of perhaps a dragging quality. There may also be menstrual abnormalities.

Treatment:

There are several treatment options for primary dysmenorrhoea. These are listed in Table 18.6 Treatment of secondary dysmenorrhoea will be of the primary condition.

TREATMENT	TREATMENT LEVEL	COMMENTS
Analgesics, usually non-steroidal anti-inflammatory drugs	1	These are described in detail in Chapter 10 - Musculoskeletal System.
Oral contraceptive	2	Suppresses menstruation and ovulation.
Dilatation of the cervix	3	This requires a general anaesthetic and reduces symptoms in about one third. May damage cervix leading to premature labour in pregnancy.

TABLE 18.6: CONVENTIONAL TREATMENT OF PRIMARY DYSMENORRHOEA

Alternative Management:

In terms of Chinese medicine, the common pattern seen is Stagnation of Liver Qi which is commonly associated with emotional disturbances. In this type there will be associated symptoms of pre-menstrual syndrome with perhaps painful breasts, irritability, headache.

Another pattern is exposure to Cold and Damp which lodge in the uterus usually associated with Deficiency of Kidney Yang. Here, pain at the beginning of menstruation will be associated with perhaps diarrhoea, cold and faint feelings.

Further patterns include Deficiency of Qi and Blood due to Deficiency of Liver and Kidneys. Some cases of Liver Qi Stagnation may lead to Flaring of Liver Fire.

It is important to take each case individually and treat accordingly. Emotional factors, sexual activity and diet are all important here. In China, it is well known that the ingestion of cold foods or drinks during menstruation may cause stopping of the menstrual flow and thence pain. This may be the origin in the West of ideas such as not washing your hair or having a bath during the period. These are not simply 'old wives' tales' or superstition but have a basis in truth. This is not to be misunderstood as saying that women are inherently weak and need to avoid certain activities. It is merely a recognition of the changes occurring during menstruation.

The treatment of painful menstruation by alternative medicine is usually successful but clearly the underlying disturbances are of importance. It is more difficult to treat if structural abnormalities are present such as endometriosis.

ENDOMETRIOSIS

This is the existence of endometrium in situations where it is not usually present. The usual sites, in decreasing order of frequency, are ovaries, uterus, fallopian tubes, general pelvic area, umbilicus and lower abdominal scars particularly after hysterectomy. The endometrium bleeds at menstruation and so these areas also bleed. However, the blood cannot escape as it can from within the uterus. There are symptoms of lower abdominal pain which may be severe in nature. There may be the occurrence of intestinal symptoms as adhesions and scarring of pelvic masses interfere with intestinal function. Eventually, quite large collections of old blood develop in the areas affected, the so-called "chocolate cysts" as they are full of dark sticky material.

The cause in conventional medicine is not well understood. There seems to be a correlation with the use of tampons, intercourse during menstruation and the use of the intrauterine contraceptive device (the 'coil'). It is commoner in women who have had few or no children.

Symptoms

Twenty or so years ago it was unusual to see this condition in anyone below the age of 30 years. Nowadays it is more common to see endometriosis in younger age groups. The main clinical feature is pain on menstruation - dysmenorrhoea. Menstrual irregularities such as heavy periods and irregular bleeding are common. Infertility is an association since the existence of inflammation, scar tissue and adhesions in the pelvis may obstruct the passage of an egg along the fallopian tube.

Typically, the pain is severe beginning before the menstruation and continuing almost to the end. There may be associated symptoms of diarrhoea and vomiting. Fainting may occur in some. In extreme cases where disease is widespread there may be the development of intestinal obstruction.

Complications

COMPLICATION	SYMPTOMS TO LOOK FOR
Infertility	Inability to become pregnant
Intestinal obstruction	Abdominal distension, constipation, colicky abdominal pain

TABLE 18.7: COMPLICATIONS OF ENDOMETRIOSIS

Diagnosis:

This is primarily by means of the clinical history. Confirmation is usually obtained by laparoscopy.

Treatment:

It must be said that the conventional treatment of endometriosis is not particularly successful since the cause is ill understood. The main aim is to produce a state of 'pseudo pregnancy' where menstruation is halted. In this way cyclical endometrial bleeding is prevented and any areas of endometrium outside the uterus may have an opportunity to recede.

There are two main drugs used. Danazol affects the release of hormones by the pituitary gland and thereby inhibits ovulation and the normal hormonal cyclical change. It also affects adrenal gland function. Common side-effects include masculinisation such as deepening of the voice, reduction in breast size, oily skin and acne, development of hair in a male distribution and occasionally enlargement of the clitoris. It is a powerful drug as can be estimated by its side-effects and by the site of its action, the pituitary gland.

The other drug which may be used is a progesterone compound, norethisterone. This is given continuously in an effort to suppress ovulation and prevent menstruation. The side-effects are those of the progesterone group in general.

Alternative management:

At menstruation the blood should normally flow down and out and endometriosis would seem to suggest that the opposite is happening. There may be several preceding events which lead to this development. The associations mentioned above of tampon use, intercourse during menstruation and the use of the intra-uterine contraceptive device are all associated with energy and blood flowing upwards rather than downwards. Tampons block the normal downward flow of menstrual blood[6]. Intercourse leads to energy flowing upwards and the "coil" is also associated with a backward flow in the reproductive organs since ectopic pregnancy (pregnancy developing in a fallopian tube) is much commoner in this situation. It has also been noted that peristalsis along the fallopian tube is often reversed in cases of the coil. In terms of prevention, it would seem that certain measures may be helpful. The use of sanitary towels rather than tampons, abstinence from intercourse during menstruation and the use of alternative methods of contraception may go a long way to reducing the incidence of endometriosis.

---

[6] This may be the genesis of toxic shock syndrome. This is an unusual occurrence of high fever and the development of shock which may be fatal. It has been related to the use of tampons. In terms of Chinese medicine, stagnation of the flow of Qi or Blood may lead to the generation of heat manifesting as fever.

As for treatment of the condition once it has developed, it is important to consider the underlying energetic diagnosis. In terms of Chinese medicine, endometriosis usually corresponds to Stagnation of Blood in the Lower Jiao.

AMENORRHOEA

This is absence of menstrual periods. The importance of amenorrhoea is that it does not always denote disease. There are times when the absence of periods is normal. The commonest cause of amenorrhoea between the ages of 15 and 45 years is pregnancy. This may seem obvious but when practitioners see people with various symptoms the first thing to jump to mind is often a pathological situation. Normal absence of periods is also seen before puberty, during pregnancy and lactation and after the menopause.

Conventionally amenorrhoea is divided into two types. The primary type is where the woman has never menstruated. This is unusual and usually associated with rare endocrine disturbances. Secondary amenorrhoea is where menstruation has occurred previously and then stopped. Women with this seek help in the clinic and alternative practitioners quite commonly see such cases.

Investigations:

I would repeat again that pregnancy is the commonest cause of amenorrhoea in the fertile years and this should always be remembered. Stopping the contraceptive pill is another common cause and may result in no periods for a variable length of time. The oral contraceptive actually stops menstruation as its primary action and bleeding only occurs because it is not taken for seven days each month. Therefore, when it is finally removed, it takes the body a length of time to recover and for normal menstruation to resume.

General health and psychological factors also need to be taken into account as part of the general case-taking. Menstruation is commonly connected to nutritional state, emotions or may be disturbed in association with chronic diseases. Hormone estimations may be done by means of blood test but most cases reveal no abnormality. The majority of cases of secondary amenorrhoea are temporary and recover with no conventional treatment.

Two specific conditions to mention here are anorexia nervosa and polycystic ovarian disease. Anorexia nervosa is described in Chapter 16 - Psychological Disorders. Amenorrhoea is a feature of severe cases where weight loss is present. There are strong mental symptoms of disordered perception where the woman thinks or perceives herself as being overweight.

Polycystic ovarian disease, sometimes known as Stein-Leventhal syndrome, is a particular group of symptoms which include amenorrhoea. There is also hair growth on the face and in a male distribution up the central line of the lower abdomen as well as cysts on the ovaries. It is treated conventionally by surgical resection of part of the ovary or by hormonal suppression of ovulation.

Alternative management:

In terms of Chinese medicine, amenorrhoea usually corresponds to one of several possible syndromes. There may be Blood Stagnation where the Blood does not move usually due either to Qi stagnation or exposure to cold. The most common situation is Blood Deficiency associated with Spleen or Kidney deficiency which is. This is seen in athletes particularly those who are vegetarian. It is an indication of the weakness which may result in the Blood as a result of overexercise. This connection was discussed in Chapter 10 - Musculoskeletal System in relation to joint disorders. Some cases of amenorrhoea are due to Phlegm obstruction.

OTHER MENSTRUAL SYMPTOMS

There are several types of menstrual disturbances including heavy or light periods, early or late periods, and irregular periods[7].

In conventional medicine, the aim is always to distinguish between those causes of menstrual abnormality which are physical in nature and those which are not. The term, dysfunctional uterine bleeding is used to describe those cases of abnormal bleeding which are not due to complications of pregnancy or structural disease of the uterus or ovaries.

In terms of dysfunctional uterine bleeding, the assumption is that there is a degree of endometrial abnormality associated with a hormone imbalance. This is usually an excess of oestrogen in relation to progesterone. Despite this statement, investigations are normal in the majority of cases. It is true to say that conventional medicine finds this group of diseases difficult to classify. It is therefore grouped according to age of onset of symptoms. I will continue to do the same as this is a helpful way of categorisation.

PUBERTAL CASES

The first menstrual cycles are usually not associated with ovulation and consequently no progesterone is produced. The endometrium becomes thickened and overactive leading to heavy and perhaps painful periods. This situation is extremely common in young women just after the onset of periods and it frequently settles with no treatment. The conventional approach is either to wait and see or to give progesterone supplements in the second half of the menstrual cycle. A frequent prescription is the oral contraceptive pill in an attempt 'to regulate the menses'. This is clearly impossible using the oral contraceptive pill since this suppresses ovarian function and stops periods completely. The only reason why women bleed when they take the pill is because they stop for seven days so this is more accurately termed 'withdrawal bleeding'.

DURING THE REPRODUCTIVE PERIOD

During this age group, irregular or cyclical excessive bleeding may occur. It is treated in a similar way to the pubertal cases. Either progesterone is given in the latter half of the menstrual cycle or the oral contraceptive pill is used. It is very difficult in conventional terms to determine a cause of these symptoms in most cases. Some women have normal hormone estimations (by far the commonest finding), some have reduced progesterone levels and yet others have a lack of ovulation. There is no consistent finding and an empirical approach is taken.

Dilatation and curettage is a surgical procedure where the cervix is dilated and the inside of the uterus is scraped to remove endometrium. This may be done as a diagnostic procedure to determine the state of the endometrium but is more commonly performed, at least at this age, in an attempt to prevent heavy periods. It has been noted that heavy menstruation may be moderated after such an operation. The rationale behind this is difficult to determine. It may be considered to be similar to kicking the television set when it does not work. Certainly repeated D & Cs may lead to permanent damage of the endometrial lining of the uterus. It is a considerably invasive procedure which I would reserve only for those cases where perhaps cancer is suspected. The operation is performed under general anaesthesia.

In some hospitals, a small plastic cannula may be inserted through the cervix to obtain samples of endometrium without any anaesthesia. The effects of this are similar to surgery on the cervix of the uterus, the consequences of which are discussed later in this Chapter.

In many cases of heavy menstrual bleeding a hysterectomy may be performed where the woman has had children and there is no desire for more. There were 20,000 hysterectomies in the United Kingdom in 1985. Most are performed for irregularities in menstruation. Up to 45% of women develop infections of the wound or urinary tract in the post-operative period. Even if the ovaries are left alone, the woman is likely to pass through the menopause four years earlier than normal.

It is important to remember that the uterus is not merely a useless organ once childbirth has finished. Hysterectomy disrupts the energetic connection between the Heart and the uterus and may

---

[7] Technical terms abound here as in other areas. Menorrhagia is heavy periods. Metrorrhagia is uterine bleeding but not at menstruation. Epimenorrhoea is a shortened menstrual cycle.

lead to mental and emotional disturbances. If a hysterectomy is performed for heavy bleeding, the woman will feel somewhat better after the operation since the cause of the blood loss has been removed. However, this may well turn out to be a short-term effect as the energetic imbalance at a deeper level remains. The practice of hysterectomy is another aspect of the general treatment of women by a male gynaecological profession and these issues are discussed fully at the beginning of this Chapter.

     A more recent technique is that of endometrial ablation. In the UK there are between 8000 and 12000 performed each year. A tube is inserted into the uterus and an electrically heated loop or laser is used to burn the endometrium. A general anaesthetic is necessary but women stay in hospital for only one or two days. There is concern about the risks of such a procedure particularly as it may be performed by inexperienced surgeons. At least four women have died as a result of the operation[8].

PRE-MENOPAUSAL CASES

Around the time of the menopause, ovulation and thence progesterone production ceases. For a time, oestrogens are still produced. Their unopposed action may overstimulate the endometrium leading to irregular or heavy periods. This is usually short-lasting although blood loss can be severe at this time. The main issue conventionally is that cancer of the body of the uterus becomes more common at this age. Dilatation and curettage is used to investigate such cases. In the absence of cancer, the use of hysterectomy is relatively common in an attempt to merely remove the symptoms. Hormone replacement therapy is a common prescription at this time.

Investigations:

Most cases are treated with investigation on the assumption that a 'hormonal imbalance' is the cause. Routine investigations which may be performed are:

- full blood count - to check for anaemia
- hormone level estimations - pituitary hormones, oestrogen, progesterone
- dilatation and curettage - particularly around the time of the menopause (this is an example of investigation and treatment combined)

Alternative management:

The four main situations of vaginal bleeding which may indicate a serious underlying condition are:

- pre-pubertal bleeding
- inter-menstrual bleeding
- post-coital bleeding
- post-menopausal bleeding

     Pre-pubertal bleeding is rare and, in these days of increased awareness of child sexual abuse, this must always be considered first as a possibility.

     Inter-menstrual bleeding is relatively common and may be part of the supposed hormonal imbalance and so included in the category of dysfunctional uterine bleeding listed above. I would refer you to the details of each in the relevant sections. Usually, if inter-menstrual bleeding is persistent or recurrent, investigation will be performed to exclude structural diseases. These include examination of the cervix, cervical smear, dilatation and curettage.

     Bleeding after the menopause (post-menopausal bleeding), is relatively uncommon and may arise from the uterus, cervix, vagina or vulva. At this age, cancer is a more common diagnosis and this is always the underlying physical problem which conventional practitioners seek to exclude. Inflammation is relatively common since the reduction in oestrogen secretion leads, in some cases, to marked degeneration of the mucous membranes and the endometrium. Inflammation may develop in these areas as a consequence. Investigation of this age group is similar to that described above for abnormal bleeding during the reproductive years.

---

[8] New Scientist, 7 November 1992.

In terms of Chinese medicine, there are three main syndromes associated with menstrual disturbances. These are Heat in the Blood leading to reckless bleeding, injury to the Chong and Ren channels and Deficiency of Qi not able to hold blood in the circulation. The actual pattern of symptoms and associated symptoms can lead to a differentiation between these three conditions.

Patterns due to Heat are usually associated with early menstruation, excessive menstruation of a bright red nature and perhaps symptoms of general heat in the body such as constipation, restlessness and anxiety.

Deficiency of Qi may lead to difficulty holding Blood in the circulation. It is usually associated with pale menstrual loss which can on occasion be heavy. There may be flooding. Spotting is common and there may be associated symptoms of Qi deficiency such as tiredness, pallor, poor appetite, diarrhoea, and uterine prolapse.

It is important to bear in mind that a more serious situation may be present in some cases. This is more likely with symptoms which occur with older women or if the symptoms are persistent or recurrent. In these cases, it is important to consider that the underlying physical abnormality may be serious and that further investigation may be warranted. This is something that needs to be raised with women that you are treating. I would refer you to the comments made in Chapter 6 - Cancer which are relevant here.

EXTRA-UTERINE PREGNANCY (ECTOPIC PREGNANCY)

This is the presence of a fertilised egg in a site other than the endometrium of the uterus, usually a fallopian tube. The cause in conventional medicine is not well understood except to say that the passage of the fertilised egg is clearly delayed along the fallopian tube. The two main situations which are associated are the use of the intra-uterine contraceptive device and pelvic inflammatory disease. The ovum embeds in the wall of the fallopian tube and starts to develop. There is no endometrium here and the thin wall of the tube is eventually eroded and ruptured by the developing embryo.

Symptoms:

There is a late menstrual period of between 6-8 weeks and there may be a positive pregnancy test or symptoms of early pregnancy. The woman presents with lower abdominal pain and the loss of dark blood from the uterus. This may be mistaken for a late period and further confusion may result from negative pregnancy tests[9]. It is important to have a high awareness of the possibility of such a condition in women where pregnancy is a possibility. Eventually the bleeding continues with increasing lower abdominal pain. There is then rupture of the fallopian tube with death of the embryo and possible death of the mother.

Complications:

COMPLICATIONS	SYMPTOMS TO LOOK FOR
Rupture of fallopian tube into abdominal cavity	Severe lower abdominal pain, guarding, rigidity, immobility, low blood pressure, rapid pulse, sweating, pallor
Miscarriage - rupture into lumen of fallopian tube	Lower abdominal pain but less than the above. Uterine blood loss, pallor, slight fever. There may be retention of urine

TABLE 18.8: COMPLICATIONS OF ECTOPIC PREGNANCY

Treatment:

It is important to recognise that unless the embryo dies before rupture the only treatment which is possible is surgical removal. This condition is considered to be a gynaecological emergency as rupture may lead to death of the mother due to massive blood loss. The embryo and fallopian tube on the affected side are removed. Ectopic pregnancy is more likely after any surgery to the pelvis so a subsequent ectopic pregnancy is a possibility. Ultrasound is helpful in diagnosis.

---

[9] A negative test does not, of course, mean that pregnancy does not exist

Alternative management:

This is a condition where surgical treatment is inevitable and there must be no delay in instituting it. Alternative medicine will centre on treatment after the necessary surgery has been performed. Blood loss may occur unless diagnosis is made early and so anaemia will be seen. Also, loss of a baby has taken place and issues around bereavement need to addressed. The after-care of such a case is described on Page 129.

- OVARIAN CYST -

A cyst is an example of a tumour. It is defined as an abnormal sac or closed cavity lined with epithelium and filled with liquid or semisolid matter[10]. There are many different types but essentially the distinction is made, conventionally, between benign and malignant. Ovarian cysts are not particularly common but occasionally women seek treatment in the alternative medicine clinic.

The symptoms depend upon the size of the cyst and whether or not it secretes hormones.

Symptoms:

Frequently, cysts are symptomless and only found on examination for some other reason.

Cysts which produce oestrogens may become evident through abnormal uterine bleeding. There may be postmenopausal bleeding, amenorrhoea or irregular bleeding.

Cysts which become markedly enlarged produce symptoms due to pressure within the pelvis. Abdominal swelling is the first thing to be noticed and eventually abdominal discomfort. Frequency of urination and even retention may develop with large cysts.

Pain can also be experienced with relatively small cysts due to the underlying energetic diagnosis which is described below.

A specific situation is that of Stein-Leventhal syndrome. This is the development of amenorrhoea with hairiness on the face. There are multiple cysts on both ovaries (polycystic ovaries). Treatment for this condition is by means of clomiphene or gonadotrophins. I have known some women to be given the oral contraceptive for this syndrome.

Investigations:

Ultrasound scans and laparoscopy are commonly used to diagnose ovarian cysts.

Treatment:

All cysts larger than 5 cm in diameter tend to be surgically removed. This is because of the possibility of malignancy. The whole ovary is usually removed. A small section of the ovary may be left if the cyst is benign. In women over 45 years, both ovaries may be removed if there is any evidence of abnormality in them.

In the case of malignancy, the ovaries, uterus and fallopian tubes are removed. Radiotherapy and chemotherapy are routinely used afterwards. Cisplatin, based upon platinum, is commonly given as a form of chemotherapy. It has many toxic side-effects but is an example of conventional medicine stumbling across the appropriate energetic remedy by chance. Platinum, in its homoeopathic provings, produces ovarian tumours. The difficulty in conventional medicine is that high doses are used leading to toxicity.

Alternative management:

In terms of Chinese medicine, ovarian cysts usually correspond to Stagnation of Qi and/or Blood. They are relatively easy to treat at an early stage where they are usually Stagnation of Qi. You need to bear in mind the underlying cause of the Stagnation in your diagnosis and treatment plan. The case is more difficult when Stagnation of Blood is apparent. It is valid to treat by means of alternative

---

[10] "Concise Medical Dictionary" (Oxford Medical Publications, 1980).

medicine and monitor progress of the cyst by means of ultrasound scans every 6 months. There is not likely to be much change in the size of the cyst in a shorter time.

Women with such syndromes may have evidence of other Stagnations in the body such as breast lumps, premenstrual syndrome symptoms and so forth. There may also be factors in the medical history which indicate the cause of such Stagnations. Common ones include emotional stress and frustration, surgery to the pelvic area particularly termination of pregnancy and the use of female sex hormones such as the oral contraceptive and treatments for infertility.

- FIBROIDS -

These are an example of a benign tumour and are known as fibromyomas. The cause of their development is unknown in conventional medicine. They are unusual before the age of 30 years and do not begin to develop after the menopause. They are commoner in women who had not had children.

Symptoms:

Most fibroids are symptomless and may only be found at routine examination, operation or post-mortem.

Heavy menstrual bleeding is the classical symptom associated with fibroids. The period is prolonged and the cycle may be shortened. Pain is unusual with the fibroid itself although the heaviness of the menstruation may be associated with discomfort.

Large fibroids may be felt on abdominal examination. Smaller tumours are detected by vaginal examination.

Investigations:

Ultrasound scan will reveal the presence of fibroids.

Treatment:

Small, symptomless fibroids are not treated conventionally. Large ones are removed surgically by means of hysterectomy. Occasionally, a myomectomy is performed where the fibroid alone is removed from the wall of the uterus. This is to be favoured in those women who wish to have children. Fibroids may recur later.

Alternative management:

In terms of Chinese medicine, fibroids usually correspond to Stagnation of DampPhlegm, Qi or Blood. The causes are considered to be emotional stagnation, overconsumption of dairy products, sexual intercourse at too early an age[11] and emotional imbalance especially in the teenage years.

---

[11] In Chinese medical thought this is considered to be before the energies are mature at around the age of 18 years.

- CANCER OF THE UTERUS -

There are two types as the uterus has a body and cervix (neck). They differ in their symptoms and age of commonest presentation and so are considered separately.

CANCER OF THE BODY OF THE UTERUS

This is not common before the menopausal period. The main incidence is between the ages of 50 and 65. It occurs more often in women who have had no children. There is no evidence that fibroids predispose to cancer. The cancer spreads locally through the wall of the uterus and there is frequently involvement of ovaries and other organs at the time of diagnosis. Cancers of this type spread locally within the pelvis via lymphatics.

Symptoms:

The classical appearance is of post-menopausal bleeding. At first, this may be fairly non-descript and infrequent but becomes commoner and heavier with time. Eventually the haemorrhage can be severe. If the woman is still pre-menopausal then intermenstrual bleeding is seen. Pain is late and signifies advanced disease.

Diagnosis:

This is confirmed by dilatation of the cervix and curettage of the endometrium (D & C).

Treatment:

The main treatment, if the cancer has not spread too far, is by surgery. The usual operation is hysterectomy with oophorectomy and removal of lymph glands within the pelvis. There may be a post-operative course of hormonal treatment with progesterone. The latter may be the only treatment given in cases not suitable for surgery.

     Radiotherapy may also be applied if surgery is not possible. The five year survival rate is 60%.

Alternative management:

The main issue for an alternative practitioner is to recognise the importance of post-menopausal bleeding as an early symptom of cancer. In terms of treatment, I would refer to the comments made in Chapter 6 - Cancer.

CANCER OF THE CERVIX OF THE UTERUS

This disease provides a classical example of the principle of staging by the conventional profession. Conventional thought is that the cells on the outside surface of the cervix begin a change towards abnormality which eventually may become malignant after several years. Each stage that the cells pass through is designated a number. The classification currently used is CIN[12] 1 to 3 - cervical intraepithelial neoplasia - otherwise known as dysplasia. Their meaning is shown in Table 18.9.

---

[12] This is pronounced 'sin' which reflects Western philosophical views of the origin of women and their symptoms.

CERVICAL INTRAEPITHELIAL DYSPLASIA	MEANING
1	Mild dysplasia
2	Moderate dysplasia
3	Severe dysplasia. May be sufficiently abnormal to be labelled 'carcinoma-in-situ[13]'.

TABLE 18.9: CONVENTIONAL CLASSIFICATION OF CELL CHANGES ON THE CERVIX (CERVICAL DYSPLASIA)

The condition of the cervix is discovered by means of a cervical smear. This is recommended to be performed every three years or so. This is the vital prerequisite to future conventional management and treatment. The current belief is that these stages lead onto each other in a progressive way and so treatment at the earlier points will stop development.

The commonest age at presentation with cancer of the cervix is between 40 and 50 years. However, increasing numbers are seen in younger women. 95% of women have had children. There is a relationship with the frequency of intercourse and number of partners. It is rare in nuns and commoner in women who have had intercourse from a relatively early age and with different partners. It is suspected that there may be a male factor as it is very rare in Jewish women - Jewish men of course are invariably circumcised. The virus of genital herpes is associated with the cancer although the significance of this is not known.

The cancer spreads by various means. These include local spread to vagina and uterus, by the lymphatic system to the glands of the pelvis, by blood spread late in the disease and by implantation of malignant cells further down the vagina.

Conventionally, there is held to be a need for routine cervical smears every three years or so although this time span keeps changing. Some women have a normal smear and then quite advanced disease one or two years later. It was always considered that there was at least 5 years between each stage so making the development of actual carcinoma about 25 years. This now seems to be very much an overestimate.

Symptoms:

Once ulceration of the cervix has occurred there is slight irregular bleeding especially on examination or intercourse and diagnosis can be made at this stage by examination or earlier by cervical smears. Pain is a late symptom and is due to spread of infection or to extensive spread of the growth.

Treatment:

The main aim of conventional treatment is to remove abnormal cells and so surgery is the considered choice. For cancer itself, the preferred operation is hysterectomy with removal of ovaries. Radiotherapy may be used with the insertion of radioactive rods into the cervical canal and the upper vagina.

In the case of dysplasia, treatment depends upon the particular stage and the preferences of the gynaecologist. There are wide varieties of approach. Generally, Stages 1 and 2 may be left alone and checked every 3 months. For some women with Stage 1 and signs of inflammation, antibiotics may be given on the assumption that bacterial infection is present. Stages 3 and above are treated surgically. This is either with lasers to remove the affected surface cells or by means of cone biopsy.

Laser treatment is performed in the out-patient clinic with no anaesthesia. The conventional belief is that the cervix has no pain sensation. This is not the experience of women who undergo these procedures. Any such treatment to the cervix is decidedly painful and certainly traumatic. Such expressions of discomfort are not dealt with seriously in most cases. Bleeding after such procedures and longer term menstrual irregularities are common.

Cone biopsy is, as its name suggests, the removal of a cone of tissue from the cervix. It is performed under general anaesthesia. This necessitates a stay in hospital of several days. Long-term problems include menstrual abnormalities and a weakened cervix which may make miscarriage more likely.

---

[13] There are many stages of cell abnormality before actual cancer may be diagnosed. Carcinoma-in-situ means that the cells have the appearance of cancer but stay in place and do not spread.

Alternative management:

One important consideration is to separate the issues of cancer and of dysplasia. Dysplasia is not necessarily cancer and does not mean that cancer is an inevitable result. Women are frightened by the whole process and words like 'cancer smear', 'smear' and 'abnormal cells' only serve to magnify this. Reassurance is helpful along with help in dealing with their current state of health.

In terms of Chinese medicine the abnormalities detected at the surface of the cervix usually correspond to Stagnation of Qi or a combination of Stagnant Qi and Blood, according to the stage of diagnosis. Alternative medicine is successful in treating stages 1 and 2 and smears return to normal usually in 3 to 6 months. Later stages can also be treated but it takes longer for the smear to show improvement. Certainly, the more abnormal the stage, the more severe the imbalance in the immune system. I would again refer you to Chapter 6 - Cancer, particularly with regard to the section on alternative management.

- PRE-MENSTRUAL SYNDROME -

This is extremely common and affects women at any age during their menstrual life. It means many different things to different people. It has only been in recent years that the conventional profession has largely accepted its existence.

Symptoms:

There are several symptom pictures and different women may have a different clinical picture. The symptoms tend to get worse before the period for a variable amount of time which in severe cases could be from the onset of ovulation. It is more common about a week to ten days before menstruation.

Emotional symptoms include irritability and depression. In severe cases, there may be personality changes which can include aggressive behaviour. Physical symptoms include breast discomfort, headaches, weight gain, desire for sweet food and lower abdominal discomfort. Lower back pain may also be a feature. Some women gain immediate relief when the period starts. With others, the symptoms gradually diminish over the course of the first two days or so of the period.

Treatment

TREATMENT	TREATMENT LEVEL	COMMENTS
Supplements such as Vitamin B_6, evening primrose oil	1	These may be suppressive in that symptoms return when they are stopped. They may not remedy the underlying energetic imbalance.
Diuretics	2	These remove fluid retention but damage the kidneys if taken regularly.
Antidepressants, tranquillisers	3	These are completely inappropriate since they rapidly lead to addiction, remove the experience of women and maintain the myth that doctors can relieve uncomfortable feelings
Female sex hormones	4	This acts by suppressing hormonal function and the menstrual cycle. Paradoxically, in some women it may worsen the symptoms for reasons discussed later

TABLE 18.10: CONVENTIONAL TREATMENT OF PRE-MENSTRUAL SYNDROME

Alternative Management:

In Chinese medicine, this condition is usually associated with Liver Qi Stagnation. There may also be evidence of Spleen Qi Deficiency. It is important to consider two main aspects in dealing with women who have such symptoms.

Firstly, the Stagnation of Liver energy leads to depression, frustration, irritability, breast discomfort, headaches and so forth.. One of the main factors which may be involved with this is an irregular life style not in keeping with natural cycles. There is a 28 day menstrual cycle in health which is affected by the weather, climate, phases of the moon and so forth. Sadly, in our society, these influences are often dismissed as being non-existent. People tend to live each week in the same way despite changes in their physiology. In the case of pre-menstrual tension, I have found that advising women to pay attention to these cycles can go a long way to relieving the symptoms. It is as if the tension is a resistance to a lifestyle which may be out of harmony. The same things happen with men but it is not so obvious. Men do not find it so easy to be in touch with their emotions and there is not the clear evidence of menstruation which reveals the presence of these physiological cycles.

Secondly, diet is important because of Spleen Qi Deficiency. This is outlined in more detail in Chapter 13 - Gastrointestinal System.

- INFERTILITY -

Although this term is in common usage it is sometimes labelled subfertility or impaired fertility which perhaps does not have so many negative associations. It is defined as inability to conceive (or in the case of the man, to induce conception). It is becoming more common in the Western world with around 1 in 8 couples having difficulty conceiving.

There are many causes - both male and female. I will consider these together since you cannot isolate most cases. It is rare to find solely a male or a female problem. Despite this, in the vast majority of cases, around 95%, it is the woman alone who will be investigated and treated conventionally.

Male factors include impotence, premature ejaculation and abnormalities in the number or quality of sperm[14]. Impotence and premature ejaculation are described in Chapter 9 - Urinary System. Abnormal or few sperm are usually considered to be due to congenital factors, mumps, irradiation or poor general health. However, in the majority of cases of abnormal sperm count, there is no significant cause which may be determined. There is often an automatic assumption that a normal sperm count is equivalent to normality. Comments such as, "Your sperm count is like that of a Greek God" reveal more about the doctor's psyche than the particular case being dealt with. Frequently, conventional doctors give the cause of infertility as unknown and then list methods of treatment to be applied. The absence of logic here seems to escape them.

Female factors include lack of ovulation, blocked fallopian tubes, endometrial dysfunction and disease of the vagina or cervix. The same comments are true here about investigation because most are normal. Most women ovulate, have patent fallopian tubes and there is little or no sign of uterine dysfunction.

Conventional medicine divides cases into primary infertility where there have been no children and secondary where children have been born but now there is a difficulty in conception. In women who have had no children yet have had a miscarriage, this is still classed as primary infertility.

---

[14] The sperm count which is considered to be normal has fallen over the past 40 years. Formerly it was 60 million per ml and now is 20 million.

Symptoms:

Apart from the obvious lack of pregnancy there may be no abnormal signs or symptoms although clearly if there is an associated condition, this will be noted. This is the conventional view. When faced with people in real life, however, there are frequently symptoms such as menstrual irregularities and abnormal menstrual flow which are difficult to classify conventionally. This is because they do not fall into one or other of the gross disease labels.

Investigations:

Investigation of infertility is now quite complex. It certainly involves intricate technology as revealed by the development of recent techniques of in-vitro fertilisation. There are four basic investigations which are performed.

In the case of the male, a sperm count and estimation of their normality are done. This may not be done if it is a case of secondary infertility and the father of the previous children is still the current partner. This assumes a certain permanence of testicular function and it is always wise to have a recent seminal examination. Certain religious groups, e.g. orthodox Jews, may be prohibited from masturbating to produce a sample of sperm and so testing is done by means of a post-coital examination. The remaining investigations are all performed on the woman.

Ovulation can be checked in several ways. At ovulation there is a slight fall in body temperature and then a persistent rise. The basal body temperature in the second half of the cycle is 0.5°C higher than that in the first half of the cycle. This simple and effective method is less popular these days with gynaecologists and usually more invasive investigations are performed. Dilatation and curettage in the second half of the menstrual cycle obtains a sample of endometrium. Ovulation must have occurred if it has been affected by progesterone. Direct ovarian examination by laparoscope around ovulation may reveal the presence of an egg about to be released. Blood levels of progesterone taken in the second half of the cycle will determine the amount of progesterone secreted and are an indication whether ovulation has occurred.

Post coital tests are performed within a few hours of intercourse to check on the condition of sperm in the vagina. In some situations, sperm die off relatively quickly and cannot make it past the vagina through the cervix. This situation which is often known by the term 'hostile vagina' is relatively uncommon. The mere labelling in this way infers a certain sexist bias on the part of the gynaecologists. I have never seen the term 'wimpy sperm' used, for example.

Investigations are performed to ensure that the fallopian tubes are not blocked. There are two methods. Dye may be injected through the cervix at the time of laparoscopy to see whether it comes through the abdominal end of the fallopian tubes. Otherwise, hysterosalpingogram is performed which is the injection of radio-opaque dye through the cervix. No anaesthetic is used. Subsequent pelvic x-rays can also reveal the same. Neither of these investigations are infallible since mere spasm of the fallopian tube may prevent the passage of dye. Therefore, the failure of dye to pass does not necessarily mean scarring by pelvic inflammatory disease or other permanent situation. A hysterosalpingogram is clearly much less invasive than a laparoscopy although lower abdominal cramps are common after this procedure. Laparoscopy is described in detail in Chapter 4 - Investigations.

CHECK FOR -	INVESTIGATION	DEGREE OF INVASIVENESS[15]
Ovulation	Temperature chart	1
	Progesterone blood test	1 (more than above)
	Dilatation and curettage	3
	Laparoscopy	3
Sperm function	Sperm count	1
	Post-coital test	1 (more than above)
Fallopian tube blockage	Hysterosalpingogram	2
	Laparoscopy	3

TABLE 18.11: INVESTIGATION OF INFERTILITY

---

[15] These criteria are discussed in Chapter 4 - Investigaions.

QUESTION TO ASK	COMMENTS
Previous pregnancies	Pregnancy is possible. Sperm count, endometrium, fallopian tubes and ovulation satisfactory at least at that time. Check for subsequent changes in health.
Previous pelvic surgery[16], ectopic pregnancy, intra-uterine contraceptive device, pelvic inflammatory disease	Possibility of blocked fallopian tubes

TABLE 18.12: IMPORTANT QUESTIONS TO ASK IN CASES OF INFERTILITY

Treatment:

This may be given to women who fail to conceive although in the vast majority of cases there is little evidence of abnormality. This is one of the reasons why treatment failures are so common since it is difficult to treat rationally if the causes are unknown.

A specific abnormality such as lack of ovulation or reduced progesterone levels in the second half of the cycle is treated directly. Ovulation can be stimulated by drugs including clomiphene, tamoxifen and pituitary hormones to stimulate the ovary. These are powerful agents which force the ovary to produce several eggs at once. One side-effect is multiple pregnancy. All drugs which are used to alter hormonal balances may have devastating psychological effects. Lack of libido is common. Anxiety and depression are almost universal. It is true to say that these are rarely addressed conventionally and are an added factor to deal with by alternative practitioners.

Progesterone may be given in the second half of the cycle if there is evidence of deficiency. A similar situation may occur here as with dysfunctional uterine bleeding. That is, progesterone may be given with normal hormone estimations just because it can be considered to be 'a good thing'.

Blockage of the fallopian tubes by scar tissue after ectopic pregnancy, pelvic inflammatory disease and so on may be corrected surgically. The success rate is relatively low.

Artificial insemination has been available for several decades and this may be done using either the sperm of the sexual partner or a donor. This procedure is the exchange of body fluids and carries a risk of infection such as hepatitis or HIV. There are also ethical issues in the case of artificial insemination by donor since the child invariably is unaware of their biological father.

The procedure which has received much attention recently is that of in-vitro fertilisation (IVF). This is bringing the egg and sperm together in a test tube, allowing fertilisation to take place and at some later stage implanting the embryo into the uterus. It is an expensive procedure costing £2000 per treatment cycle, i.e. per month of treatment. It has attracted attention far out of proportion to its success rate. It involves the stimulation of ovulation since several eggs are removed and fertilised. A number, depending upon the clinic, is placed into a fallopian tube. Progesterone supplements may be given in an attempt to maintain the pregnancy. Several fertilised eggs may be held in reserve for later insertion. These embryos are stored in cold conditions awaiting later use.

The overall success rate of in-vitro fertilisation, in terms of how many women leave the programme with a live baby, is variable. Overall, it is in the order of around 10%, with some centres having a lower success rate and some as high as 30%. There is an increased risk of foetal abnormality, miscarriage and stillbirth. In-vitro fertilisation is merely the first stage in a whole series of invasive medical techniques throughout pregnancy. Since several embryos are implanted together, multiple pregnancy is a risk.

Clearly this whole area raises ethical and moral issues, very few of which are addressed by the medical profession. In my experience, most of these are actively dismissed. It certainly is important for couples with religious or moral beliefs, particularly Catholics and Buddhists, who believe that life begins at conception. Medical practices such as multiple fertilisation, freezing of embryos, medical experimentation on embryos and selective termination of implanted embryos are viewed as unacceptable. This is an increasingly important issue in medicine as more people are offered such treatments.

A new procedure is known as gamete intra-fallopian transfer (GIFT). This is the placing of an egg and sperm into the fallopian tube without prior fertilisation in the hope that getting them

---

[16] Pelvic surgery is any surgery to the lower abdomen and pelvis. It would include appendicectomy.

together in the same place will aid conception. It is difficult to see why this should be any more successful than the normal procedure of attempted conception. A possible practical reason for this would be if the fallopian tubes are obstructed and the sperm cannot physically actually contact the egg. It is less expensive than in-vitro fertilisation but hardly more successful.

As medical techniques advance, seemingly more and more bizarre treatments will be developed. The latest to appear is the idea that ovaries from aborted foetuses can be matured and these eggs used to create embryos. It is only possible to guess at the subtle psychological and energetic consequences of this action. This is not just a case of children being born to biological mothers who have died but whose biological mothers were actively killed. It seems that medical scientists, none of whom learn or are taught morals or ethics as part of their training, find that whatever they can do they will do. This may be scientific curiosity. On the other hand it may be a desire for a reputation or large amounts of money. Whatever the underlying motivation, I have a very strong feeling we are treading a dangerous path. There seems to be not only a basic disrespect for life but also a frantic anxiety to produce a human being at any cost.

Alternative management:

In Chinese medicine, infertility is a complex issue. It is not made any easier by the great anxiety surrounding the problem or by the efforts of conventional medicine in attempting to obtain fertilisation. The usual conditions seen in women are Kidney Deficiency, Cold uterus, Blood Deficiency, Liver Qi Stagnation, Stagnant Heat and PhlegmDampness. Most cases are due to either Kidney Deficiency or Liver Qi Stagnation.

It is important to consider the timing of intercourse which needs to be adjusted to the optimum moment. Ovulation conventionally always occurs 14 days before the menstrual period but in real life this is not so certain. I have known women who have regular 28 day cycles and consistently ovulate at around 11 days of their cycle. This is seen as being impossible conventionally. I treated a woman who always ovulated at 11 days, some 17 days before her period, but the hospital always insisted on artificial insemination at 14 days.

Constitutional treatment for both partners is the most beneficial course of action although it may be difficult to persuade a couple that the man may also require attention. Normal sperm counts may be taken by the man as indicating that there is no problem to be addressed. Certainly a joint approach is much more helpful since issues around fertility are joint ones.

Psychological factors are very important to bear in mind. I have treated several couples for infertility where the woman had a previous termination or miscarriage and there is clearly still some energetic blockage in the pelvis. Whilst this remains there is little possibility of another conception taking place. These issues need to be resolved perhaps with psychological counselling or support as well as whatever constitutional treatment is undertaken.

A case of infertility is described on Page 279.

- CONTRACEPTION -

This is the prevention of conception. Although, conventionally, methods such as oral contraception and the intra-uterine contraceptive device are included in this they mainly act by preventing implantation of the fertilised embryo. It would be more accurate, therefore, to describe them as abortifacients. This has moral implications for those who believe that life begins at conception

Those methods used are assessed according to failure rate which is expressed as the number of pregnancies per 100 women using the method for the year. In the case of oral contraception, this is 0.1, the intra-uterine device 2, diaphragm with spermicide 6, condom with spermicide 8 and spermicide foam 24.

Oral contraception has many side-effects although it seems to be one of the most effective ways of preventing pregnancy. It is as if the greater the effect in preventing pregnancy, then the more hazardous to the woman. Although the oral contraceptive in use today is known as the low dose pill, this is because of the comparison with the doses used in the 60's and 70's. It does not mean that there are few side-effects. I discuss the side-effects of contraception more fully with hormone replacement therapy since these chemicals are the same.

As an aside, I see many people who take a prescribed drug and tell me that they are taking a low dose of a particular chemical. It is important to remember that a low dose is not the same thing as a mild effect. Low doses of some chemicals can be very hazardous.

Oral contraception is either by means of a combined pill (oestrogen and progesterone) or the so-called mini pill (progesterone only). The use of the oral contraceptive is an attempt to prevent ovulation. The administration of female sex hormones will interfere with the negative feedback mechanism mentioned in Chapter 15 - Endocrine System. Ovarian function is suppressed and so ovulation does not occur. However, with oral contraceptives of recent years where dosages are much lower and certainly with the progesterone-only pill, ovulation does still occur in some cases. It may be that pregnancy is prevented not merely by the suppression of ovulation but usually by the prevention of implantation of the fertilised ovum. In the latter situation, oral contraception is as likely to be a method of termination as a method of contraception. It is difficult to know how many women still ovulate who use the oral contraceptive. It is almost certainly more common than generally realised.

The intra-uterine contraceptive device (the 'coil') is a metallic or plastic shape placed inside the uterine cavity. It acts as an irritant and prevents implantation of the fertilised embryo. Common complications include heavy periods, infection leading to pelvic inflammatory disease and ectopic pregnancy. It is more commonly used in women who have already had children.

Sterilisation is a permanent method of preventing pregnancy by surgical means. Few can be reversed although this may be attempted. In women, this means an abdominal operation under general anaesthetia of tying of the fallopian tubes (also known as tubal ligation). This necessitates a short stay in hospital and is clearly more invasive than any equivalent operation on the male. There is an association with heavy periods after this operation although this connection is rarely seen in conventional textbooks. A significant number of women will then go on to have treatment for heavy periods and some may require hysterectomy.

Vasectomy in men is tying of the sperm ducts. Psychological difficulties may manifest as loss of libido or impotence. There seems to be an association with an increased risk of other health problems[17]. Certainly in terms of Chinese medicine, the operation will lead to Stagnation of Liver Qi which can lead to tumours.

Barrier methods of contraception are relatively common since they carry less moral objections. The methods available are of vaginal diaphragm, condom and spermicidal foam. Barrier methods can be messy and certainly not as effective as oral contraception. However, with correct use I feel that the success rates are far higher than those quoted above which are conventional data. Local allergic reactions can occur.

---

[17] There is an increased risk of prostate cancer. Giovannucci E, et al JAMA. 1993; 269:873-877 and Giovannucci E, et al JAMA 1993;269:878-882.

Letters to the Journal later revealed the way in which conventional pracititioners dismiss data they do not agree with. "Concern about recent studies linking vasectomy and prostate cancer has been tempered by the absence of any clear biologic rationale for the association". Daniel W. Cramer, MD, ScD, Brigham and Women's Hospital, Boston, Mass.

The rhythm method and related methods[18] use information about natural cycles. They work best for those women who have regular menstrual cycles but can be used by anyone and there are teachers who will instruct couples in their correct application. They are of varying efficiency and clearly depend upon co-operation between the couple and abstinence from intercourse around ovulation.

Retention of semen by various practices is a useful method to consider. It is cheap, has no side-effects and 100% effective. It has to be taught by a qualfied teacher and belongs to the tradition which includes Qi Gong (or Chi Kung) and other Qi exercises[19].

- BREAST DISEASE -

Disorders of the female breast are common. Any woman who has lumps or discomfort in the breast is also worried about the risk of breast cancer. With anatomy and physiology, you should certainly know the normal lymphatic drainage of the breast. I would remind you that the lateral part of the breast drains to the axilla whilst the medial side drains internally. Therefore, enlarged lymph glands in the axilla may be due to lumps in the lateral half of the breast. This area of the lymphatic system also drains the pectoral region of the upper abdominal area and the upper back.

I spend much time and space here discussing breast disease. It is a useful illustration of the conventional approach to such diseases, the conflicting evidence which is available and the pressure exerted by conventional practitioners for people to undergo the accepted forms of treatment.

LUMP IN THE BREAST

This is a common condition and 95% of cases will either be cancer, a benign tumour such as fibroadenoma or chronic mastitis. I discuss each in turn below.

Any general observations about lumps can be related to the section on Page 81. Lumps (tumours) may be either benign or malignant. It is difficult in the early stages to determine, definitely, whether a lump is cancerous or not. This leads to great anxiety for doctors and for women. Emphasis is placed on detecting the presence of lumps which are malignant. This leads to screening programmes such as routine mammography. The consequence, for an individual woman, can be traumatic and stressful. This, in itself, can generate disease.

I would remind you of the comments I made in Chapter 6 - Cancer. The type of tumour a person has, the degree of its abnormality (and malignancy), its rate of growth and its propensity to spread are all a direct result of the condition of the person's immune system. They are not dependent upon time. The emphasis for any system of medicine which is curative, therefore, is on the immune system rather than the precise presenting symptom.

Sadly, conventional medicine is obsessed by lumps and their histological type. It directs its energies at removing the lump itself without addressing its cause. This approach has the effect of magnifying any anxiety. It depersonalises people's symptoms, denies inner processes and necessarily produces brutal and brutalising treatments to remove symptoms *at any price.*

In practical terms, it is possible to gain some idea about whether a lump is serious or not. Most lumps in the breast are found by self-examination or by accident. Ask questions about its size, shape, mobility, regularity and whether it is painful. Malignant lumps tend to be hard, irregular, fixed and non-tender but in the early stages are indistinguishable from benign ones. If the lump changes with the menstrual cycle, it is more likely to be benign. If it remains the same throughout the month, it is more suspicious of malignancy.

It may be possible for a sympathetic conventional practitioner experienced in palpating breast lumps to give an opinion without frightening the woman into a particular course of action. A mammogram may give another opinion about the nature of the lump. There are several reasons to be careful about mammography and its interpretation and these are discussed fully below.

Finally, all women with a breast lump have to make a decision about their course of action. There are many possibilities and some of them are covered later when I detail some case histories. Unfortunately, the conventional profession has little time for women who wish to discuss or pursue

---

[18] "Natural Birth Control" by Katia and Jonathan Drake (Thorson's, 1984).
[19] Reference to Mantak Chia

alternative methods and great pressure is placed on them. This can only make the situation worse as stress and tension serve to deplete the immune system further. Lumps in the breast, and certainly cancer, are treated as surgical emergencies. In my opinion, this is never the case and women can gather information over some weeks and months whilst formulating their decision. It is wise not to make decisions in a state of shock but this is what women are asked to do every day of the week by surgeons and oncologists. A time of appraisal is helpful and allows some calming of the situation. In my experience, this panic and urgency is a reflection of the fear which *doctors* experience rather than the fear which women experience. It is not usually therapeutic to decide upon a course of treatment because of the emotional state of the practitioner.

CANCER OF THE BREAST

This is common, leading to 10,000 deaths per year in England and Wales. It is rare in men and unusual before the age of 30 years. There seems to be a rapidly increasing incidence of breast cancer and this may be related to the widespread use over the past 30 years or so of female sexual hormones. Cancer spreads direct to the skin where it may cause dimpling and tethering. It spreads by the lymph system to glands in the axilla and by blood to the lung, liver and bone, as well as skin.

Cancer in older women in the US is 40% commoner than in the UK and this may reflect different rates of hormone replacement treatment (HRT). In the US, about half of women take HRT whilst it is around one in twenty in the UK. Breast cancer in England and Wales increased by 36.8% in the years 1962-84. There was a sharp increase in 25-54 years old. There was an increase of some 35-45% in the 1970's. It is clear from several sources, that the use of such hormones directly increases the risk of breast cancer. This connection is discussed later in this Chapter.

In the US today a woman has twice the chance of developing breast cancer than in the 1940. Breast cancer is the most common cancer in women living in the US, causing about 44,300 deaths in 1990.

Only 30% of breast cancer cases are now linked to identifiable causes and most of these have to do with diet or constitutional factors. There have been two recent studies, one from Israel and the other from Vermont, suggesting that women with breast cancer may have been exposed to more toxic chemicals than cancer-free controls. A common toxic chemical, of course, is the use of prescribed female sex hormones.

Symptoms:

There may only be a lump found, usually on bathing or self examination although it may be discovered by a medical practitioner at routine examination. There may be prickling sensations or occasionally breast pain which may pre-date the appearance of a lump.

Depending upon the extent of growth of the cancer there may be nipple retraction of recent history, fixation to overlying skin or fixation to an underlying muscle. As stated in Chapter 6 - Cancer, these types of lumps tend to be hard, fixed and irregular in nature. It is important to acknowledge that the early detection of a lump may find it at a stage where this has not yet occurred. Discharge from the nipple of blood-strained appearance may indicate cancer.

Investigations:

It is usually diagnosed by a combination of clinical examination and mammography and aspiration or biopsy. Mammography is an X-ray of the breast requiring it to be squashed between two X-ray plates. It is uncomfortable and requires exposure to significant amounts of radiation. This is an issue particularly for those women who have repeated examinations and screening.

It is interesting to note the historical (some would say hysterical) development of mammography services[20]. In 1973 the National Cancer Institute in the US and the American Cancer Society began a national screening programme. There was no evidence of benefit to screening women under the age of 50. All women aged over 35 years were encouraged to take part.

In 1973, John C. Bailar, III, M.D., then deputy associate director for cancer control in the National Cancer Institute, expressed concern that the inclusion of women under the age of 50 in the

---

[20] HealthFacts, June 1992 v17 n157 p5(1).

screening project could cause more cancers than were being detected. His concern was based on several factors. The breast has a known sensitivity to radiation's cancer-causing effect. There is a relatively high radiation dose used. The effect of radiation damage is cumulative. Mammography has a known inaccuracy in finding cancer in the denser breast tissue of younger women.

The Annals of Internal Medicine in 1976 published Dr. Bailar's analysis showing more risks than benefit to screening young women.

In 1977 the Health Research Group made a Freedom of Information Act request for the inspection reports from the 27 cancer centres participating in the screening project. Sixteen of the mammography machines were found to be exposing women to unacceptable levels of radiation.

In the same year there were reports in the US of 48 women whose tumours were mistakenly diagnosed as cancer as a result of the screening project. The cell types were re-examined read by an independent panel of pathologists which deemed them "not classified as cancer." Thirty of these women have already had a mastectomy.

In 1991 the National Cancer Institute issued a press release showing the breast cancer rate has risen steadily over the years. They stated that the rise is consistent with the increasing acceptance of mammography. It was noted at the same time that the incidence of cancer-in-situ[21] has increased three times in the last 10 years. Many conventional medical practitioners are doubtful that cancer-in-situ is true cancer but women are still treated with mastectomy.

Also in 1991, a US General Accounting Office report found *no* progress in reducing the rate of breast cancer deaths since the 'war on cancer' was begun some 20 years earlier. Despite this, women are continually told of the various percentage rates of success they can expect from mammography, surgery, chemotherapy and radiotherapy[22]. This an example of media and medical hyperbole and has no basis in reality. It is obvious to anyone with a knowledge of energetic medicine, that such conventional treatments can only cause more ill-health. Conventional statistics however are presented as a competition with the prizes only available to those who have conventional treatment.

The use of mammography is definitely helpful for women who have a breast lump. This may have been detected either by self-examination or by a medical practitioner. It can provide information about the likely pathological process but is not infallible. It should be used as one of several methods of assessment. It is, however, less invasive than biopsy or needle aspiration. Of course, any damage to the lump may lead to increased risk of spread. There is also the issue of traumatic and stressful investigations and their effect on the immune system. These are all things to be taken into account before deciding upon a course of action.

Mammography screening, particularly in those under the age of 50 years is not only wasteful[23] it is positively harmful. Only 15% of breast cancers arise in those under the age of 50 years. The widespread use of screening exposes these women to three times the number of biopsies[24] and investigations as older women[25].

Dr Shapiro of Johns Hopkins University, said on May 5,1992 that he had reviewed data from a controversial large Canadian study about to be published. This found that women in their 40's who had annual mammograms were *more* likely to die of breast cancer than those who had only physical examination.

---

[21] There are various stages of cancer which are dependent upon its 'aggressiveness'. Cancer-in-situ is a type which remains in its site and does not spread. This indicates that the immune system is relatively strong and can maintain the cancer in that local area.

[22] At a news conference a group of over scientists and physicians released a statement condemning the U.S. National Cancer Institute (NCI) for ignoring or trivializing evidence of how carcinogens in air, food, water and workplaces are major factors in the cancer epidemic in America.

In addition, Dr. Samuel Epstein, professor at the University of Illinois School of Public Health, presented data indicating significant cancer risks in mammograms and their lack of effectiveness for pre-menopausal women. He also accused the American College of Radiology (ACR) with misrepresenting data on mammography risks. Cancer Weekly, Feb 17, 1992 p2(4).

[23] "Women under 50 years of age may not benefit from mammographic screening for breast cancer, despite screening recommendations". Davis, Devra Lee; Love, Susan M. JAMA, Jan 12, 1994 v271 n2 p152(2).

[24] 90% of biopsies are not malignant and these women are subjected to the stress and worry of invasive investigations.

[25] The Journal of the American Medical Association, Jan 12, 1994 v271 n2 p152(2)

The Canadian researchers speculated that the squeezing of the breast in the mammography machine might force cancer cells from tiny tumours into the blood stream, speeding their spread. This is also the danger with biopsy of breast lumps. The traumatic injury to the breast may lead to increased risk of spread[26].

There are hazards from the use of radiation with one cancer caused per 25,000 mammograms. The difficulty is, of course, is that no individual woman can possibly foretell if they are going to be the susceptible one.

A mammography examination of both breasts exposes a woman to a dose of radiation 20 to 25 times greater than that of a typical chest x-ray. The American Cancer Society guidelines recommend a mammogram at age 35, followed by others once or twice each year between the ages of 40 to 50, and a yearly examination after age 50. If these guidelines were followed, a woman would be absorbing significant doses of radiation. The breast is considered to extremely sensitive to the effect of radiation. Before a mammogram, a 35 year old woman has a statistical risk of 1 in 4,999 of developing breast cancer. After mammography it increases to 1 in 660[27].

An international workshop in February 1993 indicated that for every 1000 women under 50 years of age screened with mammography, 700 would require some sort of diagnostic procedure to detect fewer than 15 tumours. Seven tumours would be missed completely.

Before a cancer is detectable by a mammogram, it has been present and growing in the breast for 8 to 10 years. Statistics show that up to one in four breast lumps may not even be detected on the X-ray film. Misdiagnosis of lumps may also occur, with an average of one in three benign conditions identified as malignant[28].

Current imaging technology may also not be the best method for young women because of the density of their breast tissue. It is a relatively new technique with the difficulties of interpreting any new method. The American Board of Radiology has included questions on mammography in the past three examinations only. In 1993, the US Congress passed the National Mammography Standards Quality Assurance Act following reports that over half of clinics and operators failed to meet minimal quality assurance standards. Another serious flaw in the use of mammography is the lack of proper training for those administering the tests. Only 20 states require that an X-ray operator be certified by the American Registry of Radiological Technologists, through a two year training program[29].

In many southern states of the US, less than a third of radiology centres complies with the American College of Radiology guidelines for safety and effectiveness. An assessment of screening films in one practice found that false images[30] accounted for more than half of cases recommended for biopsy[31].

It has been said about the mammography debate, "...if our society had been oriented towards finding out whether new technology is efficacious as soon as possible after its introduction there would not be much left to debate more than 30 years later...."[32].

The investigations carried out on a woman with a breast lump are shown in Table 18.13.

INVESTIGATION	DEGREE OF INVASIVENESS
Clinical examination	1
Mammography	2
Aspiration	2
Biopsy	3 (general anaesthesia)

TABLE 18.13: INVESTIGATION OF BREAST LUMPS

[26] Special Delivery, Summer 1992 v15 n3 p12(1).

[27] Special Delivery, Summer 1993 v16 n3 p11(1).

[28] Special Delivery, Summer 1993 v16 n3 p11(1).

[29] Special Delivery, Summer 1993 v16 n3 p11(1).

[30] These are known in medical parlance as 'imaginomas'.

[31] Gillian Newstead, MD, director of Breast Imaging, New York University Medical Center, August 6,1993.

[32] Chalmers TC. "Mammography after 30 years". Online J Curr Clin Trials. May 28, 1993.

Treatment[33] [34] [35]:

The majority of cases of breast cancer are treated by surgery, either of the lump at more progressive centres using the most recent conventional treatments or by mastectomy (removal of the breast). The mastectomy performed nowadays is usually a simple mastectomy where merely the breast and axillary lymphatic glands are removed. In previous years, operations such as a radical mastectomy and super-radical mastectomy were used which remove underlying muscle and even part of the rib. There has never been any difference in outcome between any of the surgical procedures so now conventional surgeons tend to take a more conservative approach[36]. Even in lumpectomy, some axillary lymph glands will be removed for examination. If cancer has spread to any of these, clearance of lymph glands from the axilla will be performed. This commonly leads to severe oedema of the arm.

Fortunately, the practice of frozen sections are becoming less favoured by surgeons. This is the situation where a woman goes to the operating theatre and the lump or part of it is removed. A 'frozen section' of this is sent for examination. If the result shows cancer, the surgeon would remove the breast and whatever lymph glands they considered necessary. The woman, therefore, would not know whether she would wake up from the anaesthetic with her breast removed.

Following surgery there may be radiotherapy and/or chemotherapy. The vast majority of women now are advised to have these in sequence. The use of radiotherapy and chemotherapy is detailed in Chapter 6 - Cancer. The side-effects of both can be extreme but particularly with chemotherapy[37] [38].

---

[33] Although annual mammograms improve the chances that breast cancer will be detected, early detection and treatment do not decrease the mortality rate for women under 50 years old.

The Canadian National Breast Screening Study tested 90,000 Canadian women, ages 40 to 59. The major finding of the first seven years of the study is that no reduction in mortality in the 40-49 age group can be attributed to mammography screening.

"There is no evidence, either from this study or other studies, that mammograms save lives in women under the age of 50," study chief Dr. Anthony Miller, chairman of the Department of Preventive Medicine at the University of Toronto, said.

More women from the mammogram group died of cancer after seven years. Cancer Weekly, Nov 23, 1992 p2(2).

[34] The National Cancer Institute in the US has spent more than $1 billion on breast cancer alone over the past two decades. According to their figures, 26.9 women out of every 100,000 died of breast cancer in 1973; by 1988, the number had grown to 27.5 per 100,000, and the trend seems to be heading upwards.

The National Cancer Institute has spent $22 billion in the past two decades with remarkably few results. Overall death rates from many common cancers remain stubbornly unchanged--or even higher than before the NCI much-advertised 'war on cancer'. Only a few years ago, NCI leaders were setting optimistic goals, such as aiming to reduce the cancer death rate within the next decade by 50%. Any targets have now been dropped from NCI literature. Marshall, E - Science, Dec 20, 1991 v254 n5039 p1719(2).

[35] The number of women diagnosed with breast cancer has risen steadily, and the death rate has remained virtually unchanged. A 15 year review of cases of breast cancer have revealed there is no benefit from early diagnosis or changing conventional treatment.

There were was a peak of breast cancers diagnosed in the U.S. in 1974. This was the year when the wives of the President of the US and his vice-president were both diagnosed. A large number of these were followed-up for 15 years but it shows no decline in the breast cancer death rate in the U.S. HealthFacts, Sept 1991 v16 n148 p3(2).

[36] In the last 40 years, there has been only slight improvement in breast cancer survival rates, according to a 1987 GAO report. At a 1980 cancer conference, George Crile, Jr., M.D., of the Cleveland Clinic, was asked to name the advances in breast cancer treatment. "The major advances in the treatment of breast cancer have actually been retreats," he responded. "Physicians are performing less aggressive surgical treatments and finding the survival rates unaltered or sometimes improved." HealthFacts, April 1990 v15 n131 p1(2).

[37] Many patients receiving cancer chemotherapy develop infections and/or ulcerations of the mouth. The combination of mouth ulceration and infection is not only distressing for the patient but can also be life-threatening. G.M. McCarthy, et al: Cancer Weekly, April 22, 1991 p5(2).

The standard conventional belief is that chemotherapy and radiotherapy improve survival rates. There is conflicting evidence for this[39] [40] [41] although women themselves will only be told one side of the story[42]. One clinical trial published in 1976 showed that combination chemotherapy benefited women with premenopausal breast cancer and evidence of spread to lymph nodes in the axilla. The findings drew rapid acceptance and, by the end of 1976, the percentage of women receiving chemotherapy for this type of breast cancer had almost doubled. Usage continued to increase steadily until 1982. By then, the survival rate should have reflected the benefit shown in the clinical trial but, in fact, no improvement was found. This was determined in a report by the US General Accounting Office.

Such treatment would be expected to increase death rates as they severely damage the immune system. There is some evidence to suggest that this is true[43].

---

[38] There is an increased frequency of second tumours, mainly leukaemias, in women treated with chemotherapy. Rosner F, et al: Am F Hematol 1978; 4: 151-72, Geller RB, et al: Cancer 1989; 64: 629-34 and Kaldor J Acta Oncol 1990; 29: 647-55. It may also lead to an increased frequency of cancer of the oesophagus - Cancer Weekly, March 11, 1991 p4(1).

[39] "The relative efficacies of cytotoxic chemotherapy regimens in the treatment of advanced breast cancer are generally assessed by comparing response rates achieved in randomized trials. Treatment ideally prolongs survival as well as achieving successful palliation. Trials rarely demonstrate a statistically significant survival advantage". Ebbs, S.R. et al, NCI Cancer Weekly, Feb 20, 1989 p16(1).

[40] A conference of cancer specialists in the US in 1990 failed to show that chemotherapy gives any benefit to women with breast cancer. HealthFacts, August 1990 v15 n135 p6(1).

They agreed that for most women the lumpectomy plus radiation therapy is preferable to mastectomy for early-stage cancer because it preserves the breast without jeopardizing a woman's chances of survival.

[41] Until 1988, either mastectomy or lumpectomy and radiation constituted the complete treatment for women with cancer confined to the breast. Despite such treatment about 30 percent of all such women will suffer a recurrence and die of their disease. The prescription of chemotherapy or hormone drugs for these women would mean that the vast majority will endure side effects without benefit.

For the past 15 years, postoperative chemotherapy has been used to treat premenopausal women with cancer that has spread to the lymph nodes by the time of diagnosis and treatment. There has never been a subsequent study performed, which makes the basic assumption questionable. A review of five studies was conducted There is now evidence that challenges the original conclusion that premenopausal women with affected lymph nodes should undergo chemotherapy. The authors suggest that the recommendation of chemotherapy as the standard treatment for these women should be seriously reconsidered and most probably be withdrawn. Mueller, C. et al: Annals of Surgery, Sept 1991 v214 n3 p206(7).

[42] Virtually all women with breast cancer will at least have some discussion with their physicians regarding the wisdom of taking chemotherapy or the anti-estrogen drug tamoxifen. Many have received inappropriate recommendations to undergo chemotherapy. See "Women and Cancer Conference" Healthfacts, December 1985.

[43] Although postoperative radiotherapy is widely used to reduce the rate of local recurrence after treatment for early breast cancer, no significant increase in rates of survival have been shown in those who undergo the procedure.

An overview (Cuzick et al., Cancer Treatment Report, 1987; 71:15-29) of 10 randomized trials studying surgery with radiotheraphy versus surgery alone showed radiotheraphy had no significant effect on survival up to 10 years after treatment. There was, however, a significantly increased mortality amongst those who had received radiotherapy by the time of 10 years after treatment.

A total of 1,376 of the women had simple mastectomies followed by post-operative radiotheraphy. Another 1,424 had simple mastectomies with no post-surgical irradiation.

The authors confirmed the Cuzick et al. finding that mortality increased slightly in the irradiated patients roughly a decade after treatment. They found that this was due to an excess of deaths from causes other than breast cancer The most frequent cause of excess mortality was due to other cancer and cardiac disease.

It is common for women to be given tamoxifen which blocks the effect of oestrogen. It was originally developed as a contraceptive but found to be unsatisfactory. The rationale of such treatment is that as the breast is under the influence of oestrogen the cancer may also be stimulated by oestrogen. Tamoxifen interferes with the effects of oestrogen and so the cancer will not be stimulated.

It is a very powerful drug although there has been no long-term follow-up to check for side-effects[44]. It is known to produce symptoms of tiredness, heat in the body, flushing and restless legs. It may also cause hepatitis[45] and pre-cancerous conditions of the uterus[46] [47]. It may also damage the eyes[48].

In terms of alternative medicine, it should be viewed as similar to chemotherapy as it has a heating effect in burning the Blood. More recently it has been suggested that it can be given to healthy women in an attempt to prevent the development of breast cancer. This is the pharmaceutical equivalent of prophylactic bilateral mastectomy to prevent breast cancer which has been used, particularly in the US, for some years.

Alternative management:

There are several categories of Chinese medical syndrome seen in connection with breast disease manifesting as lumps. The immediate cause of the symptoms is Liver Qi Stagnation. This is very much related to emotional states and common in the West. This may be particularly true around the menopause when women may have difficulties with being appreciated and society tends to undervalue women unless they are of child-bearing years. The conflicting emotions which can occur at this difficult phase in life as children grow up and leave may lead to such conditions.The underlying diagnosis may be Spleen Deficiency, Kidney Deficiency, Blood Deficiency, Liver Qi Stagnation affecting the Chong and Ren channels and Fire Flaring.

The general comments I made in Chapter 6 - Cancer are of relevance here. They outline the multiple approach to take with a specific treatment, counselling[49], dietary therapy and meditation or visualisation. I describe cases below as an illustration of the above discussion. A case is also described on Page 91.

In the total follow-up period (up to 1988) of the Cancer Research Campaign trial 65.9 percent (783/1376) of the irradiated group died, compared with 55.5 percent (791/1424) of the group allocated to a wait-and-see policy. Haybittle et al, NCI Cancer Weekly, July 24, 1989 p18(1).

[44] In one study, 75% of women taking tamoxifen were not told of the possibility of side-effects.

[45] It has been linked with the formation of liver cancer in animals and there is currently a fierce debate as to the risks or benefits of giving it to healthy women.

[46] The authors of a study recommended that routine periodic endometrial sampling is performed on all post-menopausal patients receiving tamoxifen. In those women receiving tamoxifen in this study who had examination of their endometrium, 100% had evidence of endometrial abnormality. Cohen, I et al, British Journal of Obstetrics and Gynecology, June 1993;100(6):567-570.

Women taking tamoxifen developed cancer of the body of the uterus at a rate of over 6 per thousand. Women on placebo developed no such cancers. This has implications for trials giving tamoxifen to healthy women. Cancer Researcher Weekly, March 28, 1994 p4(1).

[47] Women who had used tamoxifen for more than 2 years had more than twice the risk of endometrial cancer than those who had never taken the drug. Vanleeuwen, F.E.; et al: Cancer Researcher Weekly, March 28, 1994 p 23(1). Also see summary in American Family Physician, Feb 1, 1994 v49 n2.

[48] Low-dose tamoxifen treatment can induce ocular toxicity. Pavlidis, NA, et al: Cancer, June 15, 1992 v69 n12 p2961(4).

[49] Researchers at the Stanford University School of Medicine and the University of California, Berkeley, found that breast cancer patients survived an average of 18 months longer if they participated in a psychological support group.

"I was quite stunned, since it was so contrary to what we expected to find," says David Spiegel of Stanford. This comment reveals the stunning ignorance of conventional medicine.

The study reviewed 86 women whose breast cancer had spread to other parts of their bodies. Fifty of the women were given the opportunity to participate in a weekly support group for one year. Survival times of the two groups were compared ten years later, and the rate for women offered support was 36.6 months, compared to 18.9 months for the other women. NCI Cancer Weekly, May 22, 1989 p3(1).

CASE ONE

A woman of 28 years came for treatment who had developed a breast lump after administration of a homoeopathic remedy. This had also brought into consciousness traumatic emotional events from her childhood. The lump was over 4 cm in diameter and rubbery in consistency. This could, conceivably, have been cancer but she knew that she did not want conventional diagnosis or treatment. We discussed her options and she decided to treat the lump as if it were cancer. In this way there would be no harmful, invasive investigations or depleting treatments. Over the course of several months when she had some further homoeopathic treatment, the lump disappeared. She has remained well and continues in her efforts to resolve remaining psychological issues.

CASE TWO

A woman of 80 years came for treatment. She had been diagnosed as having a malignant breast lump after biopsy some 4 weeks previously. She was taking tamoxifen regularly. She was being followed-up at the hospital where they had suggested that she may need further surgery to remove the lump entirely.

She had few other symptoms and her general health was good. In the elderly, breast lumps are typically slow growing and can persist for years with little or no progression. I treated her with acupuncture and herbs after making a diagnosis of Yin Deficiency with Phlegm Stagnation.

She did feel generally better after some months of treatment and the lump reduced in size. Each visit to hospital would be accompanied by renewed comments about the risk of the lump enlarging, spreading or ulcerating. She had declined further surgery and sadly the hospital doctors attempted to frighten her into accepting their treatment. She has a strong spirit, however, and she continues to take herbs and has a long-standing Buddhist meditation practice.

Some 2 years later, she remains well, her lump is unchanged in size or shape and she has just had a long distance trip to see relatives and friends. Her quality of life is good and she is happy.

CASE THREE

A woman of 33 years had a lump in the breast removed which was diagnosed as cancer. She had some glands removed from her axilla which revealed two to be involved in cancer. She decided to undergo the full course of radiotherapy and chemotherapy but declined intravenous chemotherapy at the time of the operation.

She was concerned about possible conflict between alternative medicine and conventional treatment. Some people decide to have both treatments and it is important to support them so that any adverse effects are minimised. She started herbal treatment before the radiotherapy and chemotherapy so that she was as strong as possible. Her diagnosis in terms of Chinese medicine was Blood Deficiency.

She did surprising well with few side-effects of toxicity. The main problem was with generalised aches and pains in the muscles and lymphatic glands. This arose as her Blood became weakened by the effects of the conventional treatment.

She also received healing each week and practised visualisation. She had regular psychotherapy as the cancer had developed about 18 months after emotional traumas. She recognised the relationship between these and her illness and the fact they reflected certain underlying psychological patterns.

She continues to have 'maintenance' treatments each month or so and is generally healthy about 2 years after the initial diagnosis.

CHRONIC MASTITIS

This is equivalent to fibroadenosis and the cause is not known in conventional medicine.

Symptoms

There is a discrete lump (fibroadenoma) or general lumpiness in the breast with discomfort which is worse pre-menstrually. There may be a discharge from the nipple. It is important to check the axillary area for lymphatic gland enlargement since the differential diagnosis is with cancer. Some enlargement is common which tends to vary with the menstrual cycle. Conventional treatment is either to excise the specific lump or to merely observe the patient.

Alternative Management

In terms of Chinese medicine this condition is very much associated with Liver Qi Stagnation and the comments I made earlier with regard to emotional frustration are relevant here.

DISCHARGE FROM THE NIPPLE

There are a variety of possible discharges from the nipple. Bloody discharge means either cancer or chronic mastitis. Watery discharge is seen in early pregnancy and a yellowish or greenish discharge is due to chronic mastitis. Milky discharge is known as galactorrhoea and occurs in lactation and is a side-effect of some drugs.

PAIN IN THE BREAST

This is common and may be due to several conditions. It is usually benign in nature but may herald the development of breast cancer in the future.

In conventional medicine, there may be breast abscess, mastitis or cancer. Occasionally musculoskeletal disorders affecting the chest wall may be confused with pain in the breast.

- USE OF FEMALE SEX HORMONES -

The female sex hormones of oestrogen and progesterone are produced by the ovary. They have been utilised by conventional medicine for many years now. They suppress the function of the ovary and may be used to prevent pregnancy. Since they consequently suppress menstruation, they are used in the treatment of a wide range of menstrual disorders such as dysmenorrhoea, heavy menstruation, irregular menstruation and even amenorrhoea. They are commonly said to 'regulate the periods'. This is clearly not the case since they prevent menstruation[50]. Bleeding only occurs due to their withdrawal for seven days each month. Hence the term 'withdrawal bleeding' is a more accurate one.

They may also be used to increase oestrogen levels around the time of the menopause when they are normally falling. This is an attempt to alleviate symptoms sometimes associated with the menopausal period as well as preventing or delaying the onset of osteoporosis[51] [52]. This is a thinning

---

[50] The suppression of any discharge from the body may have serious implications for health. Homoeopathic repertories provide many remedies for the treatment of disease caused by such a suppression.

[51] The extreme focus of chemical medicine on issues such as the menopause and osteoporosis leads to increases in anxiety and fear. "The promotion of hormone replacement therapy and oestrogen replacement therapy for osteoporosis and heart disease treatment is premature and being applied too generally. Research shows these therapies have serious risks that may outweigh the benefits, especially for low-risk women, but patients are rarely given the risk-benefit analysis and high-risk groups are not targeted." Worcester, N. et al: Feminist Review, Summer 1992 n41 p1(26)

[52] A recent study suggested it may be best for women with intermediate decreases in bone density to follow an exercise-calcium regime. Exercise with oestrogen is better to be reserved for those with low

of bone which may lead to fractures of bones with little injury as they become weakened. It is more common after the menopause and it is thought to be partly due to a reduction in circulating oestrogen.

It is important to recognise, as I mentioned in the Introduction to this Chapter, that the male-oriented medical profession tends to see women as inherently imperfect. The menopause is considered to be an illustration of this. I have heard gynaecologists express the view that the female menopause is a design fault of God. The use of female sex hormones at this time, by implication, is the rectifying of this mistake. I do not know whether God thinks he or she is a doctor but I know that there can only be problems when doctors think they are God.

It is also important to recognise that the menopause is not a disease state. This is true of any normal physiological stage of life such as birth, puberty, pregnancy and even death. They do not, therefore, have to be 'treated' as such to prevent them or to medicalise them.

In this discussion, I shall concentrate on the use of oestrogen and progesterone for contraception and hormone replacement treatment. These are common situations which face you in the clinic.

In terms of Chinese medicine, the time of the menopause is when Blood and Yin Deficiency with Empty Heat symptoms may develop. These lead to hot flushes, sweating, emotional imbalances, palpitations and the like. The treatment principle is to nourish the Yin and root the Empty Heat. The use of female sex hormones at this time may change the symptoms but that does not mean they are nourishing.

The energetic qualities of these drugs may be deduced from the energetic changes which occur during pregnancy. These were described in Chapter 17 - Pregnancy and Childbirth. Essentially, the female sex hormones are Yin in nature. They are Cold, therefore. They have the effect of increasing Blood although I do not think this a tonifying effect. They draw on reserves of Jing from the Kidney to increase Yin and Blood to other organs, particularly the Heart and Liver. This results in cooling of the heat symptoms sometimes associated with the menopause and any degree of anxiety.

The problem with increasing Yin but no attempt made to support the Yang is that Stagnation is likely. This is why side-effects of such drugs lead to thrombosis[53], migraine headaches, high blood pressure, breast cancer[54][55][56][57][58][59][60][61][62][63][64][65][66], uterine cancer[67], increase in weight and so

---

bone density. Prince, RL; et al: The New England Journal of Medicine, Oct 24, 1991 v325 n17 p1189(7).

[53] The most serious of those include an increased risk of heart attack, stroke, or blood clots - all of which are relatively rare conditions in women of childbearing age. Consumer Reports, August 1989 v54 n8 p498(3).

[54] The connection between oestrogen, progesterone and breast cancer is hotly debated in conventional circles. It is often stated that there is little hard evidence of such a connection. This is despite the presence of numerous trials stating that such a causal relationship exists. See the footnotes below.

The following comment, however, is typical.

Dr. Bruce Stadel, Chief of the Epidemiology Branch at the U.S. Food and Drug Administration and a coauthor of a study looking at the link between female sex hormones and breast cancer "likens the recent findings to 'blips' on an otherwise clear radar screen". These 'blips' of course are women with severe life-threatening disease!

[55] An increase in risk of 1.8. Armstrong BK: Med J Aust 148:213-214,1988.

[56] Hunt K. et al: Br J Obstet Gynaecol 94:620-635,1987 showed an increase of 1.6. This was later confirmed - Hunt, K. et al: British Journal of Obstetrics and Gynecology, Dec 1990 v97 n12 p1080(7).

[57] Ewertz M: Int J Cancer 42:832-838,1988 showed an increased risk of 2.3.

[58] Brinton LA, et al: Br J Cancer 54:825-832,1986 gave an increased risk of 1.5.

[59] There is an increased risk following the long-term use of injectable hormones. Hulka BS, Chambless LE, Deubner DC, Am J Obstet Gynecol 143:638-644,1982.

[60] Two studies have shown an increase in the risk of breast cancer for women with the largest number of recorded prescriptions. Hoover R, Glass A, Finkle WD, et al: JNCI 67:815-820,1981 and Hiatt RA, et al: Cancer 54:139-144, 1984.

[61] Scientist finds new connection between oestrogen and cancer. Liehr, JG. :Cancer Researcher Weekly, April 11, 1994 p 13(2).

[62] An increased risk of 1.5. Brinton LA, et al, Cancer 47:2517-2522,1981.

[63] An increased risk of 1.4. Ross RK, et al, JAMA 243:1635-1639,1980.

[64] A doubling in risk. Hoover R, et al, N Engl J Med 295:401-405,1976.

on[68]. The extra Yin can swamp the Yang and lead to serious consequences. These will be more severe in those women who are already Yang Deficient. Yin Deficient women will feel better in the short term but as the drugs draw upon reserves of Yin within the Kidney, the long-term effects can only be harmful. It is an almost invariable finding that women who take female sex hormones have a deep and thready Kidney Yin pulse.

The flooding of the Heart with Yin may lead to heart attack. On an emotional level it may lead to the alleviation of anxiety or the development of depression. On a mental level, it tends to produce a state of euphoria. This may be extreme and lead to psychotic features. 'Steroid psychosis' is a well-recognised complication of all the drugs whose basic make-up is the steroid molecule[69]. More commonly, a general perception of well-being exists where the woman believes they are extremely well. This is particularly hazardous as their is a lack of awareness as to the damaging qualities of these drugs.

There are also other effects as the Yang is depleted. The main one is on the Spleen. Weight gain, oedema and desire for sweet foods are common as the digestive energy is damaged by the Cold nature of the female sex hormones.

The use of such drugs for contraception is because they suppress ovarian function and thereby ovulation. There is some evidence to suggest that ovulation may still occur in some women. Pregnancy may be avoided because the drugs prevent implantation. This would suggest that they may act as an abortifacient rather than a contraceptive.

Interestingly, mung bean powder is used in China as contraception. It is effective because it is Cold in nature and has an affinity for the Kidneys and lower parts of the body. It produces a Cold Uterus so that conception is impossible. It would seem that the oral contraceptive has its effect in a similar way. Essentially, it produces a state of infertility. This 'freezing' may continue after the oral contraceptive is stopped so that amenorrhoea and infertility are well-known effects for some time.

There are conventionally several contraindications to the use of female sex hormones. These are:

- liver disease
- severe heart or kidney disease
- history of thrombosis
- tumours of the uterus or breast
- undiagnosed abnormal vaginal bleeding
- otosclerosis[70]

---

[65] Since the 1980s, there have been reports of an increased risk of breast cancer in women who received hormone replacement therapy. Hulka, Barbara S., Ca-A Cancer Journal for Clinicians, Sept-Oct 1990 v40 n5 p289.

[66] A study by a group of Massachusetts researchers indicated that long-term oral contraceptive use may quadruple the risk of breast cancer in women below the age of 45. Miller, D.R. et al, NCI Cancer Weekly, March 6, 1989 p12(2).

[67] There is a strong association between cancer of the body of the uterus and prescribed female sex hormones. Smith DC, et al: N Engl J Med 293:1164-1167,1975 and Ziel HK, et al: NEJM 293:1167-1170, 1975.

[68] There is a detailed discussion of female sex hormone side-effects in "Prescribed Drugs and the Alternative Practitioner" by Dr S Gascoigne (Ashgrove, 1992).

[69] This can be deduced from the common root of proge*sterone*, oe*strogen* and testo*sterone*. They are derived from chole*sterol* and reveal the close relationship between these drugs, the liver and fat metabolism.

[70] There is fusion of the bones in the middle ear. It is rare in blacks and occurs to some extent in 10% of Caucasians. Only 0.5-1% will have symptoms. Females are twice as likely to be affected as men. Symptoms of impaired hearing which is progressive begins in late teens and early twenties. Surgical treatment is helpful with 85% having excellent results and some improvement in 14%. 1% after the operation are totally deaf. The administration of oestrogen causes rapid, irreversible worsening of otosclerosis.

In my opinion, no woman should be given female sex hormones without at least several checks being made. I would consider the minimum to be:

- no contraindications to their use
- annual checks must be made. These will include vaginal examination, blood pressure and breast examination
- pre-selection for the prevention of osteoporosis. Only about 25% of women will develop problems. These tend to be those who smoke, are thin and slightly-built.
- a full discussion of side-effects to take place before the consideration of treatment
- oestrogens must never be prescribed without progesterone because of the greatly increased risk of cancer of the uterus. Hysterectomy obviously removes this requirement.

What can we do as alternative practitioners? We have an important role to play in education as many women are simply not aware of the problems posed by such drugs. The prevalence of well-women clinics with mammography, cervical smears and advice about the menopause and contraception are too often connected with sponsorship by pharmaceutical companies which manufacture female sex hormones. A neutral source of information is of benefit to women who are interested in taking control of their health.

Alternative medicine has an important message for women at many stages of their lives. It provides the philosophical basis and effective tools with which to regain health and maintain vitality. In this way, women can have a real choice over whether they need to take prescribed chemicals.

- HOW TO RECOGNISE A SERIOUS CONDITION IN GYNAECOLOGY -

Gynaecological symptoms are common in our society and the symptoms listed below are extremely frequent. It is important to know how to recognise if a symptom arises from a serious situation. You can use Table 18.14 as a guide to refer to when faced with a person who has one or more of these symptoms. I do not mention disease labels in the column on the right as I would not expect you to be able to diagnose conventionally. Seriousness can be assessed merely by reference to symptom pictures. However, you will be able to recognise that there are clinical appearances which would be diagnosed as a particular disease. For example, if you look at vaginal bleeding and its seriousness, you will see that these are the appearances of diseases such as cancer of the uterus.

SYMPTOMS	WHEN TO WORRY
Post-menopausal bleeding	Always - unless taking HRT
Pre-pubertal bleeding	Always - consider sexual abuse
Inter-menstrual bleeding	Persistent particularly around the menopause
Post-coital bleeding[71]	Persistent
Heavy periods	Persistent, with pallor, tiredness

TABLE 18.14: HOW TO RECOGNISE SERIOUS CONDITIONS IN GYNAECOLOGY

---

[71] Do not forget that it takes two to indulge in sexual intercourse. I know of a woman who had several invasive investigations for post-coital bleeding only to discover later that her partner had blood-streaked semen.

- SUMMARY -

Gynaecological symptoms are common in Western society.

The medical treatment of women cannot be separated from the society in which it takes place.

Conventional treatment frequently exacerbates any imbalances.

As an alternative practitioner, you need to be aware of the original imbalance and any overlying mental, emotional or physical problems caused by conventional investigations and treatment.

The alternative medical treatment of gynaecological disorders is extremely effective.

Effective healing can only occur when the woman concerned can harmonise her inner energies. This is not dependent upon changes in the outer world but can be attained through inner processes.

19 CHILDREN'S HEALTH

OBJECTIVES:

At the end of this Chapter you will be able to:
State the normal milestones of development
Describe the conventional approach to the care of children
Explain the methods for raising a healthy child
List the common disorders of childhood and their clinical features
Describe the appropriate management of each by an alternative practitioner
State the symptoms which may indicate a serious condition in a child

- INTRODUCTION -

The treatment of children can be a complex affair and is more difficult than treating adults. In Chinese medicine, it is known as the 'treatment of mutes' since they may not be able to relate their symptoms. It is said that it is ten times easier to treat a man than a woman. It is ten times easier to treat a woman than an elderly person and it is ten times easier to treat an elderly person than a child.

Disorders may arise in childhood for several reasons. There may be a problem solely with the child leading to the development of symptoms. The manifestation in the child may be a reflection of their home environment and family relationships. In most cases, there is a combination of these two factors.

Problems are minimised in infancy and childhood when the mother's health is good. The care of the woman through pregnancy, delivery and the post-natal period has important effects on the health of the developing child. Disease can, as often as not, arise from medical interference. This is an added factor to take into account today. The monitoring of children through regular health checks is of benefit in detecting abnormality early. However, the indiscriminate use of medical techniques can be damaging. I am thinking here of vaccination and the widespread use of antibiotics.

In this Chapter, I concentrate on those disorders which are specific to childhood yet are not mentioned elsewhere.

- GROWTH AND DEVELOPMENT -

In conventional medical practice, it is common to use methods of assessing progress. In the UK, it is recommended that children are seen by a doctor at 6 weeks, 2½ to 3 years and 4½-5 years. Health visitors see the child at 7-8 months and 18 months. Measurements are taken of height and weight. Note is made of developmental progress. It is also an opportunity to discuss feeding and other issues. Sadly, it may be used as an opportunity to pressurise mothers into vaccination.

There are charts of 'normal' growth. They are used to check that increases in height are in line with a perceived norm. As with most measurements, they must only be used a guide as there are many variations in a healthy population. Allowance has to be made for the height of the parents, for example. Such measurements can only be one aspect of the whole case.

Milestones are the times at which most children have attained a certain stage of development. They are useful to know so that when you are faced with a child, you can have a good idea as to its progress. Table 19.1 is a list of the normal milestones of childhood.

AGE	MILESTONE
Birth	Normal heart rate 140 per minute
6 weeks	Normal heart rate 135 per minute Head control begins to develop Moves arms and legs like swimming Neonatal reflexes present Smiles, alert
4-8 weeks	Posterior fontanelle closes
4 months	Head control
6 months	First tooth
7-8 months	No head lag Sits alone for a few seconds Beginning to move around, usually by rolling Neonatal reflexes disappeared Steady and accurate reach of hand Secure grasping in palm of hand May be interested in objects which disappear from view Able to localise sound at ear level Tuneful babbling
8-9 months	Begins to crawl
10-18 months	Anterior fontanelle closes
12 months	Normal heart rate 115 per minute May begin to walk
18 months	Able to walk alone Balance momentarily on one leg Walk upstairs Crawls backward downstairs Accurate reaching for objects Mature voluntary reach and grasp No mouthing of toys and drooling No deliberate throwing of toys in a repetitive manner - gone by 15 months Tuneful jargon, occasionally two words together Drinking from a cup and using a spoon depend upon their degree of practice
2½-3 years	Runs well in straight line Goes up and downstairs two feet to a step Can jump and climb Hand preference but can use other hand for assistance

	Visual screening possible as child can cooperate with tester Understands pictures and plays meaningfully with objects Vocabulary of at least 200 words Sentences used in speech Persistent questions such as 'What?', 'Where?' and so on are common Can skilfully feed, wash and dress Most are dry in the day and some are dry at night
4½-5 years	Normal heart rate 100 per minute Motor skills can reveal a degree of 'clumsiness'. Only a problem if severe and accompanied by other symptoms Holds pencil maturely Can copy shapes Can draw people Audiogram testing of hearing possible[1] Speech is clear, fluent and easily understood Independent in feeding, washing, toileting
5 years	20 milk teeth
5-6 years	Permanent teeth begin to erupt
10 years	Normal heart rate 90 per minute
13-15 years	28 permanent teeth
25 years	Wisdom teeth

TABLE 19.1: MAJOR MILESTONES OF CHILDHOOD

In summary, there is regular checking of babies and children to ensure they match an expected norm of growth and development. At the same time, mass vaccination is used in the belief that infectious disease will be inhibited. Vaccination is fully discussed in Chapter 5 - Infectious Disease including the vaccination schedule in the UK for children.

- CONVENTIONAL MEDICINE AND THE TREATMENT OF CHILDREN -

Most diseases in childhood are dealt with by general practitioners. Further investigation and treatment is given in hospital for more severe or difficult problems. This only occurs in between 1 and 5% of consultations depending upon the type of general practice.

The general approach to such diseases follows the general pattern of conventional medicine in that the emphasis is on physical matters. There is some recognition that psychological factors play a part but the main treatments are physical in nature.

There is no recognition in conventional medicine of the connections between certain procedures and subsequent illness. Vaccination, for example, is considered to be safe and long-term consequences are not accepted. These were mentioned in Chapter 5 - Infectious Disease. They are referred to again below with Infantile Phlegmy.

The conditions with which children present to general practitioners in the UK are summarised in Table 19.2

---

[1] The proportion of children with speech problems has doubled in the last 6 years. This may possibly be due to excessive sound levels, e.g. TV, hi-fi. Hearing problems can occur very early with babies not responding to sound. This is of relevance in special care baby units or wards in hospitals where excessive noise may affect young babies.

REASON FOR CONSULTATION	PERCENTAGE
Respiratory disease	28
Non-specific symptoms	13
Infectious disease	11
Skin diseases	10
Preventive procedures (includes vaccination)	10
Accidents	10

TABLE 19.2: MAIN REASONS FOR CHILDREN PRESENTING TO GENERAL PRACTITIONERS[2]

There are three main areas for the general practitioner. They are the recognition and treatment of episodic illness, the diagnosis of rare yet serious disease[3], disease prevention[4] and dealing with the long-term consequences of chronic disease.

- HOW TO RAISE A HEALTHY CHILD -

It may be helpful to spend some time discussing how babies and children can be given the best opportunity for health. These ideas are obtained from Chinese medical sources[5] and may be at variance with much of what is normally considered to be healthy in the West. I can only say that the philosophical ideas of Chinese medicine have been attested over several thousand years. The views we often hear in the West constantly change with time and have consequences which may not be health giving.

Babies, in terms of Chinese medicine, are immature Yang and immature Yin. This means that they are vulnerable to influences which may affect such immaturity.

The immature Yang must be protected from the application of excessive coldness. Techniques in Chinese medicine such as clearing heat, and this is the effect of antibiotics, are injurious to the Qi and Yang. Treatment must usually be directed at supporting the Yin and Blood.

Attention must be paid to diet as described in Chapter 13 - Gastrointestinal System. Most illness in childhood is the result of unhealthy diet. The ingestion of cold food and of food which produces mucus is more hazardous in children before the Yang has stabilised. Fevers flare-up quickly in children because of this immaturity of the Fire aspect. The immaturity of the Yin means that children tend to produce fluid discharges such as mucus.

---

[2] Source "Child Health: A Textbook for the DCH" by Harvey and Kovar (Churchill and Livingstone, 1985).

[3] These are primarily meninogococcal meningitis, tuberculosis, diabetes mellitus and malaria.

[4] Vaccination and developmental screening.

Screening of the newborn is performed for phenylketonuria by means of heel-prick blood test. This is a rare disease where brain damage is the result of a congenital inability to metabolise certain proteins.

A simple clinical examination will detect congenital dislocation of the hip. Failure to spot it before the child walks may lead to severe hip problems in later life.

[5] There are several books which provide further information about children's health and Chinese medicine. "Treatment of Children by Acupuncture" by Julian Scott (Journal of Chinese Medicine, 1986), "Turtle Tail and Other Tender Mercies" by Bob Flaws (Blue Poppy Press, 1985). Information was also obtained from lecture notes of Chinese Herbal Medicine course of Tinh Thong Nguyen, London Academy of Oriental Medicine.

The classical book concerning children's health and medical treatment is "How to Raise a Healthy Child.... In Spite of Your Doctor" by Robert Mendelsohn (Contemporary Books, 1984).

Specific recommendations for infant feeding are shown in Table 19.3.

At birth use a decoction of licorice to clean the tongue. This helps the energy of the Stomach. The baby cries at birth because the Stomach Qi flares up. The baby may be quiet and relaxed if the birth is trouble-free and relaxed.

Breast feed if possible

Breast feed when relaxed

Do not breast feed directly after working hard or sexual intercourse

Begin solid food with soaking rice and toast it until swollen. Powder it and add to boiling water

Start mixed feeding at about 6 months and certainly not before 3 months. The baby will let you know when they want to start solids

Avoid raw foods including raw fruit

Well cooked grains and warmly cooked vegetables are the mainstay of a healthy diet

Do not introduce more than one new food per day and then allow the child to become accusomed to the new taste

Avoid junk food, processed food, tinned food

Avoid cold, greasy and excessively sweet tastes (this means sugar and foods which have sugar added)

TABLE 19.3: DIETARY RECOMMENDATIONS FOR CHILDHOOD

For babies, there is a serious health risk from pesticides in drinking water particularly if feeds are made up with tap water. The dosage taken by children is four times that taken by adults on a weight-for-weight basis[6].

General recommendations for the care of children are shown in Table 19.4.

Do not expose to extremes of cold or heat

Do not carry the child all the time - lack of contact with the earth leads to shyness and fear

Do not overdress when playing

Keep back and stomach warm to protect Stomach and Kidney energy

Keep hands and feet warm to protect Heart and Lung

Do not let child play with dangerous toys

Do not let child watch horror, violent or pornographic films

If feels hot at back of neck, remove some clothes or may get a fever the next day

Massage the child regularly

Pay attention to diet

Do not overbathe - once weekly is fine

Do not let children be exposed to adult stress or arguments

Give appropriate treatment only[7]

TABLE 19.4: GENERAL RECOMMENDATIONS FOR THE CARE OF CHILDREN

Regarding the treatment of specific conditions in children, it is important to remember the place of the child within the family. The symptoms may manifest because of an imbalance within the child but there may be a greater imbalance within the family. This may be a relatively minor disturbance or there may be severe difficulties. The psychological issues which are important in childhood have been addressed by several people. I would recommend several sources[8].

---

[6] Report by US National Research Council, 1993.

[7] It should be clear by now that I do not classify conventional medicine as "appropriate". It should be reserved for life-threatening disease.

[8] "Childhood and Society" by Erikson (Norton, 1963), "Families and How to Survive Them" by Skynner and Cleese (Methuen, 1983), "The Inner World of Childhood" by Frances G Wickes (Coventure, 1977), "Thou Shalt Not be Aware: Society's Betrayal of the Child" by Alice Miller and "For Your Own Good: Roots of Violence in Child Rearing" by Alice Miller.

Children usually respond well to treatment with alternative medicine as their energy is relatively strong. They generally have less emotional turmoil than adults. Chinese medicine, homoeopathy, cranial osteopathy and *tuina*[9] all have an important role to play in gaining and maintaining health in childhood.

- SPECIFIC DISORDERS OF CHILDHOOD -

Children may suffer from similar diseases to adults and these are discussed in their relevant sections of the book. For example, asthma and upper respiratory tract infections may be found in Chapter 8 - Respiratory System. Epilepsy is discussed in Chapter 14 - Central Nervous System. Glue ear and otitis media are found in Chapter 12 - Special Senses.

COT DEATH

This may also be known as sudden infant death syndrome. It is the sudden death of a baby usually occurring overnight whilst in its cot of an unidentifiable cause. It can occur from a few days of age up to 2 years. Most are between the ages of 2 and 4 months. Cot death is commoner if social conditions are poor and less likely if the baby is breast-fed.

On post-mortem examination, there may be evidence of an upper respiratory tract infection, pneumonia or gastroenteritis. In about a third of cases there are minimal signs of disease and some 10% of cot deaths have no abnormal post-mortem findings.

There may be symptoms immediately before the cot death and these include skin rashes, vomiting, diarrhoea, shortness of breath and coughing.

It is true to say that conventional medicine has little understanding of the mechanism of cot death. Recent advice has included lying the baby on its back following a study which suggested that this may lead to a reduction in deaths. Interestingly, in Chinese medicine the back is Yang (related to heaven) but in young babies it is Yin. It becomes Yang later. The front is Yang in babies. It would be healthier, therefore, for babies to be placed face down so that their Yang front faces the Yin of the Earth. The observations of the conventional study may be a result of greater attention.

There are two issues to consider when discussing cot death. The first is vaccination which usually begins at about 2 or 3 months of age. There is ample evidence to connect vaccination to minor symptoms such as skin rash, vomiting, diarrhoea, crying, irritability and upper respiratory tract symptoms. It may be that such a violent shock to an immature immune system can result in serious short-term problems.

The second issue is that of separation of the baby from its mother. In Western cultures, this may be done at a very early age. It is helpful to consider the benefit of the baby sleeping with the mother for many months so that early and forced separation are avoided. The Lungs are considered in Chinese medicine to be affected by loss and separation. It is easy to see how breathing may be affected by placing a baby of a few days or weeks old in a cot away from its mother[10].

---

[9] *Tuina* is a type of remedial massage originating from China. It is simple, safe and painless. It can be used to treat a wide range of disorders in children. See "Infantile Tuina Therapy" by Luan Changye (Foreign Languages Press, 1989), "Chinese Bodywork" Edited by Sun Chengnan (Pacific View Press, 1993) and "Chinese Massage and Acupressure" (Bergh, 1991).

[10] " Continuum Concept" by Jean Liedboff (Penguin, 1986 and Arkana, 1989) is an excellent discussion of separation in infancy, its consequences and the benefits of prolonged contact between mother and baby. Also see "Three in a Bed - Why you should sleep with your baby" by Deborah Jackson (Bloomsbury, 1990).

FAILURE TO THRIVE

There is no formally agreed definition of failure to thrive. It is a general term which is applied to those children who grow and develop at a slower rate than normal. It may be noticed when the child has routine monitoring of height and developmental milestones. General practitioners and health visitors are the people are most likely to diagnose such a situation.

Growth of the child is connected to many factors including family history and constitution. The size of the child must also be assessed considering their birth weight. Most children catch up with their peers and the length it takes to do so depends upon their original weight. In severe cases, the child may always be smaller than normal.

As a rule, if the child is happy and healthy there is nothing to worry about. If the child is small but miserable and unhealthy, further investigation may be necessary.

There are several causes of failure to thrive. The commonest include chronic digestive or bowel disturbances, low grade infection, poor nutrition and chronic illness, e.g. asthma.

FEBRILE CONVULSION

This is a convulsion which occurs between the ages of 6 months and 6 years in association with a fever. It is an arbitrary definition and excludes known causes of convulsions such as meningitis, encephalitis, brain damage or epilepsy. It occurs in up to 5% of all children.

The cause in conventional medicine is not known but the association with fever is essential. Fever due to any cause may precipitate the convulsion. Common situations, therefore, are upper respiratory tract and urinary infections. An attack is more likely if one or both parents had febrile convulsions as a child. The risk is increased by a factor of 50%. Boys are affected twice as often as girls.

The convulsion occurs because of the rate of rise in temperature as well as the height of the temperature. Of the two, however, the risk has lessened somewhat by the time the height of the fever has been reached.

Febrile convulsions often occur more than once. Half of affected children have more than one attack whilst 20% have four. Up to 10% of children go on to develop epilepsy later.

Symptoms:

There is a short lasting convulsion of the grand mal type. Occasionally it may last for 30 minutes. The child typically sleeps after the attack.

Treatment:

The main treatment, conventionally, is aimed at reducing the fever. This is by means of paracetamol as aspirin is prohibited for use in children. Undressing the child and tepid sponging may also be used.

Anticonvulsants are given if the convulsion is prolonged and if they are recurrent. An EEG may be performed before treatment. The duration of treatment varies from doctor to doctor. It is usually for at least a year after the last fit.

Most children grow up and have no further attacks and seem to be no worse for the experience. A minority continues to have problems and are then diagnosed as epileptic.

UNDESCENDED TESTIS

The testes are originally an abdominal organ and they descend into the scrotum at about the eighth month of pregnancy. About 3% of male babies have undescended testes. This figure rises to 21% in the case of premature births. Virtually all testes descend with the next nine months of life.

Symptoms:

The undescended testis cannot be felt in the scrotum. It is important to distinguish this from the situation of retraction which occurs in the cold and if nervous. Occasionally the testis may be congenitally absent.

Complications:

There are various complications of undescended testis. It is more likely to twist (torsion of the testis), has an increased risk of becoming malignant at some later stage (which surgery does not change) and fertility of the affected testis will be impaired. There may be cosmetic problems later as a result of only one testis in the scrotum (or none if both are undescended).

Treatment:

Surgical treatment is performed certainly before the age of five and perhaps around the first birthday. The testis is brought down and fixed into the scrotum.

Alternative management:

In terms of Chinese medicine, this a condition related to the function of the Liver as this channel crosses the external genitalia. It is treatable by means of alternative medicine and is certainly worth delaying any operation until there has been a fair trial of treatment. Certainly, surgery can easily be postponed until the age of 5 years with no risks.

INFANTILE PHLEGMY

This is a term from Chinese medicine and has no direct counterpart in conventional medicine. It is the appearance of mucus in the child which is frequently manifest as loose stools with mucus and runny nose. In severe cases, hearing may be affected and there may be specific symptoms in the upper respiratory tract such as sore throat and cough.

The cause is weak digestive energy which cannot transform food completely. This leads to the generation of mucus which passes up to the Lungs. The digestive energy tends to be weak in children already so avoidance of factors which cause further weakening is essential. Repeated vaccination and antibiotic use are the two medical procedures which commonly damage the digestion. Also take dietary habits and emotional stresses within the family into account. Symptoms may be manifest at times of other events such as teething.

Correct diet as described above is important. If simple measures such as dietary changes do not effect an improvement, consider the application of homoeopathic remedies, herbs or *tuina*.

COLIC

This is commonly seen in babies between the ages of 2 and 6 months. The baby begins to cry in the early evening and is frequently inconsolable. The duration of the crying is variable but may be for several hours. There may be difficulty getting off to sleep and repeated waking during the night.

In terms of Chinese medicine, there are two main syndromes which lead to colic. There may be Heat in the Heart of Spleen Qi Deficiency. Effective treatments exist in homoeopathy, herbal medicine and *tuina*.

Some mothers are advised to stop breast-feeding in the mistaken belief that the milk is of 'poor quality'. Switching to infant cow's milk formulas may lead to a lessening of symptoms but this is because cow's milk, particularly the pasteurised variety, is heavy and hard to digest. There is a degree of sedation as a consequence. The baby is also likely to develop Infantile Phlegmy.

- HOW TO RECOGNISE A SERIOUS CONDITION IN CHILDREN -

In Chinese medicine, there are two sayings about children which are relevant here[11]. 'Children get illness easily, illness quickly becomes serious.' 'Zang, qi, jing, ling (spirit) - easily ill, easily cured.' The dilemma for the practitioner is which category a particular child is at any given time.

The help of the mother is helpful here since she usually knows the child best and is aware of what is and what is not normal. You must remember that the mother is also probably anxious about the welfare of her child and this may colour her opinion. You neglect a mother's concern, though at your peril.

The essential issue about treating children is the importance of monitoring. See the child frequently, every day if necessary and maintain contact over the phone. This will provide reassurance for the family and allow you to know about the progress of symptoms more easily.

Individual symptoms are dealt with in their relevant section. An alphabetical list of all these is contained in Appendix Three.

- SUMMARY -

Symptoms in children are common due to their immature energies.

Most conditions in childhood are minor and self-limiting.

Know the symptoms which may indicate a serious underlying condition.

Symptoms in children can change rapidly. Regular checking and monitoring are valuable. It enables you to observe the case closely and is reassuring for the family.

---

[11] "The Treatment of Children by Acupuncture" by Julian Scott (Journal of Chinese Medicine, 1986).

APPENDICES

APPENDIX ONE

BIBLIOGRAPHY

TEXTBOOKS OF CHINESE MEDICINE

Acupuncture: A Comprehensive Text by Shanghai College of Traditional Medicine. Translated by O'Connor and Bensky (Eastland Press)
Between Heaven and Earth by Beinfield and Korngold (Ballantine)
Blue Poppy Essays by Bob Flaws et al, (Blue Poppy Press)
BodyMind Energetics by Mark Seem with Joan Kaplan (Thorson's)
Chinese System of Food Cures by Henry Lu (Sterling)
Dragon Rises, Red Bird Flies by Leon Hammer (Crucible)
Essentials of Traditional Chinese Paediatrics Compiled by Cao Jiming et al, (Foreign Languages Press)
The Foundations of Chinese Medicine by Giovanni Maciocia (Churchill Livingstone)
Fundamentals of Chinese Medicine by Wiseman, Ellis and Zmiewski (Paradigm)
A Handbook of Traditional Chinese Dermatology by Liang Jian-Hui. Translated by Zhang Ting-Liang and Bob Flaws (Blue Poppy Press)
Mental Dysfunction as treated by Traditional Chinese Medicine Compiled by Cheung et al, (American College of Traditional Chinese Medicine)
The Path of Pregnancy by Bob Flaws (Blue Poppy Press)
Prince Wen Hui's Cook: Chinese Dietary Therapy by Bob Flaws and Honora Wolfe (Paradigm)
Something Old, Something New by Bob Flaws (Blue Poppy Press)
Traditional Acupuncture: The Law of the Five Elements by Dianne Connelly (The Centre for Traditional The Treatment of Cancer by Integrated Chinese and Western Medicine by Zhang Dai-Zhao (Blue Poppy Press)
The Treatment of Children by Julian Scott (Journal of Chinese Medicine)
Turtle Tail and Other Tender Mercies by Bob Flaws (Blue Poppy Press)
The Web Which Has No Weaver by Ted Kaptchuk (Congdon and Weed)
The Yellow Emperor's Classic of Internal Medicine (known as the Neijing) Translation by Henry Lu
Zang Fu Syndromes by John McDonald (New South Wales College of Natural Therapies)

CONVENTIONAL MEDICAL TEXTBOOKS

Cecil's Textbook of Medicine, Editd by Wyngaarden and Smith (WB Saunders)
Clinical Medicine - Second Edition - Edited by Kumar and Clark (Baillière Tindall)
Concise Medical Dictionary (Oxford Medical Publications)
Davidson's Principle and Practice of Medicine 15th Edition Edited by J Macleod (Churchill Livingstone)
Textbook of Adverse Drug Reactions, Edited by DM Davies (Oxford Medical Publications)
Textbook of Medicine by R.J.Harrison (Unibooks
Textbook of Medicine by Southam and Moxham (Churchill Livingstone
The Body at War by John Dwyer (Unwin)
Toohey's Medicine for Nurses by Bloom and Bloom (Churchill Livingstone)
Understanding disease by John Ball (Blackdown Pubs.)

ALTERNATIVE SOURCES OF INFORMATION

CHILDREN'S HEALTH

Childhood and Society by Erikson (Norton)
Chinese Bodywork Edited by Sun Chengnan (Pacific View Press)
Chinese Massage and Acupressure (Bergh)
Continuum Concept by Jean Liedboff (Penguin)
Families and How to Survive Them by Skynner and Cleese
For Your Own Good: Roots of Violence in Child Rearing by Alice Miller
How to Raise a Healthy Child .... In Spite of Your Doctor by Robert Mendelsohn (Contemporary Books)
Infantile Tuina Therapy by Luan Changye (Foreign Languages Press)
The Inner World of Childhood by Frances G Wickes (Coventure)
Thou Shalt Not Be Aware: Society's Betrayal of the Child by Alice Miller
Three in a Bed - Why you should sleep with your baby by Deborah Jackson (Bloomsbury)

URINE THERAPY

Manar Mootra - Auto-Urine Therapy by RM Patel (Bharat Serak Samaj Publications
Shivambu Kalpa by Arthur Lincoln Pauls (Ortho-Bionomy Publishing)
Water of Life by JW Armstrong

ENERGETIC MEDICINE

The Presence of the Past: Morphic Resonance and the Habits of Nature by Rupert Sheldrake (Collins)
Electromagnetic Man by Cyril Smith and Simon Best (JM Dent)
Chronic Disease by Samuel Hahnemann (Jain)
Science of Homoeopathy by George Vithoulkas (Thorson's)
Subtle Energy by John Davidson (CW Daniel)
The Tao of Physics by Fritjof Capra (Flamingo)
The Turning Point by Fritjof Capra (Flamingo)

PSYCHOLOGICAL MEDICINE

Body Centred Psychotherapy: The Hakomi Method by Ron Kurtz (Hakomi Institute)
On Death and Dying by Elisabeth Kubler-Ross (Tavistock Publications)
The Diamond Healing - Tibetan Buddhist Medicine and Psychiatry by Terry Clifford (Crucible)
Getting Well Again by Simonton and Simonton (Bantam)
The Healing Buddha by Raoul Birnbaum (Rider)
Love, medicine and Miracles by Bernie Siegl (Rider)
Love Your Disease: It's Keeping You Healthy by John Harrison (Angus and Robertson)
Mind as Healer, Mind as Slayer by K.Pelletier (Unwin)
The Natural Death Handbook, Edited by Nicholas Albery, Gil Elliot and Joseph Elliot (Virgin)
Personality Types - Jung's Model of Typology by Daryl Sharp (Inner City Books)
Rainbow of Liberated Energy by Ngakpa Chögyam (Element)
The Tibetan Book of Living and Dying by Sogyal Rinpoche (Rider)
Will To Be Well by Neville Hodgkinson (Rider)

WOMEN'S ISSUES

The Active Birth Partners Handbook by Janet Balaskas (Sidgewick and Jackson)
The American Way of Birth by Jessica Mitford (Gollancz)
The Change - Women, Ageing and the Menopause by Germaine Greer (Penguin)
The Encyclopaedia of Pregnancy and Birth by Janet Balaskas and Yehudi Gordon (Little, Brown)
Preparing for Birth with Yoga by Janet Balaskas (Element)
A Savage Enquiry by Wendy Savage (Virago)
Sex and Destiny by Germaine Greer (Secker and Warburg)
Waterbirth by Janet Balaskas and Yehudi Gordon (Unwin)

CANCER

The Bristol Diet by Alec Forbes (Century)
Cancer - The Alternative Method of Treatment by I.Bryant (Roberts)
The Cancer Cure that Worked!: Fifty Years of Suppression by Barry Lynes (Marcus)
Cancer and Leukaemia - An Alternative Approach by Jan De Vries (Mainstream)
An End to Cancer? by Leon Chaitow (Thorson's)
Gentle Giants by Penny Brohn (Cen tury)
The Healing of Cancer by Barry Lynes (Marcus)
Laetrile - Nutritional Control for Cancer by Glenn Kittler (Royal)
The Topic of Cancer by Richards (Pergamon)

PHARMACOLOGY

Cured to Death by Arabella Melville and Colin Johnson (NEL)
Prescribed Drugs and the Alternative Practitioner by Dr S Gascoigne (Ashgrove)

POLITICAL AND SOCIAL COMMENTARIES

Alternative Medicine by Robert Eagle (Futura)
Confessions of a Medical Heretic by Robert Mendelsohn
The Controlled Clinical Trial: An Analysis by Harris L Coulter (Centre for Empirical Medicine and Project Care)
Health Shock by Martin Weitz (Hamlyn)
How to Survive Medical Treatment by Stephen Fulder
Medical Nemesis by Ivan Illich (Bantam)
The Mirage of Health: Utopian Progress and Biological Change by Rene Dubos (Anchor)
Natural Medicine by Brian Inglis (Fontana)
Pasteur Exposed by Ethel Douglas Hume (Bookreal)
The Persecution and Trial of Gaston Naessens by Christopher Bird (HJ Kramer)

APPENDIX TWO

LIAISON WITH OTHER PRACTITIONERS

It may be necessary to liase with other practitioners. This may be to refer the person you have seen because you cannot treat the particular presenting problem. It may be because several treatment options are necessary. Perhaps you would like a degree of supervision from the other practitioner. Whatever the reason it is helpful to know how to go about the practical matter of liaison.

It is much more helpful if you know the practitioner. This is the value of a resource list where you know people in your locality who may help with various situations. It is valuable to have a list to hand of a homoeopath, osteopath, acupuncturist, herbalist, counsellor and so on. If you have had contact with them previously, any dealings now will be smoother.

The standard way of liaising professionally is by means of referral letter. This may not be necessary if you know the practitioner concerned and the case is not too involved. It is preferable to communicate by letter, at least initially, for other situations and particularly when dealing with conventional practitioners who you do not know.

Below is a sample letter which may be of guidance. Always type such a letter on professional notepaper. The main points to bring out are:

- state the main complaint
- say what you are intending to do about it
- describe what help or assistance you require
- offer to discuss the case further
- enclose literature about your therapy if necessary

_____

7, Alternative Avenue,
Nice-Place-to-Practise
Small Town

Tel No.

Date

Dear

Re: Mr A.N.Other, 14 Any Street, Anywhere

This man came to see me recently for acupuncture treatment. His main problem is with anxiety and depression. This is the type of problem which can respond to acupuncture and Chinese herbal medicine. I have arranged to see him for a course of treatment.

I would envisage that his improvement will be slow and that he would require help from other sources including counselling. I have given him some sources of help to contact.

He also wishes help in reducing her medication which currently consists of:

Anafranil 25mg three times daily
Nitrazepam one at night
Diazepam 5mg three times daily

I would appreciate your help later when it is appropriate to deal with these. In the meantime I shall keep in touch about his progress.

If you would like to discuss this case I can be contacted at the above address,

Yours sincerely

Arthur C.U. Puncturist

APPENDIX THREE

HOW TO RECOGNISE SERIOUS CONDITIONS

In this book, I have brought your attention to the question of serious conditions. This is discussed at the end of most Chapters. By a serious condition I mean a situation where life may be threatened or a severe degree of limitation exists. What is serious in conventional medicine is also serious in alternative medicine, the person is the same. If you understand the significance of a particular symptom, you can have confidence in your practice and know your limitations.

The seriousness of a symptom is dependent upon the degree of limitation of the person's activity or functioning. If health can be defined as freedom from limitation then disease or a symptom is a limiting factor. A serious symptom, therefore, would be one which is severely limiting, lifethreatening or indicative of a worsening situation ie progressive over a short period of time.

What do you do in a situation where a symptom may indicate a serious condition? The answer to this depends upon the degree of your experience and expertise. It is important to recognise your limitations as to what is and is not possible. You may be able to deal with such symptoms. On the other hand, you may need to refer the person to someone else. There may be a need for emergency hospitalisation. This is true in acute life-threatening conditions.

If the case is not so severe, there may be time to refer quickly to someone who may be of help. This could be a conventional practitioner or possibly an alternative practitioner. Whatever the situation, it is essential to discuss the issues with the person who has come to see you for help. You may be able to help later for the underlying problems whilst circumstances require a different approach in the short-term.

The Table below is a summary of all the symptoms I have mentioned in the text and how to recognise if they indicate a serious underlying condition.

SYMPTOM	WHEN TO WORRY
Anorexia	Severe, progressive, with mental symptoms of distorted body image
Anuria	Always
Appetite, increased	With weight loss, with mental symptoms of distorted body image
Belching	Not serious
Bleeding	Severe, persistent, recurrent, with pallor, sore throat and lymphatic gland enlargement
Bleeding, inter-menstrual vaginal	Persistent particularly around the menopause
Bleeding, post-coital[1]	Persistent
Bleeding, post-menopausal vaginal	Always - unless taking HRT
Bleeding, pre-pubertal vaginal	Always - consider sexual abuse
Bleeding, vaginal after childbirth	If heavy
Bloating, abdomen	Progressive
Body image disturbance	If associated with weight loss, amenorrhoea
Breathlessness	severe, acute, progressive, with confusion, with cyanosis, pulse rate > 120 per minute, paroxysmal attacks occurring at night
Bruising	Severe, spontaneous

---

[1] Do not forget that it takes two to indulge in sexual intercourse. I know of a woman who had several invasive investigations for post-coital bleeding only to discover later that her partner had blood-streaked semen.

Bullae	Large
Constipation	Severe, progressive, with blood, alternates with diarrhoea
Convulsions	Always
Cough	Persistent, with blood, with breathlessness
Cyanosis	Always unless cold weather only involving lips/extremities
Deafness	Short history, progressive
Dehydration	This may result from loss of fluids, e.g. diarrhoea and vomiting or lack of intake. In babies look for dry skin/lips, decreased skin elasticity, strong urine, scanty urine or even dry nappy, sleepy, lack of responsiveness. In older people there will be reported thirst also.
Delusions	Always
Diarrhoea	Severe, persistent, progressive, in the very young or old, with blood, with mucus, alternates with constipation
Dizziness	Severe, progressive
Ear, deformity	Severe
Ear, discharge	Long duration
Emotional symptoms, e.g. anxiety, fear, depression	If severe, with mental symptoms
Enuresis	Severe especially if with incontinence in the day
Eye, discharge	Not if alone. Of concern if severe, prolonged and with pain in the eye
Eye, redness	Circumcorneal, with visual disturbance
Eye, soreness	Not if mild. Of concern if *pain* rather than soreness especially with circumcorneal redness
Facial weakness	With history of ear pain
Fainting	With exercise
Fever, mild	Perhaps 99 degF. - may indicate mild disease but could be the beginning of severe disease in a weak patient, i.e. vital energy too weak to generate fever.
Fever, prolonged	Most fevers last a day or so. If several days have elapsed then this is of concern that the patient is not strong enough to throw off the problem.
Fever, very high	103 degF and above. This indicates potentially severe disease. There is strong vital energy but the process may damage the patient.
Finger clubbing	always
Flatulence	Not serious
Haematuria	Painless
Haemoptysis	Recurrent, older patient, smoker
Hallucinations	Always
Headache	Progressive, severe with short history, with other central nervous system symptoms
High blood pressure	If severe especially if associated with oedema and proteinuria
Hoarseness	Persistent (more than three weeks)
Jaundice	Unless mild in newborn
Labour, delayed onset	If more than two weeks overdue
Labour, prolonged	If cervix not dilating, with exhaustion, with changes to foetal heart rate
Loss of consciousness	With exercise, not if short duration with specific trigger (see Page 105)
Lumps, around or on the ear	Severe, if with redness, pain and deafness
Lumps, general	Short history, progressive
Lumps nodules in the skin	Short history, recent change, progressive, bleeding
Lymphatic gland enlargement	With pallor, bleeding and sore throat, progressive, moderately enlarged
Nausea	Severe
Numbness	Severe, progressive

Oedema	Acute, unilateral, severe, progressive, with cardiac symptoms, with renal symptoms
Pain	Severe
Pain, abdominal	Severe, with abdominal rigidity, with guarding, with rebound tenderness
Pain, chest	Severe, at rest, with vomiting, with rapid pulse and low blood pressure, long duration, , increasing frequency of attacks, constant and dull
Pain, ear	Severe, with fever
Pain, eye	With visual disturbance
Pain, loin	Severe
Pain, urethra	Not serious
Pallor	Severe, with fainting, with marked light-headedness or dizziness
Palpitations	Pulse > 120 or < 50, with chest pain, oedema or loss of consciousness
Paralysis	Always
Periods, heavy	Persistent, frequent, with pallor and tiredness
Placental retention	If with heavy bleeding, if prolonged (over an hour)
Pregnancy, uterine pain	Always unless at normal time for labour
Pregnancy, vaginal bleeding	Always
Proteinuria	With dysuria and backache, with high blood pressure and proteinuria
Pulse diagnosis (Chinese medicine) in acute fevers	If you treat a patient with an External Pathogenic Factor (EPF) and the pulse is superficial, floating and even overflowing you would expect the pulse to moderate after treatment. If this does not occur it indicates that the EPF may be stronger than the upright Qi. Careful assessment of the case is then necessary as treatment is likely to be difficult. The next thing to happen may be collapse of the person.
Skin, redness or weeping	Severe, large areas of skin surface
Sputum	Copious, green/yellow, blood stained, frothy
Stiffness	Severe
Stridor	Always
Suicidal feelings	Always
Suicidal thoughts	Always
Symptom, severity	The stronger the symptoms, e.g. lots of diarrhoea, lots of vomiting then this is potentially serious. However be careful since weak patients have weak symptoms, e.g. pneumonia in the elderly or patients with A.I.D.S. may present only with breathlessness - no cough and no fever. It is important to assess each case carefully.
Symptoms, progression	Assess the direction of the pathology. By this I mean is it moving to internal organs or more superficially? It is of concern if symptoms start to appear indicating pathology at a deeper level, e.g. in the case of the respiratory system this would be illustrated by sore throat with fever, cough, breathlessness and finally confusion - an effect on the deepest level (mental).
Symptoms, site	Are these in the superficial levels of the body or involving internal organs? If symptoms occur indicating pathology in the lung, kidney, liver, heart or central nervous system then these are clearly more worrying. In terms of Chinese medicine, worry more if the symptoms are at deeper levels of the Taiyin, Shaoyin and Jueyin.
Tendency to catch colds	Not serious
Thought disorders	If severe
Tingling	Severe, progressive
Tinnitus	Progressive
Tremor	Severe, progressive
Urgency	Severe, short history

Urination, dribbling	Severe, short history
Urination, frequent	Severe, short history
Vaginal discharge	Heavy, blood-stained
Veins, distended	in an abnormal site, e.g. neck when sitting up, over the chest or abdominal wall
Vertigo	Severe
Vesicles	Haemorrhagic
Vision, blurring	Progressive
Vision, double	Short history
Vision, spots or floaters	If localised area of blurring
Visual disturbance	Short history, progressive, with pain, with redness
Vomiting	Severe, persistent, progressive, in the very young or old, with blood, with food eaten days before, projectile, evidence of dehydration
Weight loss	Progressive, unexplained, with mental symptoms of distorted body image
Wheezing	If accompanied by breathlessness

APPENDIX FOUR

CORRESPONDENCE COURSE

A study guide has been written to accompany this text. It guides you through the book step by step with additional clarification and numerous practical self-assessment questions with valuable model answers. The course follows the structure of the book, but is divided into 4 study units with various topic-related sections to help you through the material. In addition to the main study, there are assignment questions at the end of each section, which will add further life to the subjects discussed, and will involve you in practical research of later benefit to you as a practitioner. If you need it, full marking of these assignments can also be provided, with expert tutor feedback and support.

Entitled **Pathology and Disease for Alternative Pracitioners**, this thorough course will very much develop your understanding of this complex subject. It follows the popular preparatory course **Anatomy and Physiology for Alternative Practitioners**. For details of both these professional courses, send an A5 sae to:

Alternative Training
8 Kiln Road
Llanfoist
Abergavenny
Gwent NP7 9NS
U.K.

Tel/Fax: 0873 856872

APPENDIX FIVE

PHARMACOLOGY

INTRODUCTION

Throughout this book, I have made references to Chinese medicine. I have attempted to translate conventional medical labels into the syndromes of Traditional Chinese Medicine. There is always a risk in so-doing that Chinese medicine may be simplified and lead to the prescription of acupuncture or herbs for a conventional diagnostic term. This is not my intention and I made the point on Page 11 that such simplification will lead to degeneration of systems of alternative medicine.

The usefulness of considering energetic syndromes is that you can understand conventional disease terms through your knowledge of alternative medicine. This is your chosen field of practice and has to be the starting point. There is no benefit in merely learning conventional medicine for its own sake. It has to be translated and interpreted into a dynamic format.

At the same time, I have also provided some information about the energetic qualities of conventional drugs. This can help practitioners of Chinese medicine decide how a particular medication may affect the case. It can change the pulse, tongue and symptoms. This can be confusing unless you understand all the influences on the person.

The information about energetic qualities of drugs is mainly my own work. I do not claim them to be the final word and I consider this to be merely a beginning.

How is it possible to gain information about conventional medicines and explain them in terms of Chinese medicine? There are several possibilities. Homoeopaths learn about the actions of substances through 'provings', that is, they gather information about symptoms produced when people take a particular substance. The actions of Chinese herbs were gathered in a similar way. Experts in Qi Gong and Chinese medicine would take a herb and know from the effect on themselves of its taste, quality and actions.

Further information may be gathered from texts of the side-effects of drugs. These are not to be considered complete lists of information but are a helpful guide. Conventional medicines are only studied on the basis of the effect they have on one symptom rather than a gathering of the totality of their actions.

Observation of people who come for treatment is invaluable in ascertaining the effect of drugs. This is particularly true if you already know, or can deduce, the original energetic diagnosis. Any changes due to the drug can be more easily assessed.

The latter two methods are those I have used to assess the energetic actions of drugs. The personal testing is the most accurate and hopefully this can be done at some time in the future.

CHINESE MEDICAL THEORY AND PRESCRIBED DRUGS

Yin and Yang, as those terms are understood by Chinese medicine, are philosophical concepts to explain the nature of phenomena. There are two important principles to consider in relation to them.

- Yin and Yang are opposite and interdependent
- Yin and Yang are interconsuming-supporting and inter-transforming

The result of these principles is that Yin and Yang cannot exist on their own. This is death. The interplay of Yin and Yang is a constant dynamic and in health they are balanced. The diagram in Figure A5.1 is a representation of this[1] .

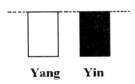

Yang   Yin

FIGURE A5.1: NORMAL BALANCE OF YIN AND YANG

Symptoms and disease are manifest when this normal balance becomes disturbed. There are several possibilities and I shall discuss them each in turn along with comments about corresponding conventional disease labels and the drugs used to treat them.

Figure A5.2 reveals the effects resulting from Invasion of Yin. This may be considered to be Cold Invasion or Damp Invasion. This is an acute syndrome and occurs in relatively strong people. Corresponding conventional medical conditions will be common cold, headache, gastroenteritis, painful joints and some causes of oedema.

Harmful Yin

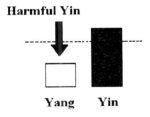

Yang   Yin

FIGURE A5.2: INVASION OF YIN

The appropriate treatment to use for such conditions is to release the exterior. This is done with warm and acrid herbs. A common conventional treatment for common cold and headaches is

---

[1] These diagrams will be familiar to most practitioners of Chinese medicine. See "Essentials of Chinese Acupuncture" (Foreign Languages Press, 1980)

aspirin. This is derived from willow bark and causes sweating and release of fever. It would seem, therefore, to be an appropriate energetic remedy in these situations. It is classed as an anti-inflammatory and it has this effect by releasing the exterior rather than cooling.

Figure A5.3 is a diagram of the situation regarding Yin and Yang which occurs with Invasion of Yang. There is excess Yang in the body with suppression of Yin. This is a common situation with fevers and counterparts in conventional medicine include common cold, acute inflammatory and   infective conditions.

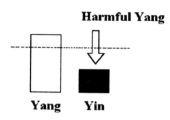

FIGURE A5.3: INVASION OF YANG

The appropriate treatment is clear or drain the heat. This is done by means of heat clearing herbs. The common drugs in conventional medicine, of course, are antibiotics. They have a powerful effect in cooling heat and rapidly reduce a fever. The difficulty with them is that they are often used in people with deficiency conditions. They are single substances and so cannot protect Qi or Blood. In a herbal formula, there will be allowances made depending upon the case. The use of cold drugs in Yang invasion is show in Figure A5.4.

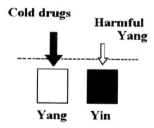

FIGURE A5.4: CONVENTIONAL TREATMENT OF YANG INVASION

From Figure A5.4, it can be seen that Yang and Yin are depleted after treatment. This is why people feel tired and weak after antibiotic treatment. Further disease is more likely now. Repeated courses of antibiotics can only lead to more illness as people become more and more depleted.

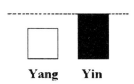

FIGURE A5.5: DEFICIENCY OF YANG

Figure A5.5 is a representation of Yang deficiency. Such conditions in conventional medicine include asthma, chronic bronchitis, cardiac failure, chronic nephritis, diabetes insipidus, enuresis, depression and so on. The appropriate energetic treatment is to tonify and warm the Yang.

Conventional medicine has a difficulty here in that it does not recognise Deficient conditions. It only sees the manifestations. In terms of Ben and Biao, it can see the Biao (the manifestation) but not the Ben (the root). All treatment is, therefore, directed at symptom relief. This can only ever be suppressive.

The exact drugs used will depend upon the precise manifestation. In general, drugs which are warm in nature are used. For example, drugs used in cardiac failure include digitalis which is derived from foxglove, the old herbal remedy to warm Heart Yang and Qi. Drugs used in chronic bronchitis and asthma include corticosteroids and salbutamol. Corticosteroids are a Yang rescuing drug which may be of value in acute situations but can only lead to severe damage if given long-term. Salbutamol is related to ephedrine which is derived from ephedra. This herb is warm and releases the exterior. It is helpful for acute conditions but dangerous if used long-term. The effect of hot drugs in cases of Yang Deficiency is shown in Figure A5.6.

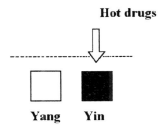

FIGURE A5.6: USE OF HOT DRUGS IN DEFICIENCY OF YANG

Symptoms are relieved by such symptoms because a relative balance of Yin and Yang is obtained. I would suggest however that the situation in Figure A5.6 is worse than that in Figure A5.5 and certainly worse than that in Figure A5.1. The continual use of the hot drugs will suppress the symptoms but removal of the drugs can only be followed by a flare-up of symptoms.

The precise clinical picture will depend upon the individual but it is possible to discuss what is likely. The key here is that Yin and Yang is continually in a state of dynamic flux as they are interconnected and intertransformable. Figure A5.5 reveals an excess of Yin over Yang. There is, in some respects, a transformation of Yang into Yin. This is the underlying process which must be remedied for health to be attained. Conventional drugs do nothing to affect this underlying process. Withdrawal of hot drugs, therefore, lead to a flare-up of Yin as the suppression is removed. This is depicted in Figure A5.7.

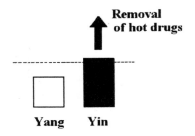

FIGURE A5.7: REMOVAL OF HOT DRUGS

The flare-up of Yin may be manifest physically as oedema or emotionally as sadness, weeping or depression. It is essential when reducing drugs that it is done slowly so that such flare-ups do not overwhelm people. In serious disease such as cardiac failure and some cases of asthma, death may be the result. The method to use is to gently tonify Yang deficiency whilst treating any manifestations of Yin excess. Gradually it is possible to reduce the drugs when the person's own Yang energy has recovered sufficiently. How far it is possible to progress depends upon the individual case.

Figure A5.8 is a represenation of Yin Deficiency. Conventional medical diseases which correspond include anaemia, Parkinson's disease, anxiety, emphysema, osteoarthritis, hyperthyroidism and hypertension.

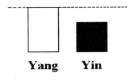

FIGURE A5.8: YIN DEFICIENCY

The appropriate energetic treatment for such a condition is tonify the Yin. As mentioned above, conventional medicine cannot recognise the root of any condition and will generally treat the manifestation, i.e. the relative excess of Yang. Drugs such as betablockers and tranquillisers are used in Yin Deficiency conditions. These are Cold in nature and their effect is shown in Figure A5.9.

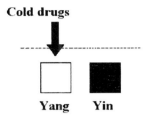

FIGURE A5.9: USE OF COLD DRUGS IN DEFICIENCY OF YIN

For the reasons discussed above in relation to Yang Deficiency, withdrawal of cold drugs leads to a flare-up of Yang which may overwhelm the person. Care must be taken to tonify Yin, support Yang and transform any excess energy. Slowly, drug withdrawal is then possible. The situation which may occur with withdrawal of cold drugs is depicted in Figure A5.10.

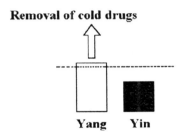

FIGURE A5.10: WITHDRAWAL OF COLD DRUGS IN DEFICIENCY OF YIN

The foregoing discussion is an attempt to illustrate how to interpret the effects of drugs in terms of Yin and Yang. In the final analysis, the effect of any drug depends upon its qualities but also on the individual consitution of the person.

– SUMMARY OF ENERGETIC QUALITIES OF DRUGS DISCUSSED IN THIS TEXT –

DRUG	ENERGETIC ACTION	ORGANS MAINLY AFFECTED
Anti-Parkinsonian drugs	Hot	Liver, Heart
Antibiotics (except sulphonamides)	Cold, damp	Lung, Spleen
Antidepressants	Hot	Heart, Liver
Antifungal	Hot	Spleen, Liver
Aspirin	Warm, dispersing	Lung, Blood
AZT	Hot	Liver, Kidney
Betablockers	Cold	Heart, Lung, Liver, Kidney, Spleen
Bronchodilators	Warm, dispersing	Lung
Cancer chemotherapy	Hot	Liver
Codeine	Hot	Heart, Lungs, Large Intestine
Corticosteroids	Hot	Lung, Spleen, Kidney
Digoxin	Warm	Heart, Kidney
Diuretics	Cold	Kidney
Female sex hormones	Cold	Kidney, Liver, Heart, Spleen
Insulin	Cold	Spleen, Lung, Kidney
Nitrates	Hot	Heart, Liver
Non-steroidal anti-inflammatory drugs	Warm, dispersing	Liver, Kidney
Sulphasalazine	Warm, dispersing	Lung
Sulphonamide	Warm, dispersing	Lung, Kidney
Tranquillisers	Cold	Heart, Liver

TABLE A5.1: SUMMARY OF ENERGETIC ACTIONS OF DRUGS

APPENDIX SIX

This is an article I was asked to write for the newsletter of a homoeopathic college. I know that many students feel overwhelmed by conventional medical information. This article outlines my ideas about the aims of learning such a subject and the general approach which must flow from this if students are to be inspired rather than bored (or perhaps 'expired' would be more appropriate!).

POURQUOI ETUDIEZ VOUS LA MEDICIN CONVENTIONELLE?

'Why study conventional medicine?' is a question which has troubled students and colleges of alternative medicine for a long time. Why, when the aims of the course are to produce a homoeopath, i.e. one who prescribes homoeopathic remedies, should Western medical sciences be included at all? After all, homoeopaths do not investigate conventionally, they do not diagnose conventionally and certainly do not treat conventionally. So what is the point? Wouldn't it be better to spend this valuable time doing something more useful or more enjoyable or both!

It may be helpful here to relate a story as an illustration. One day whilst out walking with her children, mother mouse was confronted by a fierce cat which was about to leap on the young family. Standing her ground, the mother mouse drew herself up to her full 4 cm in height and barked ferociously. At this the cat, clearly frightened, jumped back and ran away. Turning to her children she said, "There you are children. That shows the advantage of learning another language."

So it is with conventional medicine. There may be some value in learning its language. However, unless you intend to be a medical practitioner there is no need to become fluent. Just as a visit to France is more enjoyable if we know how to ask for bread, cheese and wine, we do not have to study French for 5 years. A phrase book is fine. Similarly the study of conventional medicine does not have to lead to fluency. The ONLY requirement is to learn aspects (phrases) which are relevant to the needs of the homoeopath.

What is necessary for the homoeopath? Ideally this needs to be defined by practising homoeopaths of experience since they deal with cases daily and know what is useful and what is not. However, as a non-homoeopath I shall be presumptious enough to make a few suggestions.

The essence is to be practical, to know that which is useful in clinical practice. Most information is available in textbooks and can be looked up so principles are more important than facts.

I would suggest that the general aims would be to increase the skill of the homoeopath in dealing with cases complicated by conventional investigation, diagnosis and treatment.

Specifically this could include:

- warning signs - when a symptom indicates a serious condition which may necessitate urgent intervention
- legal restrictions on practice
- how to liase with medical staff
- how to understand medical terms
- how to understand conventional disease labels in terms of levels of health, hierarchies and direction of the pathology
- how to minimise and possibly overcome or prevent the effects of conventional investigation and treatment
- how to manage people who take prescribed drugs and eventually reduce or withdraw them
- learn diagnostic skills useful in the management of cases eg auriscope, sphygmomanometer

I make no mention here of increasing confidence. I strongly believe that confidence as a homoeopath arises out of your skill and competence at homoeopathy. Conventional medicine deals with fear and limitations not with health and freedom. Therefore, the study of conventional medicine can only ever be an addition to your practice, never a replacement.

If you learn conventional medicine to this level, I am sure you will have an appropriate perspective on its usefulness. It is helpful to tread a middle path between the extremes of over-reliance with the expenditure of large amounts of study, time or energy and outright rejection. Use conventional medicine for your practice as you need it - much the same as you would use a phrase book in the Dordogne.

Bonne chance!

INDEX

This is a cumulative index and contains entries from Volume I and Volume II.

Main entries are in **bold** type.

—C—

lymphocytes, 33
lymphoma, 37, 65, 85, 124, 125
lymphosarcoma, 124
lysergic acid diethylamide, 320

—M—

M.E., **60–62**, 136, 404
macule, 212
maculopapule, 212
magnesium, 35
magnetic resonance imaging, **41**, 285, 307, 309
major depressive illness, 347
'major' tranquillisers, 308, 351, 354, 357
malabsorption, 32, 33, 35, 102, 127, 257, 292
malaria, 51, 173, 440
malathion, 227
malignancy, 33
malignant disease, 33, 103, 125, 173
malignant hypertension, 180
malignant melanoma, 213, **229**
malignant tumours, **81–82**, 85, 125
   skin, **228–30**
malnutrition, 32, 33, 34, 35, 102, 355
malposition, 368, 386, 401
malpresentation, 368, 386, **387**
mammography, **425**, 427, 435
mania, 308, 328, 349, 353, 354, 357, 360
manic depression, 347, 348, 350, **353–55**
masochism, 347
mastectomy, 426, 428, 430
   radical, 428
   simple, 428
   super-radical, 428
mastitis, 393, 432
   chronic, 424, **432**
mastoiditis, 248, 319
mean corpuscular haemoglobin (MCH), 32
mean corpuscular haemoglobin concentration
   (MCHC), 32
mean corpuscular volume (MCV), 32
measles, 19, 52–**53**, 173, 244
   vaccination, **72**
mebeverine, 280
Meckel's diverticulum, 266
melanoma
   malignant, **229**
Ménière's disease, 232, 246–**47**, 246, 249, 250
meningeal irritation, 319
meningioma, **312**
meningism, 314
meningitis, 45, 50, 51, 54, 58, 290, 301, 305, **313**,
   319, 327, 443
   meningococcal, 440
   vaccination, **75**
meningococci, 51
meningo-encephalitis, 55
menopause, 110, 208, 397, 398, 399, 412, 415,
   416, 432, 435
   symptoms, 401
menstrual abnormalities, 400, **407–13**
menstrual cycle

in terms of Yin and Yang, 398
menstruation, 397, 398
   heavy, 406, 432
   irregular, 401, 432
   normal, 398
   painful, **407–8**
mental
   definition, 346
Mental Health Act, 352
mental impairment, 331
mental retardation, 347
mesalazine, 173
mesenteric adenitis, 58
mesothelioma, 46
metabolic encephalopathy, 348
metastasis, **85**
metformin, **339**
methimazole, **329**
methotrexate, 199, 217
methyldopa, 182, 380
methylmorphine, 160, 270
methylprednisolone, 214
methysergide, 320
metoclopramide, 263
metronidazole, 220, 404, 407
mexiletine, 104
miconazole, 225, 226
migraine, 150, 196, 213, 241, 246, 290, 301, **319–
   21**, 433
milk
   cow's, 213
mineralocorticoid, 340, **341**
'minor' tranquillisers, 308, **351, 357**
minoxidil, 221
miscarriage, 45, 368, 377, 379, 413, 417, 419, 421
   habitual, 35
   incomplete, 374, **377**
   inevitable, **377**
   missed, 374, 378
   threatened, 374, **377**, 401
mole, 229
monilia, 402
mono-amine oxidase inhibitors, 180, **360**
monocytes, 33
mononeuropathy, **317**
morning sickness, 368, **376**, 388, 401
morphine, 150
Morton's metatarsalgia, 205
motor neurone disease, 297
mouth ulcers, 254
movement
   involunatary, 298
   slow, 298
multiple personality disorder, 347
multiple pregnancy, 368, 373, 374, 375, 379, 380,
   383, **388**, 421
multiple sclerosis, 23, 41, 45, 126, 172, 179, 186,
   239, 241, 242, 250, 297, 301, **309–11**
mumps, 19, 34, 52, **53–54**, 173, 187, 272, 419
   vaccination, **73–74**
mung bean powder, 434
muscle biopsy, 375